ROYAL SOCIETY OF MEDICINE

FOUNDED 1805
INCORPORATED BY ROYAL CHARTER 1834
NEW CHARTER 1907

GIFT TO THE LIBRARY

PRESENTED BY

THE PUBLISHER

DATE OCTOBER 1993

RSM/TS/1

Viral infections of the heart

Viral infections
of the heart

Edited by

J. E. Banatvala

Professor and Clinical Director of Department of
Virology, United Medical and Dental School of
Guy's and St Thomas' Hospital (St Thomas' Campus),
London

Edward Arnold
A division of Hodder & Stoughton
LONDON BOSTON MELBOURNE AUCKLAND

1993

© 1993 Hodder and Stoughton Ltd
First published in Great Britain 1993

Distributed in the Americas by Little, Brown and Company
34 Beacon Street, Boston, MA 02108

British Library Cataloguing in Publication Data

Banatvala, J. E.
  Viral Infections of the Heart
  I. Title
  616.1

ISBN 0-340-55737-0

Whilst the advice and information in this book is believed to be true
and accurate at the date of going to press, neither the author nor the
publisher can accept any legal responsibility or liability for any
errors or omissions that may be made. In particular (but without
limiting the generality of the preceding disclaimer) every effort has
been made to check drug dosages; however, it is still possible that
errors have been missed. Furthermore, dosage schedules are
constantly being revised and new side effects recognised. For these
reasons the reader is strongly urged to consult the drug companies'
printed instructions before administering any of the drugs
recommended in this book.

Typeset in 10/11pt Linotron Times by
Rowland Phototypesetting Limited, Bury St Edmunds, Suffolk.
Printed and bound in Great Britain for Edward Arnold,
a division of Hodder and Stoughton Limited, Mill Road,
Dunton Green, Sevenoaks, Kent TN13 2YA by
Butler and Tanner Limited, Frome and London.

Preface

The role of viruses in inducing cardiac disease has been a relatively neglected area in the rapidly developing speciality of clinical virology. However, the development of molecular biological techniques and their recent application to studies relating to the diagnosis and pathogenesis of the viral infections of the heart is shedding new light in an area in which major advances are likely to occur in the near future.

This book attempts to provide an up-to-date account of current knowledge including recent developments. Chapters from authors working in different disciplines including virology, epidemiology, immunology, experimental pathology and clinical medicine are included. Although a number of different viruses have been shown to cause acute cardiac disease, a number of chapters in this book place considerable emphasis on the role of enteroviruses, particularly coxsackie B viruses as they are most frequently implicated as a cause of acute myocarditis; this group of viruses may also be involved in the pathogenesis of dilated cardiomyopathy but this has yet to be demonstrated conclusively.

The chapter on the role of the Human Immunodeficiency Virus (HIV) highlights the increasing importance of this virus in heart disease. If, with better management HIV infected patients survive longer, cardiac disease may be observed more frequently among patients with AIDS.

The role of cytomegalovirus in the pathogenesis of atherosclerosis, although perhaps more speculative, is likely to interest a broad range of readers.

The identification of existing or newly recognised viruses as well as an understanding of the mechanisms by which viruses may induce cardiac disease is dependent on a multidisciplinary approach which this book has attempted to encompass. As such it is hoped that this book will be of value, not only to medical virologists, but also to others training and practising in different disciplines in pathology as well as clinicians including cardiologists, general physicians, paediatricians and specialists in infectious diseases.

I am grateful to Dr Peter Muir for his assistance in the preparation of this book and to Miss Alice Gem for considerable secretarial assistance.

J. E. Banatvala
1992

Contents

Contributors

E. Adam, Division of Molecular Virology, Baylor College of Medicine, Texas Medical Center, Houston, Texas, USA

M. E. Billingham, Department of Cardiovascular Surgery, Stanford Medical School, CVRB, Stanford, California 943305, USA

N. A. Boon, Department of Cardiology, Royal Infirmary, Edinburgh, Scotland, UK

N Cary, Department of Pathology, Papworth Hospital, Papworth Everard, Cambridge

G. B. Clements, Regional Virus Laboratory, Ruchill Hospital, Glasgow G20 9NB, Scotland, UK

N. R. Grist, Communicable Diseases (Scotland) Unit, Ruchill Hospital, Glasgow G20 9NB, Scotland, UK

M. Herzum, Philipps-Universität Marburg, Baldingerstrasse, D-W-3550 Marburg, Germany

S. A. Huber, Department of Pathology, University of Vermont College of Medicine, Burlington, Vermont 05405, USA

A. J. Jacob, Department of Cardiology, Royal Infirmary, Edinburgh, Scotland, UK

R. Kandolf, Institute of Pathology, University of Tubingen, D-7400 Tubingen and Department of Virus Research, Max-Planck Institute for Biochemistry, D-8033 Martinsried, Germany

B. Maisch, Arztl. Leiter der Abt. Innere Medizin-Kardiologie, Philipps-Universitat Marburg, Baldingerstrasse, D-W-3550 Marburg, Germany

A. Matsumori, Third Division, Department of Internal Medicine, Kyoto University, 54 Kawaracho Shogoin, Sakyo-ku, Kyoto 606, Japan

J. L. Melnick, Division of Molecular Virology, Baylor College of Medicine, One Baylor Plaza, Texas Medical Center, Houston, Texas 77030–3498, USA

P. Muir, Department of Virology, United Medical and Dental Schools of Guy's and St Thomas' Hospitals (St Thomas' Campus), Lambeth Palace Road, London SE1 7EH, UK

W. Al-Nakib, Advanced Pathology Services, Harley Street, London W1N 1DF.

D. Reid, Communicable Diseases (Scotland) Unit, Ruchill Hospital, Glasgow G20 9NB, Scotland, UK

P. Richardson, Cardiac Department, King's College Hospital, Denmark Hill, London SE5 9RS, UK

U. Schönian, Philipps-Universität Marburg, Baldingerstrasse, D-W-3550 Marburg, Germany

H. Why, Cardiac Department, King's College Hospital, Denmark Hill, London SE5 9RS, UK

T. Wreghit, Clinical Microbiology and Public Health Laboratory, Addenbrooke's Hospital, Cambridge CB2 2QW

1

Characteristics of viruses inducing cardiac disease

G. B. Clements

Introduction

The myocardium is affected in a wide range of virus infections. In some cases the myocarditis may be the primary presenting problem, in others it may occur as part of generalized disease. Usually during active myocarditis there is also an associated endocarditis and pericarditis, and commonly the terms pancarditis and myopericarditis have also been used.[1] Myocarditis is most commonly caused by the enteroviruses, particularly coxsackie B viruses. In many cases of presumed myocarditis on clinical grounds no definite evidence of viral aetiology is obtained despite extensive laboratory investigations. Lerner and Wilson[2] have summarized the criteria for assessing the value of laboratory tests in determining the aetiology of viral myocarditis. In many cases of clinical myocarditis no pathogen is identified. The strongest evidence is provided by isolation of virus from the heart but cardiac tissue is seldom available, except at *post mortem*; even then it is rarely available. Rising antibody titres or the isolation of a suggestive pathogen from a site other than the heart, for example, the throat or stool, provides suggestive evidence of the pathogenesis. Direct evidence of involvement of the heart is available in acute infections in cases of coxsackie A4, A16 and B1–5 viruses and echoviruses 9 and 22. In about 50% of those cases where suggestive evidence for a viral aetiology is available on the basis of serology coxsackie B viruses are implicated.[3] Now that endomyocardial biopsy is becoming available more data is accumulating from direct examination of myocardial tissue of patients during episodes of myocarditis. Some degree of myocardial involvement is probably very common during viral infections, perhaps it should be regarded as the norm. Several reports indicate that about 4% of children who died accidentally had evidence of an incidental myocarditis at autopsy,[4] but it is only recently that agreed histological criteria for the diagnosis of myocarditis have begun to be widely accepted.[5] The use of nucleic acid technology may help to overcome some of these diagnostic difficulties.[6–8] Electrocardiographic (ECG) findings associated with myocarditis include sinus tachycardia, ST and T segment abnormalities, ventricular conduction disturbances and extrasystoles. Such changes have been reported in up to 50% of patients with mild influenza, 40% of cases of infectious mononucleosis, 31% of cases of poliomyelitis and 30% of cases of measles, but it is not possible to be certain that such changes provide specific evidence for cardiac disease. In many cases there are nonspecific symptoms, for example, headache or upper respiratory tract infection for several weeks before there is definite evidence of a myocarditis.

In addition to direct damage to the cardiac muscle by virus infection there may be an immunologically mediated process taking place over a longer time period and continuing after clinical evidence of the triggering infection has resolved (See Chapter 5). There is accumulating evidence linking viral myocarditis with the eventual development of dilated cardiomyopathy.[9,10]

In addition to the enteroviruses many viruses have been proposed as causing a myocarditis (Table 1.1). However, in many cases the evidence is only circumstantial and direct conclusive proof of cardiac involvement is not available. There follows a brief summary of the characteristics of these virus families. Further details can be found in standard virological texts.[16]

Table 1.1   Causes of viral myocarditis (modified from Woodruff[1]).

Virus family	Virus group	Association with cardiac disease
Picornavirus	Coxsackie B	Myocarditis in isolation or in association with other symptoms, e.g. myalgia. Pancarditis in fetus during last trimester and during the first year of life
	Coxsackie A	Myocarditis, especially in neonates
	Echovirus	Myocarditis, especially in neonates
	Poliovirus	Myocarditis as one feature
	Hepatitis A	Myocarditis as one feature[11]
Orthomyxovirus	Influenza A	Myocarditis as one feature
	Influenza B	Myocarditis as one feature
Paramyxovirus	Respiratory syncytial virus	
	Mumps	Myocarditis as one feature[12]
	Measles	Myocarditis rarely
Rubivirus	Rubella	Subendocardial fibre necrosis in the fetus during the first trimester. Myocarditis, rarely during acute rubella postnatally
Arbovirus*	Dengue	Myocarditis as one feature
	Yellow fever	Myocarditis as one feature
	Chikungunya	Myocarditis as one feature
Rhabdovirus	Rabies	Myocarditis as one feature[13]
Retrovirus	Human immunodeficiency-1 virus	Evidence for cardiac abnormalities as a primary event independently of opportunistic infections[14]
Poxvirus	Vaccinia	Myocarditis during generalized vaccinia
Herpesvirus	Varicella zoster virus	Myocarditis, may be focal, during chickenpox
	Cytomegalovirus	Myocarditis rarely
	Herpes simplex virus	Myocarditis rarely
	Epstein–Barr virus	Myocarditis as one feature[15]
Adenovirus	Adenovirus	Weak association

*The term arbovirus is no longer used in taxonomy and includes viruses in a number of different families particularly togaviruses.

Enteroviruses

Introduction

The ability to culture cells has permitted the growth of poliovirus in primate cell culture.[17] This led both to the development of polio vaccines and also to the identification of a number of related viruses which together form the enterovirus genus. Characterized variously by their ability to grow in cultured cells, their pathogenicity in suckling mice and by serological techniques the enteroviruses form a diverse collection (Table 1.2). There is an extensive overlap in respect of the disease produced in many cases; as far as myocarditis is concerned, coxsackie B1–6 are particularly important. The enteroviruses form one genus of the *Picornaviridae* (the others being rhinoviruses, aphthoviruses and cardioviruses).

Table 1.2   The enteroviruses.

Group	Disease	Comment
Polio 1,2,3	Paralytic poliomyelitis, aseptic meningitis	Grow in non-neural primate cell culture
Coxsackie A1–22,24	Aseptic meningitis, herpangina, conjunctivitis (A24)	Pathogenic for suckling mice, widespread myositis, flaccid paralysis. Some grow in culture
Coxackie B1–6	Aseptic meningitis, pleurodynia, myocarditis, pericarditis	Pathogenic for suckling mice, focal myositis. Grow in culture
Echovirus 1–9, 11–27, 29–34	Aseptic meningitis rashes, febrile illness	
Enterovirus* 68–72	Conjunctivitis (70), polio-like illness (71), hepatitis A (72)	

*Since 1983 new enteroviruses isolated have been attributed numbers.

Virus properties

The enteroviruses are small RNA viruses (Fig. 1.1a) and have been extensively studied using a variety of techniques. They are not only important model systems in their own right but also cause a variety of diseases in humans and animals. The complete RNA sequences of many of the viruses have been determined, the first being that of the Mahoney strain of poliovirus type 1.[18] The three-dimensional structure of poliovirus type 1 strain Mahoney has been determined by X-ray crystallography at an atomic level.[19] Enteroviruses have a buoyant density of 1.34 g/cm^3 in caesium chloride and are stable to pH 4 and resistant to pH 2. Poliovirus has been extensively studied and is regarded as exemplifying the characteristics of enteroviruses.

The virion is not penetrated by negative stains and is nonenveloped. Particles are generally spherical, and are 25–30 nm in diameter. Shadowed preparations show blunt-ended or pointed shadows consistent with an icosahedral structure. The poliovirus capsid comprises 60 protomers each formed from one molecule of the four virion proteins VP1, VP2, VP3 and VP4 arranged in icosahedral symmetry. Virion proteins VP2 and VP4 may be phosphorylated by cellular kinases. The 20 faces of the icosahedron are each formed

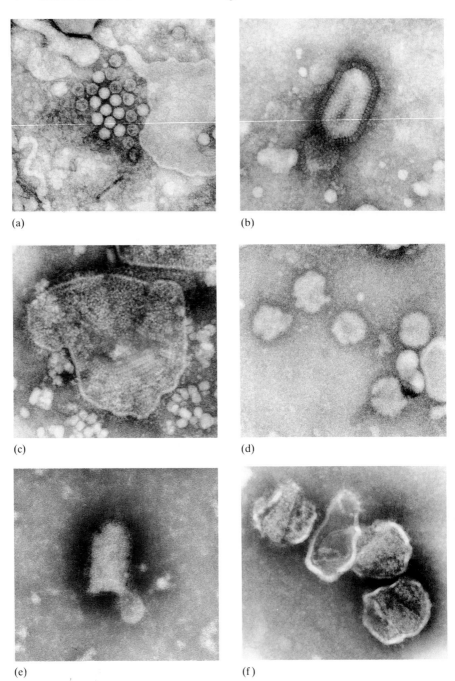

Fig. 1.1   (a) Enterovirus. (b) Orthomyxovirus. (c) Paramyxovirus. (d) Rubella. (e) Rabies. (f) Human immunodeficiency virus-2. (g) Orthopoxvirus. (h) Herpesvirus. (i) Adenovirus. All preparations were negatively stained with 3% sodium phosphotungstate at pH 6.4. × 200 000. The rabies electron micrograph was kindly supplied by Dr A. Field. The remaining electron micrographs were kindly supplied by Dr I. L. Chrystie.

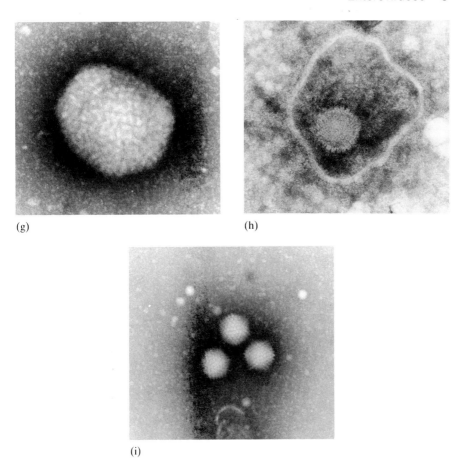

(g)

(h)

(i)

from three protomers, with VP1 at the apices. Surrounding each of the apices is a cleft or canyon within which may be the site at which the virus attaches to the cell surface, possibly by a specific receptor. However, there is also evidence that virion surface structures may be involved in cellular binding in some cases. The basic structure and organization of the core structures of the capsid proteins of other picornaviruses which have been examined in sufficient detail are extremely similar. The unique features characteristic of particular serotypes are surface loops, and the amino and carboxy termini of these regions comprise the antigenic sites. There are two other components of the capsid. Firstly, the amino terminus of VP4 is covalently linked to a myristic acid residue which, it has been suggested, may form a scaffolding for assembly of the capsid proteins.[20] Secondly, within a fold in the VP1 protein there is thought to be a 16 carbon lipid molecule which may contribute to assembly or uncoating.

Genome organization and function

The complete sequences of several strains of poliovirus and other picornavirus genomes have been published.[21] As a result the pattern of genome organization is more clearly understood. With a molecular weight of 2000–3000 kD the genomes range from 7500 to 8500 nucleotides having a total coding capacity of approximately 200 kD of polypeptide. At the 5′ end of the genome there is a small virus coded protein VPg of 22 amino acids covalently linked to the genome and at the 3′ end a tract of 40–100 adenosine residues. The map of the enterovirus genome is presented in Fig. 1.2. The first 740 or so nucleotides at the 5′ end are not translated and probably mediate a variety of essential functions including packaging, replication and initiation of protein synthesis. The genome, in effect, functions as an mRNA having a single open reading frame terminating about 70 nucleotides from the 3′ end. It is initially translated to produce a single large polyprotein which is cleaved. Following this untranslated region there is the polyadenosine tract.

The structural proteins (VP1, VP2, VP3 and VP4) are coded at the 5′ end of the genome which is the first region to be translated forming the precursor, P1, and is initially cleaved at the far end of ID from the polyprotein separating the P1 region from the remainder of the polyprotein. There is a second cleavage site of the polyprotein which produces the P2 region which consists of the 2A, 2B and 2C proteins and also P3 comprising the 3A, 3B, 3C and 3D proteins. The known functions of the proteins are indicated in Fig. 1.2. Virus-coded proteases can carry out the cleavages and poliovirus RNA translated in HeLa cell extracts yields virtually the same pattern of proteins as in the infected cell. With the accumulation of sequence data from a number of enteroviruses the conventional classification has been reviewed.[21] This classification for the three poliovirus types and the coxsackie B viruses is supported by the molecular data, there being more than 70% identity of the P1 coding region within these two subgroups. However, the correlation is less clear cut in other cases. There are at least three groups by homology among the coxsackie A viruses for which sequence data are available. Coxsackie A21 has similarities to the polioviruses while coxsackie A9 belongs with the coxsackie B subgroup and coxsackie A2 falls into neither grouping. There is little sequence data available so far on the echovirus subgroup, however, echoviruses 6 and 11 are closely related to the coxsackie B subgroup. Echovirus 22 has little similarity to any of the other enteroviruses.

Organization of enterovirus genome

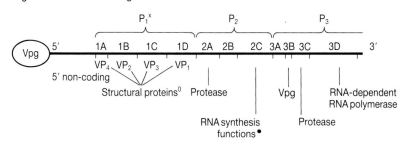

Fig. 1.2 Organization of the enterovirus genome. x, Nomenclature of Rueckert and Wimmer.[22] o, Common names. ●, Consensus NTP (nucleotide triphosphate) binding domain/helicase-like motifs.

Productive cycle

Enteroviruses enter host cells by using cellular receptor molecules on the surface of the plasma membrane. The poliovirus receptor is a protein of the immunoglobulin superfamily[23] and coxsackie A13, 18 and 21 viruses use an intercellular adhesion molecule ICAM-1,[24,25] also a member of the immuno-globulin superfamily as their receptor. The coxsackie B group and also echovirus type 6 may bind to a further receptor. After attachment it is assumed that the virus particle enters the cell by receptor-mediated endocytosis. Uncoating of the particles takes place within the host cell. The details of this process are unclear but may involve the loss of VP4 from the surface of the particles. The phosphorylation of VP2 and VP4 by cellular kinases may contribute to the destabilization.[26] The lipid-like molecule which occupies the pocket in the β barrel of VP1 may also play a role because drugs which inhibit the uncoating of rhinoviruses also occupy this pocket.[27]

Whatever the exact process, the genomic RNA is released from the virus particles into the cell where it is infectious. Since it is possible to produce infectious virus from RNA or cDNA[28] copies of the genome by transfection, the structural proteins are not required following release of nucleic acid into the cell. Protein synthesis is mediated by ribosomes which bind to the 5′ end of the RNA, which is acting as an mRNA molecule, and which scan for the initiation codon used for protein synthesis which is 743 nucleotides from the end. Unusually these mRNA molecules do not carry a 'cap' structure at the 5′ end and furthermore the molecules associated with ribosomes lack the protein VPg which is covalently linked to the virion RNA molecules. The 5′ noncoding region of enteroviruses is relatively long, highly conserved and probably has a complex secondary structure which is functionally important, for example, it may influence which internal binding site is used by ribosomes for initiation.

After viral protein synthesis has started host protein synthesis is switched off possibly as a result of virus-coded proteases cleaving the initiation factor P220 needed for the cap-dependent host cell protein synthesis. Enteroviruses express at least two proteases which are very specific in their action. These are the 3C which carries out the majority of cleavages and the 2A which cleaves the polyprotein. In some cases there may be self-cleavage and a variety of intermediates in the cleavage pathway may have protease activity. Commonly, two peptides are recognized, for example, the P1 protein of poliovirus is cleaved from the remainder of the polyprotein by protease 2A cleaving between a tyrosine and a glycine residue. Exposure of a particular peptide pair, and also its environment, seems to determine the exact site of cleavage. Protease 3C carries out the later processing steps cutting between specific glutamine – glycine residues in the P1 region of polio between VP2 and VP3 and VP3 and VP1. The cleavage in 3D is between tyrosine and glycine probably by the action of 2A. The cleavage between VP2 and VP4 occurs as the final step during maturation of the particle.

Poliovirus RNA replication takes place by means of a virus-coded RNA-dependent RNA polymerase (3D) associated with cell proteins initially to produce negative strands from the positive sense genome.[29] The negative strands are templates for the synthesis of progeny positive sense RNA molecules which are produced in great excess.[30] Within infected cells there are full-length double-strand RNA molecules, replicative forms. There are, in addition, partially double-stranded molecules consisting of a full-length template RNA, which may be of either polarity, and multiple nascent RNA molecules of opposite polarity undergoing synthesis. These nascent RNA molecules have a molecule of VPg covalently linked at the 5′ terminus. Several virus-coded proteins are needed for RNA synthesis. Protease 3D has RNA polymerase activity[31] and is the main component in replicative complexes, 3B (VPg) is both covalently linked to the nascent strands and also, as the uncleaved 3AB, is present in membrane preparations having RNA polymerase activity. The highly conserved protein 2D has consensus elements that predict nucleotide binding and it has been proposed as a helicase.

The structural proteins are synthesized and processed as a coordinated unit assembling to form pentamers of VP0, VP1 and VP3 which are 14S particles. Isolated pentamers can assemble to form procapsids, complete empty virion shells which sediment at 75S. Infected cells yield 14S on extraction which assemble to form the 75S structures. The RNA is incorporated into the virion by an as yet undetermined mechanism. The final step in virion maturation is VP0 cleavage to yield VP2 and VP4. It may be that this cleavage is facilitated by encapsidation of virion RNA and ensures stability of the mature particle. In each capsid there are one or two copies of VP0 remaining uncleaved.

Definition of antigens

The humoral arm of the immune response plays the major role in protecting from enterovirus infection. The initial classification of enteroviruses was carried out with the help of sera containing specific neutralizing antibodies. In the case of enteroviruses, such antibodies recognize structures on the surface of the virus particle, and after binding to them render the particle noninfectious. In this way individual serotypes were defined. However, it became apparent that antigenic differences occur within independent isolates of a single serotype. Examples of these differences occur in type 3 poliovirus and coxsackie B5, and have been confirmed by nucleic acid hybridization studies and by nucleic acid sequencing.

Serological studies have been given new impetus by the use of monoclonal antibodies which recognize particular epitopes. With these reagents the components of the surface structures of the virion forming the epitopes that react with antibody have been defined. This was achieved by selecting 'escape mutants' resistant to neutralization by a particular monoclonal antibody.[32,33] Sequencing the RNA of the resulting antigenic mutant virus subsequently has permitted the exact delineation of the resulting structural changes. These were found located on the surface of the particle as several separate sites where the sequence of amino acids of one or other of the structural proteins had changed. Some sites involve only one protein, for example, site 1 of polio is located to VP1 (amino acid residues 89–100, 142, 166 and 253). Other sites may involve two of the structural proteins, for example, site 2 involves VP1 (amino acid residues 220–222) and VP2 (amino acid residues 164–170 and 273). The exact sequences involved and their importance differs between serotypes. Each antigenic site forms an epitope where the conformation of the molecule brings amino acid residues together in such a way as to form a target suitable for recognition by the immune response. Although the monoclonal antibodies are raised in mice the results are entirely consistent with the information obtained from structural studies. The regions acting as epitopes are exposed on the surface of the virion and it would seem that the human immune response is broadly similar to that of the mouse. Recently, chimeric polioviruses have been produced, for example, by replacing the variable loop of poliovirus type 1 defining the major antigenic sites of VP1 with the equivalent loop from poliovirus type 3.[34,35]

Physical treatment can modify the surface structure of enteroviruses and to some extent virions are the product of their environment. For example, site 1 which is the immunodominant site as defined by mouse monoclonal antibody has a trypsin cleavage site. Virus recovered from the gut of vaccinees carries site 1 in its cleaved state and as a result the antigenic properties are modified. The virus in the gut is thus antigenically very different from that released from cell culture or present as a viraemia or within tissues.

Effects on host cells

Monolayer cultures of primate cells support the growth of polioviruses, coxsackie B viruses and the echoviruses. The cytopathic effects are generally very similar, the cells rounding up and then detaching. Some enteroviruses, particularly the coxsackie A group, do not replicate at all well in cell culture but may be isolated in newborn mice. There is accumulating evidence for the occurrence of persistent infection in culture following infection under appropriate conditions.

Orthomyxoviridae

The term 'myxovirus' was coined initially to describe an affinity for mucus and included a large group of enveloped viruses with the ability to attach to glycoprotein surface receptors. This is now separated into two families orthomyxoviridae (influenza) and paramyxoviridae (parainfluenza, mumps, measles and respiratory syncytial virus).

The influenza viruses are a major cause of respiratory infections occasionally producing worldwide pandemics with much associated morbidity and mortality. There are three types of influenza:

Influenza A   May exhibit considerable antigenically variability: cause of the majority of outbreaks of epidemic influenza
Influenza B   Antigenically variable, can also cause epidemics
Influenza C   Antigenically stable, causes little illness in humans

Influenza A infections are widespread, occurring in a number of species including, for example, pigs, horses and birds, as well as humans. Influenza formed one of the driving forces to establish the importance of clinical virology. Thus the 1918/1919 worldwide pandemic of influenza provided an urgent impetus to establish diagnostic and epidemiological methods. Much of the early work following the first isolation of the virus in 1933 used animals and the discovery that influenza viruses could be grown in fertile hens' eggs led, in due course, to the development of a vaccine. Influenza still retains the ability to produce pandemics.

Influenza virus particles are pleomorphic enveloped structures of 80–110 nm in diameter (Fig. 1.1b). The eight segmented genome of negative sense RNA has a total length of about 13 600 nucleotides and codes for at least ten proteins. If a particular cell is coinfected by two different influenza A viruses mixtures of parental segments may be assembled into progeny. Termed genetic reassortment, this phenomenon may result in abrupt changes in viral surface antigens. A lipid envelope originating from the cell surrounds the virion and floating in the envelope are many copies of the virus glycoproteins, haemagglutinin (HA) and neuraminidase (NA) which project as spikes on the surface. Being enveloped, influenza virions are sensitive to ether but they are relatively hardy and can survive without loss of viability when stored at 0–4°C for several weeks. Differences in the antigenicity of the nucleoprotein (NP) and matrix proteins (M) divide influenza viruses into the three types A B and C there being no serological cross-reactivity between them. Subtyping is carried out using antigenic variation in the surface glycoproteins HA and NA. The nomenclature for influenza isolates includes the following: type, host of origin, geographic origin, strain number and year of isolation. Antigenic descriptions of the HA and NA are in parentheses for type A. The host of origin is omitted for human isolates. In all there are 13 subtypes of HA and nine of NA of which three HA (H1, H2, H3) and 2 NA (N1, N2) subtypes have been recovered from humans.

The HA binds viral particles to cells and is the major antigen against which neutralizing antibodies are directed. As the name implies this molecule is able to agglutinate erythrocytes under appropriate conditions. The three-dimensional structure of the protein has been defined by X-ray crystallography and detailed structural functional correlations carried out.

Within the lipid bilayer, in which the haemagglutinin and neuraminidase float, there is the matrix protein within which is the nucleoprotein. The genome has been sequenced and the polypeptides assigned to appropriate segments.

Productive cycle

Influenza virus particles bind to receptors on the cell surface and enter the cell in coated vesicles and are transported to endosomes. Within these vesicles there is a low pH environment which produces a configurational change which activates fusion of virus envelope and the cell membrane. After its entry into the cytoplasm the viral RNA is transported to the cell nucleus as a virion core complex where mRNAs and negative sense progeny RNA are synthesized. The mechanism of mRNA synthesis is unique as host cell coded capped RNAs are used as primers. Following viral protein synthesis the HA and NA are inserted into the plasma membrane which is followed by budding to release particles containing cores.

Definition of antigens

Of the seven virus-coded structural protein components four can act as antigens. These are the antigenically variable HA and NA and the two major internal proteins NP and M which are conserved and shared between each influenza type. There is also a cell-mediated immune response to influenza against a variety of antigens.

Effects on cells in culture

Fresh isolates of influenza virus may not produce cytopathic effects in monkey kidney cells, but virus infection may be detected by haemadsorption.

Paramyxoviridae

All members of this family initially infect via the respiratory tract. Respiratory syncytial virus (RSV) and the parainfluenza viruses are the most important respiratory infections of infants and young children. Mumps and measles are important and common diseases of childhood, the former in association with malnutrition being a major cause of infant mortality in the developing world.

Paramyxoviridae closely resemble the myxoviridae, being enveloped, but are a little larger at 150–300 nm in diameter and more pleomorphic and more fragile (Fig. 1.1c). There is a helical nucleocapsid. The genome is one single strand of negative sense RNA approximately 15 000 nucleotides long and thus there is no possibility of reassortment. Indeed, all are antigenically stable. The six structural proteins are in broad terms analogous to those of the influenza viruses. There are two membrane glycoproteins, the larger one possessing both HA and NA activity and being involved in attachment to the host cell while the other (F) induces membrane fusion and (except for RSV) haemolysis. All share common antigenic determinants and hyperimmuniz-ation stimulates cross-reactive antibodies. The F protein is an important component mediating fusion of the viral envelope with the plasma membrane of the host cell and also fusion between host cells permitting cell to cell to cell spread of virus and the associated development of syncytia. In an analo-gous way to the influenza HA the F protein is synthesized as an inactive precursor FO which is cleaved by an extracellular protease to F1 and F2 which remain joined by a disulphide bond and in so doing activates the fusion and haemolytic functions. The presence of this appropriate protease activity probably plays an important part in virus spread. The NH_2 terminus on the Fl cleavage product is highly conserved and shares homology with the influ-enza virus HA N-terminus.

Genome organization and function

All the paramyxoviruses have the same basic organization of the genome, there being a series of genes transcribed from a single promotor near the 3' terminus. Mumps and measles viruses have seven genes in the same order with one, an internally coded nonstructural gene, being within the gene for the phosphoprotein.

Productive cycle

Following attachment by a virus envelope glycoprotein to the surface of the cell, fusion between the envelope and the plasma membrane takes place. This fusion is effected by the F protein which is proteolytically cleaved from a larger precursor molecule releasing the nucleocapsid into the cell cytoplasm. The negative sense genome is transcribed by a virion-associated RNA-dependent RNA polymerase without exogenous primers. The nucleocapsids assemble in the cytoplasm and by budding through the plasma membrane, which carries the virus-specified glycoproteins, acquire the envelope.

Definition of antigens

Humoral immunity is directed against the envelope glycoproteins and can neutralize infectivity. Internal proteins, the nucleocapsid, are targets for the cell-mediated immune response.

Effects on cell in culture

Measles and mumps can be grown in human embryo kidney, human amnion or monkey kidney cells. In both cases there is a cytopathic effect with giant cell formation.

Rubella

Although rubella had been described as a disease entity in the mid-eighteenth century and the teratogenic effects of the virus was documented by Gregg (1941), it was not until 1962 that the virus was isolated. Rubella virus is classified as a nonarthropod borne togavirus and is assigned as the only member of the genus *Rubivirus*. Rubella is an enveloped pleomorphic virus 40–70 nm in diameter with a genome of positive sense single-stranded RNA (Fig. 1.1d). The envelope which buds from the surface of the infected cell carries projecting viral glycoproteins which include a haemagglutinin. Within the the envelope is the nucleocapsid 30–40 nm in diameter which is fragile and most probably has an icosahedral symmetry and contains the core which is 10–20 nm in diameter. The RNA has a sedimentation coefficient of 40s, is 10–11 kb long, polyadenylated and can retain infectivity if extracted carefully. The genome has recently been sequenced.[36]

Productive cycle

Following entry into the cell the virion RNA is released into the cytoplasm. The genome organization and pattern of transcription appears to follow that of Sindbis and Semliki forest viruses. The 5' end of the genome is capped and the 3' end polyadenylated. The parental genome can act as an mRNA and is translated from a particular ribosome binding site to give two poly-proteins, the first being 230 kD and as a result of read through a second one of 270 kD. The two polyproteins are cleaved, producing nonstructural pro-teins which effect transcription and replication. Firstly, a full-length negative sense RNA is synthesized which subsequently acts as a template for the synthesis both of progeny full-length positive strands and also a subgenomic 26s mRNA. The latter is initiated from an internal site and is the mRNA for structural proteins. This is translated to form a 110 kD polyprotein which is subsequently cleaved to the nucleocapsid protein C and the major envelope glycoproteins E1 and E2. There are at least two glycosylated patterns of E2, E2a and E2b.

Definition of antigens

There are haemagglutinating and complement-fixing antigens. The former are associated with the spikes on the surface of the viral envelope. Several complement-fixing antigens have been described associated either with the haemagglutinin or the core. There is no evidence for antigenic variation among strains of rubella virus.

Effects on host cells *in vivo*

Rubella virus has a relatively long replicative cycle, in Vero cells virus production is maximal 48 hours after infection. There is no shut off of host cell RNA synthesis and only partial inhibition of overall cell protein synthesis. Virus also replicates well in BHK cells as it does in a wide range of primary and continuous cell cultures. In some cases a cytopathic effect is produced, in others there is no cytopathic effect, but infection can be demonstrated by haemadsorption. In some cases a noncytopathic replicative cycle is established perhaps in part mediated by defective interfering particles.

Arboviruses

The term arbovirus is used to describe arthropod-borne viruses that are transmitted to vertebrate hosts during biting to suck blood. Virus replication can take place both in the arthropod vector and the vertebrate host. In many cases the life cycle is complex involving a number of different vectors and hosts. It is now recognized that there are over 500 such viruses belonging to a number of different families and in some cases the classification remains unclear. Although in many cases the disease may be asymptomatic or mild in humans there are situations where it is severe and may be fatal. The full range of the pathology and biology of many of these viruses remains to be described but a myocarditis has been recognized in some (Table 1.3).

Table 1.3 Arboviruses clearly associated with myocarditis.

Family	Virus	Genome	Comments
Togaviridae	Chikungunya	Single-stranded positive sense RNA, 12 kb long	50–70 nm diameter, lipid envelope
Flaviviridae	Dengue	Single-stranded positive sense RNA, 11 kb long, sequenced	45 nm in diameter, lipid envelope
	Yellow fever	Single strand positive sense RNA 10.8 kb long, sequence	Approximately 45 nm in diameter, lipid envelope

Rabies

Rabies virus is a member of the *Rhabdoviridae* and is assigned to the *Lyssavirus* genus. There are four members of the genus which produce disease in humans; the prototype is classic rabies (serotype 1), Lagos bat virus (serotype 2), Mokola virus (serotype 3) originally isolated from a shrew in Ibadan and Duvenhage virus (serotype 4) which is widespread in bat populations.

Classically a bullet-like shape, the rabies virus is enveloped with dimensions of 180 × 65 nm, but large pleomorphic forms may also be evident (Fig. 1.1e). In addition, after passage at high multiplicities smaller particles are produced containing only part of the viral genome which act as defective interfering particles. The envelope carries surface spikes made from a virus-specified glycoprotein (G). The envelope is formed from the plasma membrane by budding. Beneath the envelope is a layer of the matrix protein (M). Within the particles is the RNA which is of negative sense and tightly coiled into a nucleocapsid, the major protein of which is the M protein. The minor proteins are the L (polymerase) and NS (core phospho protein) with which the RNA polymerase activity is associated. The genome of the rabies virus has been sequenced and consists of 12 000 bases with the polypeptides encoded in the following order from the 3′ end: N (nucleocapsid), NS, M, G and L.

Productive cycle

Rabies virus does not readily grow in cell culture without prolonged passage and adaptation. Virus adsorbs on to the surface of cells in culture, the virion surface glycoprotein interacting with receptors on host cells which may be phospholipid or glycolipid. The virion envelope then fuses with the host cell plasma membrane which results in ingestion of the particle. Then there is attachment to liposomes, release of the nucleocapsid, transcription mediated by the virion polymerase and subsequently RNA replication. Translation takes place, the newly synthesized L, NS and N proteins associating with the progeny RNA to produce cores. The G protein and M protein associate with both the plasma membrane and internal membranes of the cell through which the cores bud to produce virus particles which are shed from the surface.

Definition of antigens

All five proteins are antigenic and antibodies to them have been detected. Those to the N protein are group-specific while those to the G protein of the spikes are type-specific. Monoclonal antibodies have allowed a more precise definition of the epitopes recognized.

Retroviridae

There are three subfamilies of the *Retroviridae*: *oncovirinae, lentivirinae* and *spumavirinae*. As far as human viruses are concerned HTLV1 and HTLV2 are *oncovirinae* and HIV-1 (initially christened HTLV3 or LAV) and HIV-2 are now assigned to the *lentivirinae*. The human foamy viruses are members of the *spumavirinae* and as yet have no disease associations. There is a wide range of lentiviruses which cause disease in various animal species, for example, visna-maedi of sheep which in susceptible strains of animals produces a relentlessly progressive disease leading to wasting, pneumonia and paralysis.

Human immunodeficiency virus is an enveloped virus 110 nm in diameter with an icosahedral shell surrounding a conical core within which is the coiled diploid genome which is a 60–70s dimer of identical positive sense RNA strands (Fig. 1.1f) Associated with the genome in the core is the gag (p24) protein and the reverse transcriptase (pol). The icosahedral shell is made up from the gag (p18). The virus envelope is formed by budding through the cell membrane within which is the virus-coded (env) transmembrane glycoprotein (gp41) to which is loosely attached the external glycoprotein (gp120).

The genome of HIV-1 is 9.2 kb long and has been completely sequenced Fig. 1.3. The long terminal repeats (LTR) are on either side of the main structural genes gag, pol and env, but in addition there are at least five additional proteins expressed, most of which are involved in regulation of viral gene expression.

Transactivation gene (tat) codes for a 14 kD polypeptide which specifically binds to the TAR region of the LTR. After binding, full-length transcripts are produced in large amounts.

Regulation of gene expression (rev) codes for a 19 kD protein which binds to a region of the RNA in the env coding region and permits the transport of full-length spliced mRNA for the structural proteins to the cytoplasm.

Negative factor gene (nef) codes for a 27 kD protein which interacts with the LTR in such a way as to reduce transcriptional activity.

Virus infectivity factor (vif) produces a gene product which is a structural gene. Its presence in the virion is required to confer infectivity, possibly being in some way involved in uncoating.

vpu (in HIV-1) and vpx (in HIV-2) code for small proteins whose function is unclear.

HIV-1

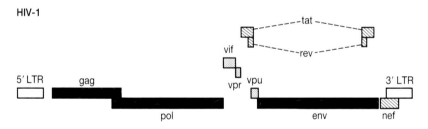

Fig. 1.3 Genome organization of HIV-1.

Productive cycle

Human immunodeficiency virus binds via the gp120 to the CD4 receptor which is expressed on helper T cells and also a variety of other cells including blood monocytes, tissue macrophages and dendritic cells. Subsequent conformational changes lead to fusion of the envelope with the cell membrane and internalization. After uncoating, the reverse transcriptase synthesizes a double-stranded copy of the RNA genome, a provirus. These may circularize and move to the nucleus of the cell where they may become integrated into the host chromosomal DNA. Following integration the genome may remain latent and the cell show no other evidence of having been infected. Alternatively, the productive cycle may be initiated immediately (or after a period of latency). Transcripts are synthesized, polypeptides are synthesized and in some cases cleaved and assembled into progeny virions which bud from the plasma membrane in a process which kills the cell.

The role of the regulatory proteins of the virus in this process is clearly important but there appears to be a coordinated interaction with cellular regulatory factors in some cases. During latency spliced mRNA that codes for tat and rev is transcribed at low level. In HIV infected dividing cells or T cells stimulated to divide by antigens HIV expression may be upregulated and a productive cycle initiated. It may be that the period of latency may extend for many years in some cases.

Definition of antigens

In the infected cell there may be a variety of antigens expressed, only some of which are incorporated as structural genes into the virion. The p24 which forms the nucleoprotein complex of the core may be shed into the serum and can be detected as p24 antigen. This antigen can be detected during the early acute phase and usually during the later phase; its presence is a useful marker for viral replication. There are in addition other gag cleavage products: p55, p25 and p18 and also some intermediates. The envelope glycoprotein precursor is 160 kD and may be detected in infected cells, and its products the envelope glycoproteins gp41 and gp120 are highly immunogenic. Some regions, particularly of gp120 are highly variable. The reverse transcriptase precursor is cleaved to a 10 kD proteinase, a 32 kD endonuclease and a 65 kD reverse transcriptase all of which are immunogenic.

Effects on host cells

The entry of HIV into cells *in vitro* is dependent on the presence of the CD4 receptor. Transfection of the CD4 gene into a range of cells has created a number of adherent productive lines, for example, HeLa. These are more tractable to work with in some ways than the suspension cultures of lymphocytes. The productive cycle after infection generally lasts 24–48 hours and leads to the formation of syncytia and eventually to the death of cells. Primary isolates may differ in their rate of replication and the extent of their cytopathic effect.

Poxviruses

Although smallpox has now been eradicated, vaccinia is still in use; both are members of the orthopoxvirus genus. Poxvirus particles are characteristically brick shape (300×250 nm) within which there is a double-stranded DNA genome (Fig. 1.1g). The virions are complex in structure with an external lipid envelope within which there is a dumb bell core and two associated lateral bodies. The genome is 15×10^4 kD long and is not in itself infectious, there being virus-coded enzymes contained within the core that are essential for transcription. The genome of vaccinia has recently been sequenced.[37] There are more than 100 polypeptides specified by the genome of vaccinia many of which are glycosylated. Some regions of the genome are not essential and can be deleted and replaced with recombinant sequences from other sources.

Productive cycle

Following entry of vaccinia into the target cells either by pinocytosis or membrane fusion replication takes place in cytoplasmic inclusions although nuclear functions are required. The core is uncoated and mRNA is synthesized in a coordinated series of steps eventually leading to DNA replication, uniquely, in cytoplasmic 'factories'. Subsequently, late mRNA is synthesized which results in the production of late proteins. Virus assembly takes place within cytoplasmic inclusions and virus is released following death of the cell. There is no evidence for persistence or latency, the host cellular DNA and protein synthesis being very effectively inhibited after infection. Multiple virus-specified polypeptide species are expressed which are antigenic, over 20 were initially detected by immunodiffusion.

Herpesviridae

There are at least seven human herpesviruses all of which are morphologically indistinguishable and capable of establishing latent infections. Three sub-families have been distinguished (Table 1.4). The recently described human herpesvirus, HHV-6, is ubiquitous and the cause of exanthem subitum of infancy.[38] Even more recently HHV-7 has been isolated from buffy coat cells of a healthy individual but to date there has been no disease association.[39]

All herpesviruses are large enveloped particles with an icosahedral capsid 100 nm in diameter (Fig. 1.1h). Between the envelope and the capsid are the tegument proteins. Within the capsid is the core comprising a cylinder of protein around which is wound the double-stranded DNA. The genome of human herpesviruses 1 to 5 have all been sequenced and range in size from Epstein–Barr virus (EBV) at 128 884 bp to cytomegalovirus (CMV) at 230 000 bp. The genomes are arranged in a variety of ways. Herpes simplex viruses HSV-1 and HSV-2 comprise a long and a short unique sequence each of which are flanked by inverted repeats. Also present is a direct terminal redundancy which is also present internally at the joint between the internal copies of the inverted repeats. The virion DNA exists as one of four equimolar isomers differing in the relative orientation about the joint. In the case of varicella-zoster virus (VZV) the general pattern of organization is similar

Table 1.4 Human herpesviruses.

Subfamily		Human herpesvirus number	Target cells
Alpha herpesvirinae	*Herpes simplex* type 1	1	Dorsal
	Herpes simplex type 2	2	Root
	Varicella zoster virus	3	Ganglia
Gamma herpesvirinae	Epstein–Barr virus	4	B lymphocytes Nasopharyngeal epithelium
Beta herpesvirinae	Cytomegalovirus	5	Buffy coat cells
	Human herpesvirus 6	6	Buffy coat cells
	Human herpesvirus 7	7	Buffy coat cells

except that the inverted repeat flanking the long unique sequence is very short and two of the four possible isomers are present in excess and furthermore there is no terminal redundancy. Epstein–Barr virus has a linear genome consisting largely of unique sequence but with tandem repeats. Cytomegalovirus has a generally similar organization to HSV but is half as big again. There is a gradual accumulation of base changes within HSV-1 and HSV-2 such that individual isolates are distinguishable by restriction endonuclease digestion unless replicate isolates from a single individual or a number of individuals infected from a common source are examined.

The enormous database derived from sequencing has allowed the genetic contents of the human herpesviruses to be identified and the organization of the genomes compared. In the case of HSV-1 more than 70 protein species are encoded, many of which have no recognized function. Genes are transcribed in both directions on both strands of the genome and are closely packed. There are several examples of transcription units comprising nested families of mRNAs having different lengths sharing a common 3′ coterminus. The arrangements of HSV-1 and HSV-2 genomes are almost identical while that of VZV is extremely similar. The EBV genome carries homologous genes of 25 of the HSV and VZV genes located in their long unique sequence arranged in three separate blocks within each of which the genes are largely colinear. Recently the sequence of the CMV genome has become available and there are many similarities with the genome of the other herpesviruses, but one feature is the large number of putative open reading frames coding for what appear to be glycoproteins. The sequence of the HHV-6 genome has not yet been published, there are, however, regions homologous to CMV.

Productive cycle

Herpesviruses can interact with cells either leading to a productive cycle or to the establishment of latency. There is some evidence in animal systems of an oncogenic potential but apart from the relationship between EBV and Burkitt's lymphoma and nasopharyngeal carcinoma and the possible involvement of HSV-2 as a cofactor in carcinoma of the cervix there is no evidence of oncogenesis in humans.

The productive cycle is organized as a cascade and ranges in length from about 16 hours for HSV to 3 days for CMV. First expressed are the immediate early genes which are transcribed by cellular mechanisms in association with, in the case of HSV-1, a transactivating virion structural gene or major tegument protein ((UL 48). There are five immediate early genes of HSV-1 and HSV-2 encoded in separate regions of the genome and the products of three of these in association with host cell proteins can transactivate promoters of early viral genes. In this way the switch from the immediate early to the early phases of the cycle is effected. In the case of VZV there are four proteins predicted that are homologous to HSV-1 immediate early genes. In the case of CMV the immediate early 1 and 2 genes are adjacent and specify multiple overlapping spliced mRNAs. In the case of EBV the protein encoded by BMLF1 can transactivate a wide range of promoters and has some sequence homology with one of the HSV-1 immediate early genes.

Many of the early proteins have functions related to virus DNA synthesis and generally differ in their characteristics from their cell homologue. Following expression of the early proteins virus DNA synthesis takes place which is followed by late phase of the cycle during which there is transcription across the whole of the genome. There are 30 or more virion proteins in the case of HSV-1 at least six of which are glycoproteins. Some of these glycoproteins are involved in the attachment and entry of virus into cells.

Definition of antigens

Immune human serum has antibody to 30 or more HSV-specified proteins. The glycoproteins gB and gD are the principal targets for neutralization in the case of HSV-1 but the other glycoproteins are also important antigens for the immune response. Antibody which does not have neutralizing activity can be detected, for example, by enzyme-linked immunosorbant assay (ELISA) or immunoprecipitation. There may be a substantial degree of cross-reaction between the immune response to HSV and VZV. The immune response to CMV is even more complex than that to HSV. There is also a cell-mediated immune response to herpesviruses which in some cases has been shown to be HLA-restricted.

Effect on host cells *in vitro*

Herpes simplex viruses HSV-1 and HSV-2 produce a rapid cytopathic effect on a wide range of cell lines. Varicella-zoster virus and CMV infect human fibroblast cell lines in culture producing a slowly developing cytopathic effect. In the case of EBV no fully permissive system is available in vitro although primary B cells can be transformed and B cell lines superinfected. Human herpesvirus-6 infects not only B and T lymphoid cell lines but a wide range of other cells.

Adenoviruses

There are 41 serotypes of adenovirus which infect humans and these have been divided into six subgenera on the basis of their haemagglutination of monkey and rat erythrocytes. Adenovirus particles are icosahedral, the capsid being 70–90 nm in diameter. Each capsid is made up of 252 capsomeres and at each of the 12 vertices there is a projecting fibre attached to a capsomere termed a penton (Fig. 1.1i). There are 12 pentons in each particle, the remaining 240 capsomeres are termed hexons. Within the capsid there is a nucleoprotein core containing the double-stranded DNA genome. The nucleic acid has a molecular weight of 20000–25000 kD and representatives of several human serotypes have now been sequenced. Within each subgroup there is more than 70% DNA homology, but between subgroups there is only 10–25% homology. The genome organization has been defined from the sequence data, the genes being tightly packed and situated on both DNA strands. There are four early genes expressed before DNA synthesis coding for proteins which have regulatory functions and five late genes which predominantly code for structural proteins. Each gene produces several different mRNA species as a result of multiple splicing sites.

Adenoviruses attach to the cell surface by means of a knob at the tip of the fibres which binds to specific receptors. Initially, following infection, DNA enters the cell nucleus where it is uncoated and regions are transcribed, about 40% of the genome, and expressed. After about 8 hours virus DNA synthesis commences and virus transcription increases in amount and extends to cover the entire genome. Throughout the late phase of the cycle increasing amounts of structural proteins accumulate and assemble in the cell nucleus and may be visualized as paracrystalline assays. In some situations under experimental conditions adenoviruses may transform cells.

There are at least 10 different structural polypeptides in the virion and antibody is detectable against a variety of determinants.

The hexon bears a group-specific determinant demonstrated by complement fixation. It also has a type-specific determinant detected by neutralization. The knob region of the fibre has a type-specific activity demonstrated by haemagglutination inhibition.

Human adenovirus strains infect a wide range of cell lines although continous or primary cell lines support growth best. The cycle usually progresses rapidly to cell lysis within 18 hours or so. Following cell transformation little if any infectious virus is produced but virus DNA sequences are integrated into the host cell genome.

References

1. Woodruff J. F. Viral myocarditis. *Am J Pathol* 1980; **101:** 425–79.
2. Lerner A. M., Wilson F. M. Virus myocardiopathy. *Prog Med Virol* 1973; **15:** 63–91.
3. Grist N. R., Bell E. J. A six year study of coxsackie B infection in heart disease. *J Hygiene* 1964; **73:** 165–72.
4. Saphir O., Simon W. A., Reingold M. I. Myocarditis in children. *Am J Dis Childhood* 1964; **67:** 294–312.
5. Banatvala J. E. Coxsackie B virus infections in cardiac disease. In: Waterson A. P. ed. *Recent Advances in Clinical Virology*. London, Melbourne, New York: Churchill-Livingstone, 1983: Volume 3. 99–115.
6. Kandolf R. The impact of recombinant DNA technology on the study of enterovirus heart disease. In: Bendinelli M., Freedman H. eds. *Coxsackieviruses – A General Update*. New York: Plenum, 1988: 293–318.
7. Kandolf R., Hofschneider P. H. Viral heart disease. *Springer Seminar Immunopathology* 1989; **115:** 1–13.
8. Bowles N. E., Richardson P. J., Olsen G. J., Archard L. C. Detection of coxsackie B virus-specific RNA sequences in myocardial biopsy samples from patients with myocarditis and dilated cardiomyopathy. *Lancet* 1986; **i:** 1120–3.
9. Caforio A. L. P., Stewart J. T., McKenna W. J. Idiopathic dilated cardiomyopathy. *Br Med J* 1990; **300:** 890–1.
10. Johnson R. A., Palacios I. Dilated cardiomyopathies of the adult (second of two parts). *New Engl J Med* 1982; **307:** 1119–26.
11. Yazu T. A case of hepatitis A accompanied by acute myocarditis. *Nippon Shokakibyo Gakki Zusski* 1988; **85:** 1304–7.
12. Broustet P., Dallochio Sagardiluz J. *et al*. Observation anatomoclinique d'une myocardite ourlienne chez un homme de 34 ans. *Arch Mal Coeur* 1964; **57:** 1457–73.
13. Raman G. V. S., Presser A., Spreadbury P. L. *et al*. Rabies presenting with myocarditis and encephalitis. *J Infection* 1988; **17:** 155–8.
14. Levy W. S., Simon G. L., Rio S. J. C., Ross A. M. Prevalence of cardiac abnormalities in human immunodeficiency virus infections. *Am J Cardiol* 1989; **63:** 86–9.

15. Tyson A. A. Acute Epstein Barr virus myocarditis simulating myocardial infarction with cardiogenic shock. *Southern Med J* 1989; **82:** 1184–7.
16. Collier L. H., Timbury M. C. In: Parker M. T., Collier L. H. general eds. *Topley and Wilson's Principles of Bacteriology, Virology and Immunity*. 8th Edition. Volume 4. Sevenoaks: Edward Arnold (Publishers) Ltd, 1990.
17. Enders J. F., Weller T. H., Robbins. Cultivation of the Lansing strain of poliomyelitis virus in 7 cultures of various human embryonic diseases, *Science* 1949; **109:** 85.
18. Kitamura N., Semler B., Rothberg P. G. *et al*. Primary structure, gene organization and polypeptide expression of poliovirus RNA. *Nature* 1981; **291:** 475–533.
19. Hogle J. M., Chow M, Filman D. J. Three dimensional structure of poliovirus at 2.9 Å resolution. *Science* 1985; **229:** 1358–65.
20. Chow M., Newman J. F. F., Filman D. *et al*. Myristilation of picorna virus capsid protein VP4 and its structural significance. *Nature* 1987; **327:** 482–6.
21. Stanway G. Structure, function and evolution of picornaviruses. *J Gen Virol* 1990; **71:** 2483–501.
22. Rueckert R. R., Wimmer E. Systematic nomenclature of picornavirus proteins. *J Virol* 1984; **50:** 957–9.
23. Mendelsohn C., Johnson B. Transformation of a human poliovirus receptor gene into mouse cells *Proc Natl Acad Sci (USA)* 1986; **83:** 7845–9.
24. Greve J. M., Davis G, Meyer A. M. *et al*. The major human rhinovirus receptor is ICAM-I. *Cell* 1989; **56:** 839–47.
25. Staunton D. E., Merluzzi V. J., Rothlein R. *et al*. A cell adhesion molecule ICAM-I is the major surface receptor for rhinoviruses. *Cell* 1989; **56:** 849–53.
26. Ratka M., Lackmann M., Ueckermann C. *et al*. Poliovirus associated protein kinase: destabilization of the virus capsid and stimulation of the phosphorylation by Zn^{++}.*J Virol* 1989; **63:** 3954–60.
27. Smith T. J., Kemer M. S., Ming L. *et al*. The site of attachment in human rhinovirus 14 for antiviral agents that inhibit uncoating. *Science* 1986; **233:** 1286–93.
28. Racaniello V. R., Baltimore D. Cloned poliovirus complementary DNA is infectious in mammalian cells. *Science* 1981; **214:** 916–9.
29. Rueckert R. R. Picornaviruses and their replication. In: Fields B. N. ed. *Virology*. New York: Raven Press, 1985: 705–38.
30. Kuhn R. J., Wimmer E. The replication of Picornaviruses. In: Rowlands D. J., Mayo M. A., Mahy B. W. J. eds. *The Molecular Biology of Positive Strand RNA Viruses FEMS Symposium No. 32*. London: Academic Press, 1987: 17–51.
31. Flanegan J. B., Baltimore D. Poliovirus – specific primer dependent RNA polymerase able to code poly (A). *Proc Natl Acad Sci (USA)* 1977; **74:** 3677–80.
32. Minor P. D., Ferguson M., Evans D. M. A. *et al*. Antigenic structure of polioviruses of serotypes 1, 2 and 3. *J Gen Virol* 1986; **67:** 1283–91.
33. Page J. G. S., Mosser A. G., Hogle J. M. *et al*. Three dimensional structure of poliovirus serotype 1 neutralizing determinants. *J Virol* 1988; **62:** 1781–94.
34. Murray M. G., Kuhn R. J., Arita M. *et al*. Poliovirus type 1/type 3 antigenic hybrid virus constructed *in vitro* elicits type 1 and type 3 neutralizing antibodies in rabbits and monkeys. *Proc Natl Acad Sci (USA)* 1988; **85:** 3203–7.
35. Burke K. L., Dunn G., Ferguson M. *et al*. Antigenic chimaeras of poliovirus as potential new vaccines. *Nature (London)* 1988; **332:** 81–2.
36. Dominguez G., Wang C.-Y., Fry T. K. Sequence of the genome RNA of rubella virus: evidence for genetic rearrangement during togavirus evolution. *Virology* 1990; **177:** 225–38.
37. Goebal S. J., Johnson G. P., Perkus M. E. *et al*. The complete DNA sequence of vaccinia virus. *Virology* 1990; **179:** 247–66.

38. Yamanaski K., Okuno T., Shiraki K. *et al.* Identification of human herpesvirus-6 as a causal agent for exanthem subitum. *Lancet* 1988; **1:** 1065–7.
39. Frenkel N., Schirmer E. C., Wyatt L. S. *et al.* Isolation of a new herpesvirus from CD4 [+]Tcells. *Proc Natl Acad Sci (USA)* 1990; **87:** 748–52.

2

Epidemiology of viral infections of the heart

N. R. Grist and D. Reid

Introduction

Information on the epidemiology of viral infections of the heart is scattered and incomplete. It requires recorded evidence from studies where virological diagnostic tests have been applied to clinically categorized cases in a systematic manner. There are few instances where this has been achieved, and even then the range of viruses for which tests have been available, let alone applied, has generally been limited.

There are various reports of particular virus infections associated with or causing heart disease, and these are discussed elsewhere in this book. This chapter deals with data available from surveillance programmes and the epidemiological impact of the various viral infections.

International data

Surveillance of viral activity at international level has been carried out for many years by reports submitted to the World Health Organization (WHO).

Table 2.1 lists the cases categorized as 'cardiovascular' in the Global Surveillance of Virus Diseases programme of the WHO from 1975 to 1985 inclusive. The statistical evidence is outstanding in the case of the coxsackie B viruses (Fig. 2.1), followed by influenza B; of possible but less certain statistical significance are influenza A, 'picornavirus not typed' (recorded by WHO where the virus type has not been specified), coxsackie A viruses, cytomegalovirus, parainfluenza virus and echoviruses; even less significant are polioviruses and rhinoviruses. It should be noted that congenital diseases form a separate heading in the WHO tabulation, so that developmental abnormalities attributable to rubella and cytomegaloviruses are excluded from Table 2.1.

Because the data listed by WHO are derived from reports supplied by many different countries, they have the merit of wide coverage, but with limitations. Thus the degree of surveillance activity in different countries varies, both in the level of participation and in the selection of cases for testing as well as the available range of tests. Tests for coxsackie B virus infections by antibody studies are more widely available and so more often used for these than many other virus infections. Results of tests may not be reported centrally or transmitted to WHO. A conspicuous gap in Table 2.1 relates to 'arboviruses', a heading not used in the WHO tabulation although

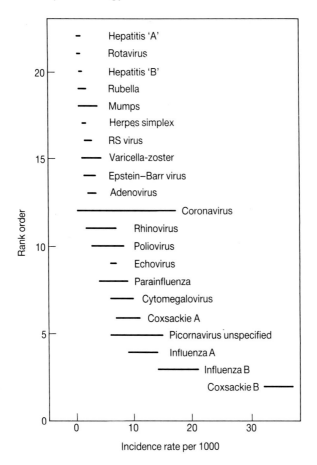

Fig. 2.1 Relationship of viral infections to cardiovascular disease (World Health Organization: global surveillance). The figure shows 95% confidence limits for the incidence rates specified in Table 2.1.

several of these (e.g. dengue, yellow fever and Chikungunya virus) have been reported in cases of myocarditis and may be important in countries where they are prevalent.

Despite these gaps, the WHO data do show major correlations, notably for coxsackie B viruses which are by far those more often recognized in cardiac disease. Some coxsackie A viruses have been identified as causing myocarditis, but knowledge of these is incomplete since classical techniques for their recognition required inconvenient and expensive tests in newborn mice; new techniques such as those based on nucleic acid hybridization, amplification by the polymerase chain reaction, and use of specific monoclonal antibodies, should facilitate further research in this area. Tests for IgM antibodies against virions and procapsid antigens of coxsackie B viruses might clarify the contribution of coxsackie A and echoviruses to cardiac disease as they have in insulin dependent (type 1) diabetes melitus.[1]

Table 2.1 World Health Organization global surveillance of viral infections related to cardiovascular disease (1975–1985).

Virus	Total	Cardiovascular disease	Rate per 1000	Rank order
Coxsackie B	19203	665	34.6	1
Influenza B	4608	80	17.4	2
Influenza A	6391	75	11.7	3
Picornavirus (unspecified)*	2071	20	9.7	4
Coxsackie A	6704	61	9.1	5
Cytomegalovirus	9666	77	8.0	6
Parainfluenza	5323	35	6.6	7
Echovirus	45921	293	6.4	8
Poliovirus	2635	13	4.9	9
Rhinovirus	2441	9	3.7	10
Coronavirus	331	1	3.0	11
Adenovirus	16921	47	2.8	12
Epstein–Barr virus	8489	20	2.4	13
Varicella–Zoster	3564	8	2.2	14
Respiratory syncytial virus	15573	33	2.1	15
Herpes simplex	62440	81	1.3	16
Mumps	2322	3	1.30	17
Rubella	6949	7	1.0	18
Hepatitis B virus	23764	17	0.7	19
Rotavirus	24064	9	0.4	20
Hepatitis A virus	11019	3	0.3	21

*The precise interpretation of the heading 'picornavirus (unspecified)' is unclear, and this category has been omitted from our analysis.

Epidemiological aspects of various viral infections

The epidemiological characteristics of the various viral infections of the heart vary with the virus involved and a range of other factors such as the age of the patient, the season of the year and the degree of contact (Table 2.2). Although the heart is exposed to infection during the viraemic phase of many of these infections, only a minority give rise to overt cardiac disease. This points to the importance of factors such as the immunological and other specific characteristics of the individual host, of temporary physiological conditions such as the adverse effects of exercise, and of strain variations in cardiopathic virulence by infecting viruses. In young children the myocardium is particularly affected and they may rapidly develop cardiac failure. Adults often present clinically with pericarditis although the myocardium is probably always affected. Both coxsackie A and B viruses are most often seen in children whereas influenza virus type A can affect all ages (Chapter 2). The season also affects the frequency with which the various viruses occur, notably influenza A and B which predominantly occur in the winter and spring. Many of the cases of viral carditis are sporadic but outbreaks (e.g. especially coxsackievirus infections), epidemics and even pandemics (e.g. especially influenza A infections) can occur. Spread may come from an infected case or from faecal–oral transmission from water, food or articles contaminated by faeces.

Table 2.2 Some epidemiological characteristics of viruses commonly associated with cardiac disease.

Virus	Age	Usual season	Occurrence	Spread
Enteroviruses: coxsackie A and B, echoviruses	Most often children (acute cardiac presentation mainly myocarditis), also adults (acute, cardiac, presentation mainly pericarditis)	Summer in temperate climates	Mainly sporadic, also outbreaks and epidemics	Faecal–oral route from water, food or articles contaminated by faeces; respiratory spread from contact with infected persons
Influenza A and B	Most often children, especially influenza B, also all ages	Winter and spring	Sporadic cases, outbreaks, epidemics and pandemics	Contact with infected persons or their respiratory discharges
Cytomegalovirus	All ages, primary infections mainly in children; reactivation at any age	All seasons	Congenital. Outbreaks of primary infection in residential nurseries. Reactivation by immune depression at any age	Maternal transmission to foetus. Intimate contact with infected person
Parainfluenza	Mainly children	Winter (summer for type 3)	Sporadic cases and outbreaks	Contact with infected persons

Enteroviruses

These hardy picornaviruses are prevalent worldwide, particularly in warm climates and warm seasons, in children and young persons, and in conditions of overcrowding with poor hygiene and sanitation. Spread is mainly by the faecal–oral route and sometimes by the respiratory route which becomes relatively more important in conditions of good hygiene and sanitation. Spread is common within families and nosocomially, mainly without symptoms. Immunity is mainly type-specific, but transient, silent reinfections can occur. Exposure to different enteroviruses, which share various antigens, builds up a broad range of antibodies within the first decades of life. The prevalent types of enterovirus vary from year to year in a community, outbreaks affecting particularly children, but also involving adults in communities where immunity is incomplete because of higher standards of hygiene and sanitation. In such communities, relative paucity of antibodies in women of childbearing age can allow outbreaks among neonates in maternity units to which an enterovirus has been introduced. Among these infants, unprotected by passive antibody, severe infections can occur with acute myocarditis as a prominent, life-threatening feature.[2,3] During the widespread epidemic of coxsackie B5 virus infection which affected many countries of Europe in 1965, a collaborative survey in the UK organized by the Public Health Laboratory Service showed that of 1160 reports 48 (5.3%) were associated with pericarditis (41), myocarditis (5) or unspecified cardiovascular disease (2). Two of those with myocarditis died.[4]

The proportion of coxsackievirus infections found among patients with acute myopericarditis varies greatly in a variety of studies carried out in different countries. Some of these are listed in Table 2.3 where, despite the difficulties in achieving virological proof, acceptable positive findings were reported in up to three-quarters of most series studied, with higher rates

Table 2.3   Proportion of coxsackie virus infection found among acute myopericarditis patients.

Group investigated	Number positive	Reference
34 pericarditis (sporadic)	1 (3%)	Johnson et al.[5]
20 myopericarditis (sporadic)	5 (25%)*	Middleton and Grist[6]
12 pericarditis (epidemic)	6 (50%)	Bennett[7]
18 myopericarditis (epidemic)	14 (78%)	Helin et al.[8]
12 myocarditis (children)	6 (50%)	Berkovich et al.[9]
57 myopericarditis (adults)	22 (39%)	Sainani et al.[10]
45 myopericarditis (adults)	10 (44%)†	Koontz and Ray[11]
8 myopericarditis (adults)	5 (63%)*	Woods et al.[12]
153 myopericarditis (sporadic, mixed ages)	59 (39%)*	Grist and Bell[13]
19 myocarditis (young adults)	4 (21%)	Madhavan et al.[14]
18 myocarditis (children)	4 (22%)	Ayuthya et al.[15]
102 myopericarditis (adults)	38 (37%)	El-Hagrassi et al.[16] (1gM pos)
11 myopericarditis (adults)	4 (36%)	O'Neil et al.[17]
1137 myopericarditis (mainly adults)	185 (16%)*	Bell and McCartney[18]

*Includes cases with static antibody titres of 256 or more.
†Includes three cases with titres less than 256.

during outbreaks of coxsackie infection (particularly types A4, A16 and B1–5).

The range of age (infancy to old age) and sex (male predominance) in a series of patients diagnosed virologically in Glasgow is illustrated in Table 2.4.[19,20] The excess of older males in the coxsackie B group may be partly attributable to availability of serological diagnosis for group B but not normally for group A infections, facilitating diagnosis in older age groups where virus isolation is most difficult to achieve and where males predominate in cardiac disease.

Table 2.4   Age, sex and clinical presentation of 27 cases of coxsackie virus myopericarditis.

	Virological Group	
	Coxsackie A	Coxsackie B
Age (years)		
0–1	3	2
2–10	0	5
11–40	0	5
>60	0	2
Sex		
Male	1	14
Female	4	7
Not recorded	0	1
Disease		
Myocarditis	3	13
Pericarditis	2	9

The predominance of coxsackie B viruses over coxsackie A and echoviruses as recognized causes of cardiovascular disease was shown in a previous analysis of international data.[21] After adding a further year's data, the relative significance of the main individual enteroviruses contributing to cardiovascular disease is illustrated in Table 2.5. This table also shows the low or negligible rates of cardiovascular disease in infections by some common enteroviruses familiar as causes of outbreaks of epidemics, notably coxsackie A9 virus and echovirus types 4 and 30. Cardiovascular diagnoses were associated with 4% of coxsackie B2 infections, with approximately 3% of infections with coxsackie B3, B6, B1 and echovirus 16 infections, and with about 2% of coxsackie A4, B4 and B5 infections. The relevance of these viruses in cardiac disease has been supported by detection of viral antigen in heart tissue or pericardial fluid of cases of acute myocarditis, and this has also been reported for echovirus 9, echovirus 22 and coxsackie A16 infections[22] of which fewer than 1% were associated with cardiovascular diagnoses in Table 2.5.

Influenza

Influenza A and B viruses are well-known respiratory pathogens spread by the airborne route and causing periodic epidemics, and occasional pandemics when a novel antigenic variant of influenza A appears. These outbreaks are well recognized to cause increased mortality from various cardiac diseases, particularly in older persons and those with already impaired hearts. Most of

Table 2.5 Association of some typed enterovirus infections with cardiovascular diagnoses (WHO data 1975–1985).

Virus	Total tests	Cardiovascular diagnoses	
		Number	Rate per 1000
Coxsackie B2	3470	140	40
Coxsackie B3	3283	105	32
Echovirus 16	239	7	29
Coxsackie B6	491	14	29
Coxsackie B1	2403	67	28
Coxsackie A4	201	4	20
Coxsackie B5	4530	87	19
Coxsackie B4	4630	86	19
Echovirus 22	3292	30	9
Echovirus 14	1487	13	9
Echovirus 11	8339	58	7
Coxsackie A9	2807	21	7
Echovirus 9	3239	20	6
Echovirus 30	5574	22	4
Coxsackie A16	1161	6	0.8
Echovirus 4	687	0	0

this is probably due to the added cardio-respiratory stress of the febrile, toxic illness, but influenza A virus has been detected in the heart of a few patients with acute cardiac disease during influenza (reviewed by Woodward *et al.*[23] and Lansdown[24]). Either direct damage or immunopathological processes may be involved in causation of disease by these membrane-bound viruses which contain host antigens. Myalgia, typical of influenza and several other acute viral infections, can be an important symptom presaging myocarditis.[25]

Other viruses

The WHO data (Table 2.1, Fig. 2.1) are suggestive but uncertain in respect of many other viruses, of which several are occasionally reported in cardiac disease, either coincidentally or sometimes causally, perhaps reflecting the interaction of different viral variants and host variability.

Of more epidemiological significance and worthy of comment are 'arboviruses' which are so prevalent and sometimes epidemic in many tropical and subtropical areas where myocardial diseases of uncertain origin are also common. Dengue and chikungunya viruses have long been known as causes of acute myocarditis,[26–28] and the largely unexplored role of such viruses in endemic areas may well be important and merits further investigation. Cardiac damage is also characteristic of yellow fever and other viral haemorrhagic fevers including those due to hantaviruses,[29] arenaviruses[30] and filoviruses.[31] The myocardium is also well recognized to be damaged in rabies, as again reported recently.[32] The contribution of the human immunodeficiency virus (HIV) to heart disease is considered in Chapter 7.

Acknowledgements

The help of Margaret McInnes, Gwen Allardice, Andrew Millar, Fiona Johnston, Patricia Cassels and Mary Graham of the Communicable Diseases (Scotland) Unit and Karin Esteves of the World Health Organization in the preparation of this chapter is much appreciated.

References

1. Frisk G., Nilsson E., Tuvemo T., Friman G., Diderholm H. The possible role of coxsackie A and echoviruses in the pathogenesis of type I diabetes mellitus studied by IgM analysis. *J Infection* 1992; **24:** 13–22.
2. Gear J. H. S. Coxsackievirus infections in the newborn. *Prog Med Virol* 1958; **1:** 106–21.
3. Gear J. H. S., Measroch V. Coxsackievirus infections in the newborn. *Prog Med Virol* 1973; **15:** 42–62.
4. Public Health Laboratory Service. Coxsackie B5 virus infections in 1965. *Br Med J* 1967; **4:** 575–7.
5. Johnson R. T., Portnoy B., Rogers N. G., Buescher N. G. Acute benign pericarditis: Virologic study of 34 patients. *Ann Int Med* 1961; **108:** 823–32.
6. Middleton P. J., Grist N. R. A serological investigation of coxsackievirus group infection in patients with cardiac disease and chest pain. *Scot Med J* 1965; **10:** 108–11.
7. Bennett N. McK. Coxsackie B pericarditis. *Med J Australia* 1966; **2:** 178–9.
8. Helin M., Savola J., Lapinleimu K. Cardiac manifestations during a coxsackie B5 epidemic. *Br Med J* 1968; **3:** 97–9.
9. Berkovich S., Rodriguez-Torres R., Lin J. S. Virologic studies in children with acute myocarditis. *Am J Dis Child* 1968; **115:** 207–12.
10. Sainani G. S., Krompotic E., Slodki S. J. Adult heart disease due to the coxsackievirus B infection. *Medicine* 1968; **47:** 133–47.
11. Koontz C. H., Ray C. G. The role of the coxsackie Group B virus infections in sporadic myopericarditis. *Am Heart J* 1971; **82:** 750–8.
12. Woods J. D., Nimmo M. J., Mackay-Scollay E. M. Adult heart disease associated with coxsackie B virus infection. *Med J Australia* 1973; **2:** 573–7.
13. Grist N. R., Bell E. J. A six year study of coxsackievirus B infections in heart disease. *J Hyg (Camb.)* 1974; **73:** 165–72.
14. Madhaven H. N., Chandrasekhar S., Agarwal S. C. Coxsackie B virus infections in myocarditis in adults – South India. *Indian J Med Res* 1974; **62:** 332–8.
15. Ayuthya P. S. N., Jayavasu J., Pongpanich B. Coxsackie Group B virus and primary myocardial diseases in infants and children. *Am Heart J* 1974; **88:** 311–14.
16. El-Hagrassi M. M. O., Banatvala J. E., Coltart D. J. Coxsackie B virus specific 1gM responses in patients with cardiac and other diseases. *Lancet* 1980; **ii:** 1160–2.
17. O'Neil D., McArthur J. D., Kennedy J. A., Clements G. Coxsackie B virus infection in coronary care unit patients. *J Clin Pathol* 1983; **36:** 658–61.
18. Bell E. J., McCartney R. A. A study of coxsackie B virus infections 1972–1983. *J Hyg (Camb)* 1984: **93:** 197–203.
19. Bell E. J., Grist N. R. Enteroviruses and heart disease. *Cardiol Dig* 1972; **7:** 11–14.
20. Grist N. R. Coxsackievirus infections of the heart. In: Waterson A. P. ed. *Recent Advances in Clinical Virology*. Edinburgh: Churchill Livingstone, 1977: 141–50.
21. Grist N. R. Epidemiology and pathogenicity of coxsackieviruses. In: Schultheiss H. P. ed. *New Concepts in Viral Heart Disease*. Berlin: Springer-Verlag, 1988: 26–32.
22. Minor P. D., Bell E. J. Picornaviridae (excluding rhinovirus). In: Parker M. T., Collier L. H. eds. *Topley and Wilson's Principles of Bacteriology, Virology and Immunity*. 9th edition. Volume 4. *Virology*. Sevenoaks: Edward Arnold, 1990: 323–57.
23. Woodward T. E., McCrumb F. R., Carey T. N., Togo Y. Viral and rickettsial

causes of cardiac disease including the coxsackievirus etiology of pericarditis and myocarditis. *Ann Int Med* 1960; **53:** 1130–50.

24. Lansdown A. B. G. Viral infections and diseases of the heart. *Prog Med Virol* 1978; **24:** 70–113.
25. Lewes D., Rainford D. J., Lane W. F. Symptomless myocarditis and myalgia in viral and *Mycoplasma pneumoniae* infections. *Br Heart J* 1974; **36:** 924–32.
26. Obeyesekere I., Hermon Y. Myocarditis and cardiomyopathy after arbovirus infections (dengue and chikungunya fever). *Br Heart J* 1972; **34:** 821–7.
27. Obeyesekere I., Hermon Y. Arbo virus heart disease: myocarditis and cardio-myopathy following dengue and chikungunya fever – a follow up study. *Am Heart J* 1973; **85:** 186–94.
28. Naragatnam N., Stripalo K., de Silva N. Arbovirus (dengue type) as a cause of myocarditis and pericarditis. *Br Heart J* 1973; **35:** 204–6.
29. Hullinghorst R. L., Steer A. Pathology of epidemic haemorrhagic fever. *Ann Int Med* 1953; **38:** 77–101.
30. Simpson D. I. H., Bowen E. T. W. Arenaviruses. In: Wetherall D., Ledingham J. C. G., Warrel D. A. eds. *Oxford Textbook of Medicine*. 2nd edition. Volume 1. Oxford: Oxford University Press, 1987: 5.134–5.139.
31. Bowen E. T. W., Simpson D. I. H. Marburg and Ebola fevers. In: Weatherall D., Ledingham J. C. G., Warrel D. A. eds. *Oxford Textbook of Medicine*. 2nd edition. Volume 1. Oxford: Oxford University Press, 1987: 5.155–5.158.
32. Raman G. V., Prosser A., Spreadbury P. L., Cockcroft P. M., Okubadejo O. A. Rabies presenting with myocarditis and encephalitis. *J Infection* 1988; **17:** 155–8.

3

The histopathological diagnosis and morphological features of acute myocarditis

M. E. Billingham

Introduction

The term myocarditis may be applied when the histological examination of the myocardium shows evidence of an inflammatory process. Used in this broad term, any inflammatory process affecting the myocardium may be caused by bacterial, rickettsial, fungal, parasitic or viral organisms (Tables 3.1–3.3). Although these organisms continue to affect the myocardium, particularly in patients receiving immunosuppressive drugs or in the case of immune deficiency syndrome (AIDS), in developed countries most cases of acute myocarditis are thought to be due to viral infection. Myocarditis has been described in a number of the common childhood viral diseases; however, in these diseases clinical myocarditis is quite rare and often benign. Certain enteroviruses such as coxsackie B[1,2] (B1–5, A4 and 16) and some echovirus serotypes (especially 9, 11, and 22) are known to be particularly cardiotropic and to cause acute myopericarditis experimentally in animals. Despite there findings, it has yet to be established conclusively that myocarditis is virally induced. Even when an organism is isolated, it is often not known whether direct invasion and tissue damage by the infectious agent or an allergic hypersensivity response or even a toxic response to this agent is responsible for the morphological and clinical manifestations of acute myocarditis. Raised titres of neutralizing antibody in the serum may suggest viral myocarditis, but this finding is not necessarily diagnostic. Viral particles have not yet been unequivocally seen in the myocardium except for cytomegalovirus in the immunocompromised host (Fig. 3.1). More recently, enteroviruses have been implicated in the aetiology, this being suggested by the finding of enteroviral RNA in endomyocardial biopsy samples from histologically proven cases of acute myocarditis.[3,4] More recent studies, however, using the polymerase chain reaction, a more sensitive technique, have demonstrated enteroviruses in control tissue from patients without myocarditis or dilated cardiomyopathy.[5,6] The inference that dilated cardiomyopathy is the endstage of virally induced myocarditis, although widely suspected, also has not yet been unequivocally proved. Work in this area continues to progress and perhaps a definite answer will be forthcoming soon. The above definition of myocarditis suggests strongly that its morphological manifestations namely, an inflammatory infiltrate of the myocardium, is due directly or indirectly to the response to an

Table 3.1 Bacterial infections known to cause myocarditis.

Staphylococcus aureus septicaemia	Gonococcal septicaemia
Streptococcal infections	Salmonella septicaemia
C. diptheriae	B. abortus
N. meningitis	M. tuberculosis
T. pallidun	P. pseudomallei
B. borgorfei	B. pertussis
B. recurrentis	B. persica

Table 3.2 Major causes of myocarditis other than viral and bacterial.

Protozoa	Parasites	Hypersensitivity
Trypanosoma cruzi (Chagas' disease)	*Trichonella (spiralis)*	Rheumatic fever
Toxoplasma gondii		Dermatomyositis
E. histolytica		Scleroderma
		Rheumatoid arthritis
		Other autoimmune diseases

Table 3.3 Viral and chlamydial infections known to cause myocarditis.

Enteroviruses	Herpes simplex	Cytomegalovirus
Mumps	Measles	Hepatitis A
Influenza	Vaccinia	Epstein–Barr
C. psittaci	Poliomyelitis	Yellow fever
Rubella	Rabies	

See also Table 1.1

infection by an organism. An inflammatory response, however, may be due to other causes as well, such as toxic or hypertensivity changes to drugs or immunological insults (transplantation rejection) and, for this reason, acute myocarditis is more accurately referred to as 'idiopathic myocarditis'.

Evidence supporting a clinical diagnosis of acute myocarditis includes a history of a preceding viral illness such as influenza, the presence of fever and myalgia, arrhythmias in a previously healthy individual, and eventually a large failing heart. These clinical changes (see chapter 4) although well described are non-specific and identical clinical features might be the result of such other diseases as myocardial sarcoidosis or idiopathic dilated cardio-mypathy. The clinical diagnosis is therefore difficult and only suggestive. For this reason, the incidence and cause of acute myocarditis has not been well established. The widespread use of the endomyocardial biopsy technique for obtaining myocardium *in vivo* raised hopes that it would be possible to diag-nose acute myocarditis more accurately if a histopathological examination showed a definite inflammatory infiltration of the myocardium. Even in the cases where the endomyocardial biopsy is positive for inflammatory infiltrates, the diagnosis of acute viral myocarditis can only be suggested when all the other diagnostic pitfalls have been ruled out. Consequently, a definitive diag-nosis of idiopathic myocarditis has to be made with caution.

Acute cardiac rejection closely resembles acute myocarditis morphologi-cally (Fig. 3.2) and in the last 20 years an enormous amount of experience has been gleaned from cardiac rejection which is in essence an acute inflammatory

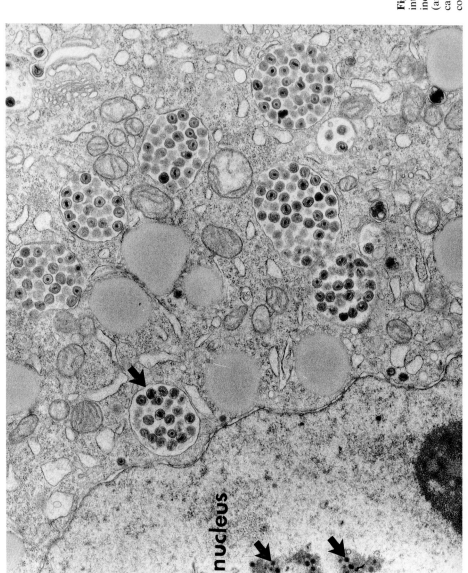

nucleus

Fig. 3.1 Electron micrograph of intranuclear and intracytoplasmic inclusions of cytomegalovirus (arrows) from the endomyo-cardial biopsy of an immuno-compromised patient. × 16 600.

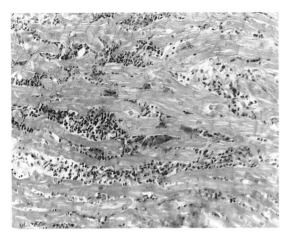

Fig. 3.2   Myocardial biopsy showing a florid interstitial infiltration of activated lymphocytes with myocyte damage in acute cardiac rejection. H&E × 185.

infiltrate of the myocardium and therefore serves, to a certain extent, as a model for acute myocarditis in humans (see Chapter 11).[7] A wealth of experience gained with the histopathology of acute rejection has shown that the heart failure does not occur with focal areas of acute rejection, but only when there is a widespread global interstitial infiltrate of inflammatory cells (Fig. 3.2); this fact confuses the understanding of clinical acute myocarditis. If the widespread infiltrate is also necessary for the presence of heart failure in acute myocarditis, it is then very probable that this entity has been overdiagnosed from the morphological standpoint since most patients are not biopsed until they are already in heart failure, many biopsies showing only focal changes.

The purpose of this chapter is to describe the histopathological changes of acute viral myocarditis and to discuss the pitfalls of diagnosis on endomyocardial biopsy as well as to present the arguments and evidence for and against the supposition that idiopathic cardiomyopathy may, in some cases, follow acute myocarditis. Since this chapter relates specifically to viral myocarditis, myocarditis resulting from bacterial, fungal and rickettsial causes will not be discussed in detail.

The gross manifestations of acute myocarditis

In acute myocarditis from all causes the heart is usually grossly enlarged with dilated ventricles. The papillary muscles and trabeculae carneae of the ventricles may be flattened. The myocardium is pale, yellow or grey, and darker areas of minute haemorrhages are also seen. Most of the myocarditidies produce essentially similar anatomical changes which will be described here as characteristic of the group as a whole. There are, however, minor variations in the morphological picture depending on the aetiology. In early, focal, acute myocarditis, the heart may be within normal limits for size grossly but more often however, it is dilated. In severe acute myocarditis the heart is always dilated, flabby and pale. On the cut surface, the myocardium is often pale with scattered haemorrhages. Mural thrombi in the atria and ventricles are much less frequent than in dilated congestive cardiomyopathy because the length of illness is usually shorter. Acute fulminating cases may have visible areas of frank myocardial necrosis similar to microinfarctions. Acute myocarditis has been described as a panmyocarditis. Not only the endocardium and myocardium may be affected but also the pericardium. Therefore, the pericardium may be seen to contain either pericardial effusion or to have a fibrinous pericarditis.

The histopathological changes of idiopathic myocarditis

Acute myocarditis has been described as a panmyocarditis as mentioned above. The histopathological changes of acute myocarditis associated with specific viruses or viral syndromes is similar. Although minor variations may occur in the morphological picture due to different specific viruses, these are slight. The morphological picture of acute myocarditis reveals an inflammatory infiltrate which varies with time. The lesions may show a predilection for the subendocardial or subepicardial regions in which case there is an associated fibrinous pericarditis. There is a varying amount of myocyte necrosis. At first the inflammatory infiltrate may be mixed with neutrophils, sometimes giant cells, eosinophils, histiocytes and even Anitschkow cells. The inflammatory infiltrate is spread throughout the interstitium involving adjacent myocytes and may also cause a vasculitis although this is not always the case (Figs. 3.3 and 3.4). Focal infiltrates and even diffuse infiltrates extend through all parts of the myocardium including the conduction system where they may cause sudden or unexpected death from arrythmias. When the myocarditis is extensive there may be enough myocyte damage to cause frank heart failure. Multiple, small myocardial abscesses, although described, are usually seen only when the disease is accompanied by pyaemia and there is a secondary bacterial infection. Patients dying after a longer interval may

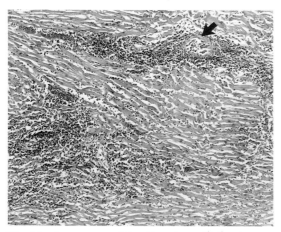

Fig. 3.3 Acute myocarditis with an interstitial and perivascular infiltrate (arrow) of lymphocytes. H&E × 60.

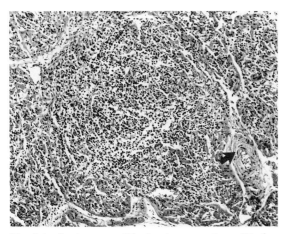

Fig. 3.4   Acute myocarditis showing no perivasculitis (arrow). H&E × 60.

show considerable interstitial fibrosis with compensatory hypertrophy (Fig. 3.5). Myocytes may show varying degrees of damage, but coagulation necrosis can occur or one may see myocyte eosinophilia and contraction bands adjacent to the inflammatory infiltrate. Although nowadays it is possible to stain for different types of leucocytic antigens, the further differentiation between the varying types of inflammatory cells is not useful diagnostically at this stage except to rule out lymphomatous infiltrates. It is important, to be able to differentiate acute myocarditis with extensive myocardial necrosis from a myocardial infarction. This is not difficult apart from the endo-myocardial biopsy diagnosis. In infarcts, there is a distinct border zone of infarction (Fig. 3.6) with central necrosis and a peripheral cellular infiltrate, whereas in acute myocarditis it is more common to find smaller areas of myocardial necrosis surrounded by inflammatory cells. It should be noted that in most cases the character of the cellular infiltrate does not permit a

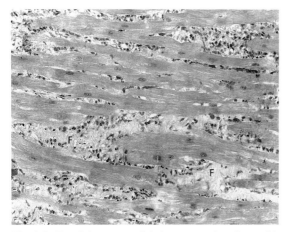

Fig. 3.5   Resolving myocarditis in a reparative phase with small, inactivated lymphocytes and newly formed interstitial fibrosis (F). H&E × 180.

specific aetiological diagnosis. As discussed later, new molecular biological techniques including *in situ* hybridization and polymerase chain amplification may help identify the presence of viral genomes within myocardial cells (Figs. 3.7 and 3.8).[5,6]

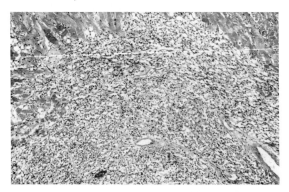

Fig. 3.6   Edge of a recent myocardial infarct with granulation tissue. Note 'punched out' border of infarct in the top portion of the photomicrograph. H&E × 60.

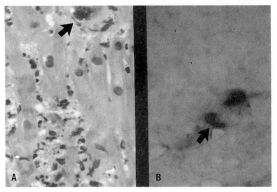

Fig. 3.7   (A) Cardiac biopsy showing cytomegalovirus (arrow) with a mixed (neutrophils, eosinophils and lymphocytes) inflammatory infiltrate in the interstitium. (B) *In situ* hybridization of panel A confirming cytomegalovirus particles (arrow). A: H&E × 210; B: × 210.

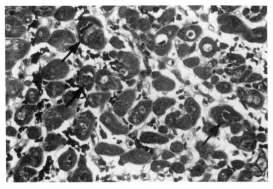

Fig. 3.8   Cardiac biopsy showing cytomegalovirus inclusions (arrows) in myocytes. Note in this case there is no significant inflammatory infiltrate, only perimyocytic oedema. H&E × 180.

Idiopathic giant cell myocarditis

Although the aetiology of this form of myocarditis is not known viruses have been implicated and it is therefore included in this chapter. The lesions in this disease are usually fulminating and extensive with large areas of myocyte necrosis with discreet serpiginous borders. The inflammatory infiltrate within the damaged myocardium is predominately lymphocytic, but large giant cells are present (Fig. 3.9). The inflammatory infiltrate in giant cell myocarditis may also include eosinophils and plasma cells; it may be either quite an admixed infiltrate or predominantly lymphocytic. The giant cells may be elongated or strap-like when seen in longitudinal sections. This condition has been known to occur with thymomas and an identical histological picture is seen in some cases of Wegner's granulomatosis.[8,9] It is thought that sarcoidosis can become confluent and generalized, however, sarcoid is usually manifested as discrete noncaseating granulomas as described below. Giant cell myocarditis is rapidly fatal, but cardiac transplantation has been successful in several cases. In one case, recurrence of the giant cell myocarditis occurred in the donor heart within 3 months of cardiac transplantation.[10] The giant cells may be multinucleated giant cells derived from muscle fibres attempting to regenerate (Fig. 3.10) or giant cells of a foreign body type. Thus far, organisms have not been demonstrable.

The purpose of this chapter is to describe the histopathological changes of viral idiopathic myocarditis, but as some of the other causes of granulomatous myocarditis need to be excluded they will be described very briefly: In tuberculous myocarditis, localized masses (tuberculoma) or miliary lesions may be seen within the myocardium. The tuberculomas are firm, yellow lesions which are usually discrete and which contain acid fast bacilli. These lesions may occur in the interventricular and interatrial septae and may therefore involve the conduction system. Fungal myocarditis is seen nowadays, especially in immunosuppressed patients is the result of opportunistic infections (Fig. 3.11). Cryptococcus, aspergillus, monilia and other fungal lesions are readily seen when stained with silver stains (Fig. 3.12) and can be distinguished from other forms of myocarditis. Syphilitic myocarditis is rare although it is re-emerging in some inner cities. Localized gumma usually involve

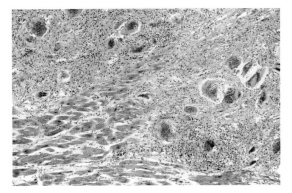

Fig. 3.9   Giant cell myocarditis illustrating the serpiginous border of necrotic myocardium and multinucleated giant cells from an explanted heart. H&E × 60.

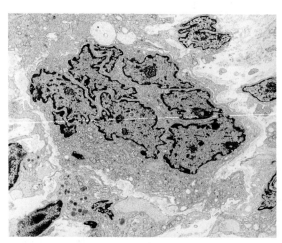

Fig. 3.10 Electron micrograph showing a multinucleated cell in giant cell myocarditis in a 56-year-old patient. × 2650.

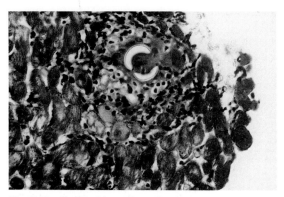

Fig. 3.11 Cardiac biopsy in an immunosuppressed patient showing a small granuloma with a cyst of coccidioidomycosis. H&E × 60.

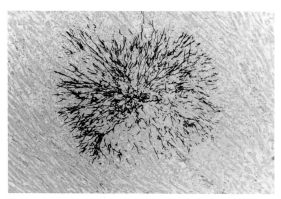

Fig. 3.12 Aspergillus myocarditis in an immunocompromised patient showing the frond-like colony. Methanamine silver × 37.

the interventicular septum and therefore may also produce arrythmias. A diffuse interstitial myocarditis of the newborn has been described with syphilis.[11]

Sarcoidosis

Myocardial involvement by sarcoidosis is a serious complication and conduction disturbances of all types may occur. Sudden death has been described and arrythmias are common. Thirty per cent of patients with myocardial sarcoid die in heart failure. However, cardiac transplantation has been successful, and in these cases recurrence has not been reported.[12] The myocardial manifestations of sarcoidosis usually show discreet noncaseating granulomas containing giant cells and epithelial cells, and there may also be a surrounding lymphocyte infiltration (Fig. 3.13). This disease, although of unknown aetiology is included in this section as a viral aetiology has not been entirely ruled out. Nevertheless this type of myocarditis does not usually provide a diagnostic problem.

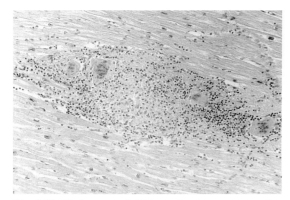

Fig. 3.13   Endomyocardial biopsy showing a noncaseating granuloma with giant cells typical of sarcoidosis. H&E × 60.

The acute myocarditis of Chagas' disease

The acute myocarditis of Chagas' disease (Fig. 3.14) has been well described before[13–16] and since this disease is not caused by virus it will not be included in this chapter.

Thus it can be seen that the diagnosis of acute myocarditis can in most cases be established histopathologically at autopsy or in an explanted heart. The diagnosis is much more difficult when examining endomyocardial biopsies. If treatment is to be attempted, accurate diagnosis of myocarditis in the living patient becomes particularly important. The widespread use of multiple endomyocardial biopsies has raised hopes that it may be possible to diagnose acute myocarditis more accurately and earlier if histopathological examination show the presence of a definite inflammatory infiltration of the myocardium. The next portion of this chapter deals with the role of endomyocardial biopsy in the diagnosis of viral myocarditis.

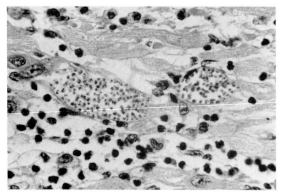

Fig. 3.14   Intact cysts of *Trypanosoma cruzi* (Chagas' disease) in the myocardium. H&E ×
280.

The role of endomyocardial biopsy in the diagnosis of acute idiopathic myocarditis

Endomyocardial biopsy is now an established and safe procedure in experienced hands which has been well described many times in the literature.[17,18] Although the development of the technique of myocardial biopsy raised hopes that it would be possible to diagnose myocarditis more accurately if the endomyocardial biopsy showed a definite inflammatory infiltration of the myocardium, unfortunately, the size of the biopsies (usually not more than 2 mm in maximum dimension), often made the interpretation of the finding difficult.

The role of the endomyocardial biopsy in establishing a diagnosis of acute myocarditis may be summarized as: (1) To identify the inflammatory infiltrate within the myocardium. (2) To exclude other causes of myocardial disease which might clinically mimic viral myocarditis; and (3) to follow the development of acute myocarditis in the chronic stages. Dilated cardiomyopathy is a sequel long suspected to have resulted from acute myocarditis, but has as yet not been satisfactorily proved. (4) To monitor the effect of treatment.[19]

The treatment of acute myocarditis with corticosteroid induced immunosuppression is controversial. There are anecdotal results suggesting that patients improve with a reduction in the inflammatory infiltrate,[20] however, there are other reports, particularly involving viral-induced myocarditis, in animals, suggesting that immunosuppression might, in fact, increase the spread of the virus so that encephalitis or other sequelae may ensue. It was therefore decided in 1984 to institute a Multicenter Myocarditis Trial in the USA in an attempt to clarify the incidence of acute myocarditis in the general population and also determine whether treatment with immunosuppression was effective. The Trial includes only patients with positive endomyocardial biopsies for acute myocarditis. The question then arose as to what constitutes a 'positive biopsy'. There existed a wide spectrum of opinions regarding the interpretation of inflammatory infiltrates amongst pathologists themselves. The reported frequency of 'biopsy-proven' myocarditis from various centres ranged from 3 to 63%. This caused difficulty, not only for clinicians treating patients, but also because the results of studies undertaken on patients supposed to have 'biopsy-proven' myocarditis could be misinterpreted. Concern about such misinformation, together with the need to do a meaningful randomized multicentre study on the possible beneficial effects of immunosuppression on acute idiopathic myocarditis led to a meeting in Dallas, Texas in March, 1984, of eight cardiac pathologists with experience and interest in the interpretation of the endomyocardial biopsy specimen. The so-called Dallas' criteria for a histopathologic definition and classification of myocarditis were formulated at this meeting.[21] The goals of the group were: (1) to define myocarditis from the morphological standpoint on endomyocardial biopsy; (2) to develop histopathological criteria for the diagnosis of acute myocarditis; (3) to establish a simple reproducible working classification that most pathologists could follow; (4) to outline the problems and pitfalls relating to establishing the diagnosis of endomyocardial biopsy; (5) to assess the applicability and reproducibility of the classification system; and (6) to make the information available to pathologists and clinicians. The first requirements were to have adequate endomyocardial biopsies diagnosis.

Technical considerations

Since myocarditis is often focal, a minimum of three, but preferably five separate biopsy specimens should be obtained to rule out acute myocarditis. It has been shown on other studies where myocardial inflammatory infiltrates are being assessed that four pieces of biopsy tissue may result in a 2% false negative biopsy.[22] If not clinically contraindicated, more tissue samples are therefore desirable to increase the sensitivity of the technique, especially if one of the smaller bioptomes or a femoral approach is used. If four or more pieces of tissue are obtained, then special studies, such as immunohistochemistry, electron microscopy or immunofluorescence can be performed, but each of these tissue samples should also be examined by light microscopy to ensure adequate sampling.

To avoid errors, biopsy sections should be cut at a maximum of 4μ thick as thicker sections, even when negative, artifactually appear as 'cellular' and may be mistaken for acute myocarditis (Fig. 3.15).

Each of the sections from the biopsy specimen should be examined carefully in order not to miss focal lesions; the tissue in paraffin block should be sectioned through the block (usually in 'step sections') and unstained slides for additional special stains saved in between the stained slides. The sections should be stained well with haematoxylin and eosin and a connective tissue stain, preferably Masson's trichrome stain, not only to highlight fibrous tissue, but also to help in the identification of early myocyte damage or degeneration and necrosis.

It was also suggested that an adequate history should be obtained and the final diagnosis should not be rendered until the clinical history and physiological data were available. At a minimum, this should include the age, sex, duration of illness where known, and the status of the coronary arteries in older patients (preferably determined by angiography), ventricular function, drug history (particularly the use of pressor amines) immunosuppressive agents, illicit drugs or other known cardiotoxic or hypersensitivity-provoking agents. Infectious ill-

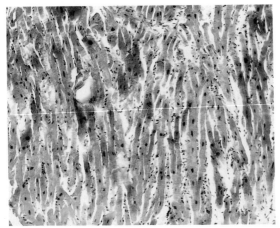

Fig. 3.15 A very thick section of myocardium which appears to have an interstitial infiltrate which is spurious and is not due to lymphocytes. H&E × 60.

nesses and other pertinent information on a previous biopsy should also be made known to the pathologist. For the purpose of the Multicenter Myocarditis Trial, it was required that a minimum of five pieces of tissue should be obtained for the follow-up biopsies to minimize false negative results.

Immunoserological markers of myocarditis (see Chapter 9)

The accurate diagnosis of acute 'viral' myocarditis can only be established with identification of virus and associated inflammation in the myocardium (Fig. 3.16). In order to establish a viral aetiology of myocarditis, it is necessary to isolate the virus from the myocardium by culture or from the pericardial fluid or by identification by immunofluorescence, peroxidase-labelled antibody or ferrtin-labelled antibody of type-specific virus localized in the myocardium that correlates with the pathologic changes. Isolation of a virus from the pharynx or faeces are only suggestive evidence. A fourfold rise in type-specific neutralizing, haemagglutination-inhibiting or complement-fixing antibodies or a titre of 1:32 or greater of type-specific IgM neutralizing or haemagglutination-inhibiting antibodies are associations, but not definitive evidence of acute myocarditis. Most patients with acute myocarditis present to the clinician after the phase of active viral replication. Patients with chronic dilated cardiomyopathy may have elevated titres of type-specific enteroviral antibodies including virus specific IgM antibodies when compared with patients showing other forms of cardiac disease or normal controls. These high antibody titres have been cited as indirect evidence supporting the hypothesis that a viral illness initiated the immunopathologic events that led to chronic inflammation and subsequent dilated cardiopmathy. Although early studies suggested that detection of anti-heart antibodies (AHA) would be useful as a screening test for establishing the presence of immune-mediated inflammation in patients with cardiomyopathy (see chapter 6), further studies have emphasized the lack of specificity of these antibodies. Abnormalities in suppressor cell function have been demonstrated in some patients with idio-

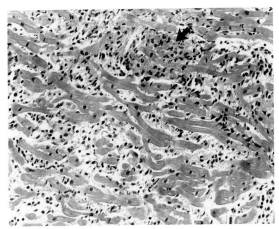

Fig. 3.16 Endomyocardial biopsy showing acute myocarditis with myocyte damage (arrow). Note normal background morphology of myocytes. H&E × 60.

pathic dilated cardiomyopathy and acute myocarditis,[23] but, in a different population of cardiomyopathic patients, this immunoregulatory defect could not be confirmed.[24] In summary, immuno-serologic testing has not shown the reliability necessary for use as a screening tool in the identification of patients with myocardial inflammatory disease.

There is a considerable difference of opinion regarding the diagnosis of acute myocarditis with what is called 'chronic myocarditis' or features of cardiomyopathic histopathology that included lymphocytes. Because of this, the incidence of acute myocarditis in the literature varies from 5 to 16%[25–28] of patient studies, whereas others have found chronic inflammatory cells in 25%[29] of biopsy specimens and yet another report indicated 63% of biopsies had inflammatory changes in patients with unexplained heart failure.[30] It was quite clear that rigid morphological criteria had to be established and adhered to if a useful diagnosis of acute myocarditis was to be made for the purpose of the Multicenter Myocarditis Trial. Accordingly, in March, 1984, the so-called 'Dallas criteria' for the diagnosis of acute myocarditis on endomyocardial biopsy were established.

The Dallas criteria (see p. 43)[21]

(see p. 43)

By consensus, the authors defined acute myocarditis as 'a process characterized by an inflammatory infiltrate of the myocardium with necrosis and/or degeneration of adjacent myocytes which was not typical of the ischaemic damage associated with coronary artery disease'. Idiopathic (presumed viral) myocarditis would be termed 'primary myocarditis', whereas acute myocarditis due to other causes, for example, toxoplasmosis or Chagas' disease, would be termed 'secondary myocarditis'. As mentioned previously, the Dallas criteria were defined for the myocarditis trial, therefore, separate terminology was adopted for the first diagnostic biopsy and for the subsequent biopsies. The three diagnostic categories of acute myocarditis for the initial biopsy were (Table 3.4):

Table 3.4 The Dallas' criteria for endomyocardial biopsy diagnosis.

First biopsy	Subsequent biopsies
Myocarditis (inflammatory infiltrate with myocyte damage) ± fibrosis	Ongoing (persistent) myocarditis ± fibrosis
Borderline myocarditis (rebiopsy may be indicated)	Resolving (healing) myocarditis ± fibrosis
No evidence of myocarditis	Resolved (healed) myocarditis ± fibrosis

Modified from Aretz *et al*.[25]

1. Active myocarditis with or without fibrosis: both an inflammatory infiltrate and damage of the adjacent myocytes were required for this diagnosis (Fig. 3.16). The myocyte damage ranged from frank necrosis to subtle cellular disruption with closely applied lymphocytes to the cell surface (Fig. 3.17). In general, the uninvolved myocardium was within normal limits.
2. Borderline myocarditis: (not diagnostic and requiring a repeat biopsy). This term implies that the inflammatory infiltrate is too sparse or that the myocyte damage is not seen on light microscopy (Fig. 3.18). Additional

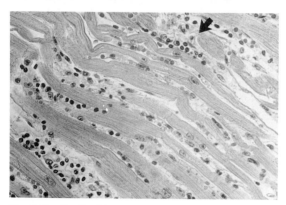

Fig. 3.17 Cardiac biopsy showing myocyte disruption by inflammatory lymphocytes in acute myocarditis. H&E × 185.

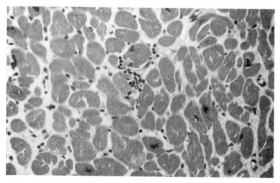

Fig. 3.18 Cardiac biopsy showing a small central aggregate of lymphocytes without adjacent myocyte damage. H&E × 185.

sections of the original biopsy specimens might demonstrate diagnostic changes in which active myocarditis can be diagnosed without a repeat biopsy.
3. No evidence of myocarditis: a biopsy in which there is no interstitial inflammatory infiltrate or myocyte damage.

Diagnostic categories for all subsequent biopsies were divided into three categories (Table 3.4).

1. Persistent or ongoing acute myocarditis: this diagnosis is made when the degree of interstitial infiltrate is the same or worse than that of the original biopsy specimen.
2. A resolving myocarditis: this diagnosis is made when the inflammatory infiltrate is less than in 1 above and reparative changes of fibroblasts and scar tissue are evident (Fig. 3.5)
3. Resolved myocarditis: where there is now no inflammatory infiltrate remaining and no evidence of ongoing cellular necrosis. Scar tissue may be present with adjacent compensatory hypertrophy.

It should be emphasized that the formulation of the Dallas criteria was prompted, convened and implemented by pathologists who were to take part in the Multicenter Trial. It was not meant to establish a definite classification of acute myocarditis in general, but rather the purpose was to test some of the problems of diagnosis by endomyocardial biopsy, for example, are the small focal inflammatory infiltrates in the heart a manifestation of myocarditis or not? The Dallas criteria have been misunderstood and misrepresented as a classification that sometimes is used as a *sine qua non* of the histological diagnosis of acute myocarditis. Pathologists using the Dallas classification should be aware that it was devised to achieve a more uniform diagnosis and the classification itself has yet to be tested.

As mentioned before, the biopsy tissue should be well fixed, thinly sectioned and well stained and the general guidelines outlined in Table 3.5 adhered to. If possible, and if acute myocarditis is suspected, it is wise to save serum at the time of the endomyocardial biopsy and also to freeze biopsy tissue for further studies, as mentioned above. Electron microscopy may be useful, although not essential (Fig. 3.19). It goes without saying that the biopsy should be obtained as soon as possible following the acute illness, and many difficulties have probably arisen as a result of biopsies being taken 6 to

Table 3.5 Requirements for optimal biopsy diagnosis of idiopathic myocarditis.

1. Adequate tissue (minimum of 3, 4–6 pieces preferred)
2. Sections cut at 4–6 µm thick in 'ribbons' at 3 step levels.
3. Adequate staining (haematoxylin and eosin + connective tissue stain). Electron microscopy, immunohistochemistry and eosinophil stains helpful, but not required.
4. Save serum and freeze biopsy tissue.
5. Obtain biopsy during or as soon as possible following the acute illness.
6. Drug history and coronary artery status should be obtained.
7. Rule out secondary myocarditis with an identifiable cause, e.g. Chagas' disease, toxoplasmosis-simulating viral myocarditis.

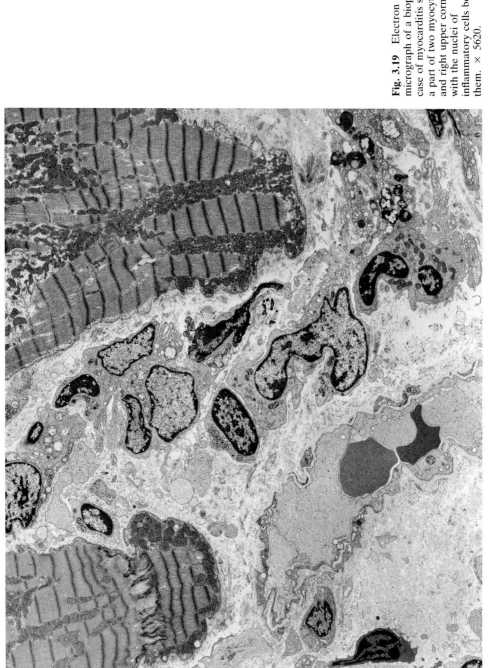

Fig. 3.19 Electron micrograph of a biopsy of a case of myocarditis showing a part of two myocytes (left and right upper corners) with the nuclei of inflammatory cells between them. × 5620.

8 weeks following the acute clinical illness. It is important at the time of the biopsy to take a careful drug history, not only of illicit drugs that the patient may be on, but also of therapeutic drugs which could cause toxic or hypersensitivity myocarditis. This information should be available to the pathologist reading the biopsies. The coronary artery status of the patient is also of major importance as it alerts the pathologist to possible ischaemic damage which could be mistaken for acute myocarditis. A history to rule out secondary myocarditis with an identifiable cause such as Chagas' disease (Fig. 3.14) or toxoplasmosis (Fig. 3.20) (the infiltrate of both of which could simulate acute idiopathic myocarditis at certain stages) should also be obtained. It is clear that the handling of the endomyocardial biopsy and its processing should be done with extreme care, bearing in mind the problems of sampling error as well as artifacts and pitfalls of diagnosis.

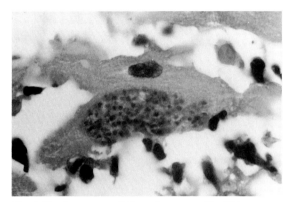

Fig. 3.20   Intact cyst of *Toxoplasma gondii* within a myocyte. H&E × 310.

Pitfalls in the endomyocardial biopsy diagnosis of idiopathic Myocarditis

The caveats and pitfalls in the diagnosis of acute myocarditis[32] from endomyocardial biopsy are enumerated in Table 3.6. Some of these pitfalls have already been covered. It is important that the timing of the biopsy in relation to the acute symptoms is known to the pathologist. Some pathologists may find themselves too readily influenced by a 'classical clinical history' of acute myocarditis in a previously young, healthy adolescent, for example, who suddenly goes into heart failure following a 'flu-like' syndrome. There is a tendency for some pathologists to want to 'fit in' with the clinical findings and, or course, a lymphocyte or two can nearly always be found if looked for hard enough! It is essential for the pathologist to interpret only what is present on the biopsy, even if this does not fit the clinical picture. It is very important to review the background morphology of the biopsy. Thus, if there is marked hypertrophy and fibrosis with large, bizarre-shaped nuclei, particularly in a younger patient or in a patient who has had coronary disease ruled out by angiography, then the biopsy better supports a diagnosis of idiopathic dilated cardiomyopathy, even if a few residual lymphocytes are seen (Fig. 3.21). The pattern of the inflammatory infiltrate is also important,

Table 3.6   Caveats in the endomyocardial biopsy diagnosis of idiopathic myocarditis.

1.   Timing of biopsy in relation to acute symptoms
2.   Bias from clinical diagnosis
3.   Size and sampling error
4.   Quantitative criteria (how many lymphocytes are normal?)
5.   Lymphocytes in other conditions, e.g. cardiomyopathy
6.   Drug-related myocarditis
7.   'Tip of the iceberg' effect
8.   Secondary myocarditis
9.   Mistaken identity, e.g. lymphomas, leukaemias

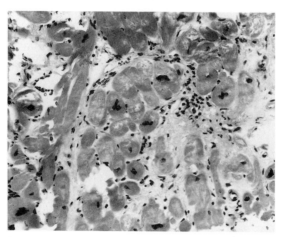

Fig. 3.21   Cardiac biopsy showing markedly hypertrophied myocytes, interstitial fibrosis, and with an interstitial aggregate of lymphocytes in a patient with endstage dilated cardiomyopathy. H&E × 215.

and if the patient is in heart failure a more florid interstitial infiltrate rather than small, focal aggregates of lymphocytes would be expected. The size and sampling error of the biopsies has already been discussed.

The quantitative criteria for the number of lymphocytes required to establish a diagnosis of acute myocarditis is of importance. In the study by Edwards *et al.*[33] it was shown that up to five lymphocytes per high-power field in any biopsy were considered within normal limits. Large autopsy studies listed in Table 3.7 show an average of 4–5% of lymphocytes in the heart of patients without acute myocarditis. Therefore the question arises, in an endomyocardial biopsy as to how many lymphocytes are within normal limits? As a rule, random lymphocytes within the heart which are within normal limits do not show adjacent myocyte damage. However, sometimes this can be difficult to assess due to tangential sectioning. It is for this reason that the category in the Dallas criteria of 'borderline myocarditis' was made as this requires a follow-up biopsy which should answer the question of whether the small aggregate of lymphocytes, as seen in Fig. 3.18, really is myocarditis or not.

A difficult diagnostic condition arises in the case of endomyocardial biopsies in idiopathic cardiomyopathy. In these patients, the clinical history is often very similar to that of acute myocarditis. In these cases also, the background morphology is usually of myocyte hypertrophy with large,

Table 3.7 Lymphocytes in normal myocardium.

Percentage of lymphocytes		Reference
4.2% (total 5626)	Unselected autopsies	Saphir[25,34]
5.0% (total 61)	Accidental death in healthy airmen	Stevens et al.[26]
2.9% (total 1402)	Autopsies from AFIP*	Gore and Saphir[35]
5.5% (total 4782)	Consecutive autopsies	Kline et al.[36]
9.3% (total 86)	'Normal' donor hearts	Tazelaar and Billingham[37]

*Armed Forces Institute of Pathology.

bizarre-shaped nuclei and mature fibrosis (Fig. 3.21). Previous studies have shown that aggregates of interstitial lymphocytes (usually small and not the activated cells seen in acute myocarditis) are present in up to 83% of random sections taken from endstage idiopathic cardiomyopathy specimens.[37] In our series of acute myocarditis biopsies as well as autopsies at Stanford University, we have not seen any cases of unequivocal acute myocarditis with a background of hypertrophy and fibrosis, even in older patients. In this case, there is a semantic dilemma as to whether 'endstage cardiomyopathy' is the same as 'endstage chronic myocarditis'. The reader should be aware that endstage cardiomyopathy, if sampled sufficiently, does show a high proportion of lymphocytic infiltrates. A study performed at Stanford, where a mean of six random sections from the left ventricle, right ventricle and interventricular septum were examined in 108 cases of endstage idiopathic dilated cardiomyopathy coming to cardiac transplanation between 1968 and 1984, checked carefully for lymphocytic infiltrates, showed 14 of 108 (13%) without any infiltrate, whereas 87% of cases did show an inflammatory infiltrate, predominantly lymphocytic.[38] Caution is required in distinguishing acute idiopathic myocarditis from 'chronic' myocarditis or, preferably designated, idiopathic cardiomyopathy, since immunosuppressive treatment is not likely to improve the latter and may make it worse.

Drug related myocarditis

Drug-related myocarditis has been well-described previously.[39,40] This may, however, present considerable diagnostic difficulties unless a careful history of drugs taken by the patient is obtained. Many drugs can cause both toxic-related myocarditis as well as hypersensitivity myocarditis. Drug-induced toxic changes in the myocardium have become an increasing problem and the list of drugs causing these changes is added to frequently. The more common of these drugs is shown in Table 3.8. Drugs causing acute myocarditis with an inflammatory infiltrate and sometimes vasculitis can be divided into:

1. Toxic myocarditis
Lesions in toxic myocarditis are usually dose related; the more drug that is given, the greater the number of lesions and the greater the amount of myocardial damage. The inflammatory lesions, if not focal, are often of different ages and while some of the lesions may be early and acute, others may show repair and scarring in the same field. In general, the inflammatory infiltrate (which is either perivascular or interstitial) is mixed, showing a polymorphous inflammatory infiltrate, and if a vasculitis is present (Fig. 3.22), haemorrhage

Table 3.8 Drug-related myocarditis.

Hypersensitivity myocarditis	Toxic myocarditis
Penicillin	Anthracyclines
Sulphonamides	Cyclophosphamide
Tetracyclines	Arsenicals
Streptomycin	Fluorouracil
Phenylbutazone	Lithium carbonate
Isoniazide	Phenothiazines
Tetanus toxoid	Catecholamines
Diphtheria toxin	Theophylline
Horse serum	Quinidine
Amphotericin B	Barbiturates

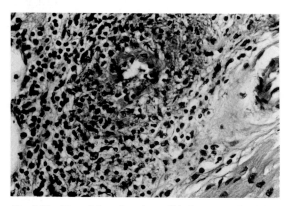

Fig. 3.22 Vasculitis and perivasculitis from a cardiac biopsy of a patient on cyclophosphamide. H&E × 185.

may also be present. If the lesions are severe, frank myocyte necrosis may occur.

2. Hypersensitivity Myocarditis

Hypersensitivity or allergic myocarditis may also be confused with idiopathic myocarditis. In contrast to toxic myocarditis; the lesions are generally of the same age. They are sometimes focal and may appear granulomatous, for example, lesions caused by isoniazide therapy. Vasculitis is not prevalent as in toxic myocarditis. Myocytolysis may be present, although frank necrosis is unusual. As lesions are potentially reversible and there is no vasculitis or necrosis, it follows that fibrosis is not a feature of hypersensitivity myocarditis, although it may follow massive degranulation of the eosinophils. This is unusual in drug-related disease. The inflammatory infiltrate is sometimes mixed, but the predominant cell is the eosinophil, of which very large numbers may be present (Fig. 3.23). If the offending drug is withdrawn, and steroid therapy administered, the eosinophilia may disappear rapidly, leaving only reparative changes. In general, toxic myocarditis is not difficult to distinguish from idiopathic myocarditis except when only small portions of the lesions are available, as in some endomyocardial biopsies.

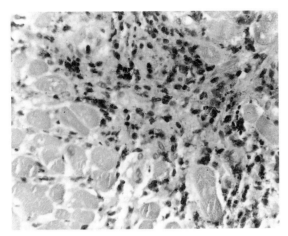

Fig. 3.23   Cardiac biopsy showing infiltrate of granular eosinophils in hypersensitivity myocarditis. H&E × 250.

'Tip of the iceberg' effect

'Tip of the iceberg' effect may be a pitfall in the diagnosis of acute myocarditis. It stands to reason that if there is a granulomatous infiltrate or a myocardial infarction deeper in that portion of myocardium biopsied, and only the edge of one of these lesions is seen, it may be represented as a focal area of acute myocarditis (Fig. 3.24). 'Tip of the iceberg' effect should always be uppermost in the mind of the pathologist screening biopsies for acute myocarditis. In order to ensure that there is no underlying lesion, it is important to section the whole block of the biopsy.

Secondary myocarditis

Secondary myocarditis may sometimes be confused with idiopathic myocarditis if the pathognomic features of fungi or other organisms are not readily

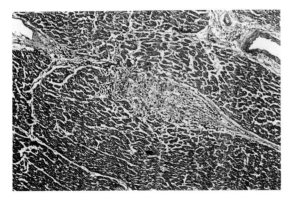

Fig. 3.24   Myocardium showing an apparent focal myocarditis (centre) which on further sectioning proved to be a sarcoid granuloma illustrating the 'tip-of-the-iceberg' effect. H&E × 37.

seen on the biopsy. In the appropriate setting, where there is a possibility of secondary myocarditis, the biopsy should be carefully stained with silver stains (Fig. 3.12) to rule out fungus or any other organism likely to cause an inflammatory infiltrate. In the case of myocarditis caused by Chagas' disease (Fig. 3.14) or *Toxoplasma gondii* (Fig. 3.20) a good haemotoxylin and eosin stained slide is often better than special stains, especially periodic acid solution (PAS) stain, because the myocardium is full of glycogen and the positively staining glycogen will mask and make the finding of organisms much more difficult.

Malignant 'Look-alikes' of acute myocarditis

There, is also the question of mistaken identity of lymphocytes, for example, lymphomatous infiltrates which, if focal, may be mistaken for acute myocarditis. This is because lymphocytes due to virus often appear atypical and a distinction between the atypical inflammatory cells and lymphomatous cells may present a diagnostic problem (Fig. 3.25). The history, of course, is helpful in these cases, as are the more modern techniques of polymerase chain

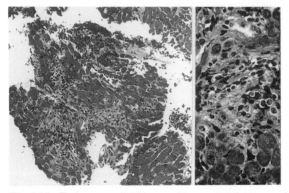

Fig. 3.25   Endomyocardial biopsy with myocyte damage and 'lymphocytic' infiltrate suggesting acute myocarditis. The right panel showing malignant T-cell lymphoma. Left panel: H&E × 55. Right panel: H&E × 155.

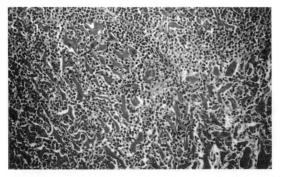

Fig. 3.26   Section of myocardium showing a florid interstitial infiltrate from malignant cells of mycosis fungoides. H&E × 60.

reaction (PCR) and *in situ* hybridization (Fig. 3.7) as well as specialist immunohistochemical techniques.

Massive leukaemic or malignant infiltrates such as those seen in mycoses fungoides are usually not a diagnostic problem for the diagnosis of acute myocarditis (Fig. 3.26). Last, but not least, the pathologist should be aware of any instrumentation to the right ventricle, for example, pacemaker placement, which could account for an inflammatory infiltrate (Fig. 3.27).

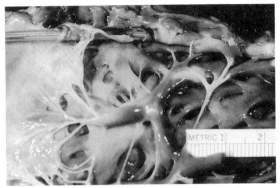

Fig. 3.27 Photograph of pacemaker passing through the tricuspid valve and embedded in the right ventricular septum.

Progression of viral myocarditis to dilated cardiomyopathy

It has long been suspected that viral myocarditis may lead to idiopathic dilated cardiomyopathy. There is a growing body of evidence associating serological findings consistent with coxsackie B virus serotypes and the development of acute myocarditis, and a smaller number also associating infection with the virus with idiopathic cardiomyopathy. Recent reports have shown that the morphologic demonstration of acute myocarditis is much lower than that suspected clinically, so despite the availability of adequate follow-up series in active myocarditis, there is a paucity of reports documenting morphological progression from biopsy-proven viral myocarditis to idiopathic dilated cardiomyopathy. This transition is regularly seen in controlled animal experiments,[41] but in humans documentation has been varied. In most cases, not all the documented myocarditis progresses; however, a large series is difficult to obtain since often the patients are either treated or end up receiving a heart transplantation. It does seem as though, in some cases at least, there is a progression from acute viral myocarditis with an inflammatory infiltrate and a normal myocardial background to the hypertrophy, fibrosis and dilation of endstage cardiomyopathy.[42,43] It is possible that only some patients are affected this way, whereas others who have 'subacute' myocarditis do not progress to cardiomyopathy. The question of whether acute myocarditis can progress to endstage dilated cardiomyopathy raises some provocative questions. It is known that cases of acute myocarditis will show a panmyocarditis

– pericarditis syndrome at autopsy. Acute myocarditis is also known to present with pericarditis and pleural effusions. It would be reasonable to expect, therefore, that in the endstage of an acute myocarditis, in this case idiopathic cardiomyopathy of the dilated type, there would be evidence of chronic pericarditis and a thickened pericardium. It is interesting that cardiomyopathies do not, in fact, have any evidence of previous pericarditis and the pericardium is usually smooth and glistening without adhesions despite the remarkable destruction of the underlying myocardium.

There have been some criticisms of the endomyocardial biopsy as a tool for diagnosing acute myocarditis, especially when negative biopsies occur in the light of a good clinical picture. Is sampling error a contraindication to diagnostic biopsies, as some have suggested?[44,45] Until a better technique for diagnosing acute myocarditis is established, it is not constructive to criticize the value of the endomyocardial biopsy on the basis of sampling error without at least offering an alternative solution.[46] The endomyocardial biopsy carefully performed and intelligently examined (bearing in mind the obvious pitfalls) is still a useful diagnostic tool for the study and management of acute myocarditis as well as many other cardiac disease states. It is interesting to note that the biopsy has been described as the 'gold standard' for making the diagnosis of acute rejection (which is a myocarditis) for over 20 years and, despite many efforts to supercede it with noninvasive studies, it has stood the test of time and sampling error has not been a major problem. Like every other diagnostic technique, the biopsy has its limitations, and these have been well documented and are frequently re-emphasized in the literature. Interpretation of acute myocarditis by endomyocardial biopsy remains difficult because not all lymphocytic infiltrates within the heart are necessarily the result of viral myocarditis, as discussed above. Although sampling error may reduce the sensitivity of active myocarditis, the specificity should be quite high. Careful analysis of reports of histological myocarditis in patients with unexplained heart failure, however, demonstrates a great variability in incidence in the past, and this wide discrepancy is in large part a result of lack of a uniform histological criteria. The Dallas criteria defining myocarditis have been useful in standardizing more recent reports. The results of the Multicenter Myocarditis Trial will be key in directing future investigation regarding the immunopathogenesis and treatment of active myocarditis.

The histopathological changes in idiopathic (presumed viral) myocarditis have been described. The pitfalls of diagnosis and differential diagnosis in the endomyocardial biopsy evaluation of acute myocarditis have been reviewed and described. Our understanding of the morphological changes in acute myocarditis and our diagnostic ability is greatly improved; however, the progression to idiopathic dilated cardiomyopathy is still not satisfactorily proven and more work needs to be done.

References

1. Grist N. R., Bell E. J. Coxsackieviruses and the heart (editorial). *Am Heart J* 1969; **77**: 295–300.
2. Helin M., Savola J., Lapinleheu K. Cardiac manifestations during a coxsackie B5 epidemic. *Br Med J* 1968; **3**: 97–9.
3. Archard L. C., Bowles N. E., Cunningham L. *et al.* Molecular probes for detec-

tion of persisting enterovirus infection of human heart and their prognostic value. *Eur Heart J* 1991; **12** (Suppl D): 56–9.

4. Archard L. C., Bowles N. E., Cunningham L., *et al.* Enterovirus RNA sequences in hearts with dilated cardiomyopathy: A pathogenetic link between virus infection and dilated cardiomyopathy. In: Baroldi G., Camerini F., Goodwin J. F. eds. *Advances in Cardiomyopathies*. Heidelberg: Springer-Verlag, 1990: 194–8.

5. Weiss L., Movahed L. A., Billingham M. E., Cleary M. L. Detection of coxsackievirus B3RNA in myocardial tissues by the polymerase chain reaction. *Am J Pathol* 1991; **138:** 497–503.

6. Weiss L. M., Lui X.-F., Chang K. C., Billingham M. E. Detection of enteroviral RNA in idiopathic dilated cardiomyopathy and other human cardiac tissues. *J Clin Invest* 1992; **90:** 156–9.

7. Billingham M. E. Is acute cardiac rejection a model of myocarditis in humans? *Eur Heart J* 1987; **8:** 19–23.

8. McCrea P. C., Jagoe W. S. Myocarditis in myasthenia gravis with thymoma. *Irish J Med Sci* 1963; 444–53.

9. Burke J. S., Medline N. M., Katz A. Giant cell myocarditis and myositis associated with thymoma and myasthenia gravis. *Arch Pathol* 1969; **88:** 359.

10. Yacoub M., personal communication.

11. Davies M. J. Myocarditis. In: Pomerance A., Davies M. J. eds. *The Pathology of the Heart*. Oxford: Blackwell Scientific Publishers, 1975: 193–210.

12. Valantine H. A., Tazelaar H. D., Macoviak J. *et al.* Cardiac sarcoidosis: Response to steroids and transplantation. *J Heart Transpl* 1987; **6:** 244–50.

13. Datta B. N. Parasitic diseases of the heart. In: Silver M. D. ed. *Cardiovascular Pathology*. New York: Churchill Livingstone, 1991: 1279–96.

14. Puigbo J. J. Chagas' heart disease. *Cardiologia* 1968; **52:** 91.

15. Prata A. Chagas' heart disease. *Cardiologia* 1968; **52:** 79.

16. Koberle F. Chagas' heart disease – pathology. *Cardiologia* 1968; **52:** 82.

17. Ursell P. C., Fenoglio J. S. Jr. Endomyocardial biopsy: Established diagnostic procedure. *Chest* 1983; **84:** 122–3.

18. Mason J. W. Endomyocardial biopsy: the balance of success and failure (perspective). *Circulation* 1985; **71:** 185–8.

19. Billingham M. E. Acute myocarditis: A diagnostic dilemma. Editorial. *British Heart Journal* 1987; **58:** 6–8.

20. Mason J. W., Billingham M. E., Ricci D. R. Treatment of acute inflammatory myocarditis assisted by endomyocardial biopsy. *Am J Cardiol* 1980; **45:** 1037–44.

21. Aretz H. T., Billingham M. E., Edwards W. D. *et al.* Myocarditis: A histopathologic definition and classification. *Am J Cardiovasc Pathol* 1986; **1:** 3–14.

22. Spiegelhalter D. J., Stovin P. G. I. An analysis of repeated biopsies following cardiac transplantation. *Stat Med* 1983; **2:** 33–40.

23. Fowles R. F., Bieber C. P., Stinson E. B. Defective *in vitro* suppressor cell function in idiopathic congestive cardiomyopathy. *Circulation* 1979; **59:** 483–91.

24. Anderson J. L., Greenwood J. H., Kawanishi H. Evaluation of suppressor immune regulatory function in idiopathic congestive cardiomyopathy and rheumatic heart disease. *Br Heart J* 1981; **46:** 410–14.

25. Saphir O. Myocarditis – A general overview, with an analysis of two hundred and forty cases. *Arch Patholol* 1947; **32:** 1000–51.

26. Stevens P. J., Underwood, Ground K. E. Occurrence and significance of myocarditis in trauma. *Aerospace Med* 1970; **41:** 770–80.

27. Noren G. R., Staley N. A., Bandt C. M., Kaplan E. L. Occurrence of myocarditis in sudden death in children. *J Forensic Sci* 1977; **22:** 118–96.

28. Mills A. S., Hastillo A., Hess M. L. Lymphocytic infiltration of the myocardium in idiopathic dilated cardiomyopathy: Underestimation of myocarditis with endomyocardial biopsy. *Circulation* 1984; **70** (Suppl II): 1604 (abs).

29. Baandrup U., Olsen E. G. J. Critical analysis of endomyocardial biopsies from

patients suspected of having cardiomyopathy, I. morphological and morphometric aspects. *Br Heart J* 1981; **45:** 475–86.

30. Chi-Sung Zee-Cheng, Cheng Chang Tsai, Palmer D. *et al.* High incidence of myocarditis by endomyocardial biopsy in patients with idiopathic congestive cardiomyopathy. *J Am Coll Cardiol* 1984; **3:** 63–70.
31. Aretz H. T. *et al.* Myocarditis: the Dallas criteria. *Hum Pathol* 1987; **18:** 619.
32. Billingham M. E. The diagnostic criteria of myocarditis by endomyocardial biopsy: In: Sekiguchi M., Olsen E., Goodwin J. eds. *Myocarditis and Related Disorders.* Heidelberg: Springer-Verlag, 1985: 133–7.
33. Edwards W. D., Holmes D. R. Jr., Reeder G. S. Diagnosis of active lymphocytic myocarditis by endomyacardial biopsy: quantitive criteria for light microscopy. *Mayo Clin Proc* 1982; **57:** 419–425.
34. Saphir O. Myocarditis: A general review. *Arch Pathol* 1942; **33:** 88–137.
35. Gore I., Saphir O. Myocarditis: Classification of 1402 cases. *Am Heart J* 1947; **34:** 827–30.
36. Kline I. K., Kline T. S., Saphir O. Myocarditis in senescence. *Am Heart J* 1963; **65:** 446–57.
37. Tazelaar H., Billingham M. E. Myocardial lymphocytes (Fact, fancy or myocarditis?). *Am J Cardiovasc Pathol* 1986; **1:** 47–50.
38. Tazelaar H. D., Billingham M. E. Leucocytic infiltrates in idiopathic dilated cardiomyopathy: A source of confusion with active myocarditis. *Am J Surg Pathol* 1986; **5:** 279–85.
39. Billingham M. E. Morphologic changes in drug-induced heart disease. In: Bristow M. R. ed. *Drug Induced Heart Disease.* New York: Elsevier, 1980: 127–49.
40. Billingham M. E. Pharmacotoxic myocardial disease: An endomyocardial study. In: Sekiguchi M., Olsen E., Goodwin J. eds. *Myocarditis and Related Disorders.* Heidelberg: Springer-Verlag, 1985: 282.
41. Matsumori A., Kawai C. An animal model of congestive (dilated) cardiomyopathy: Dilatation and hypertrophy of the heart in the chronic stage with DBA/2 mice with myocarditis caused by encephalomyocarditis virus. *Circulation* 1982; **66:** 355–60.
42. Billingham M. E., Tazelaar H. D. The morphological progression of viral myocarditis. *Postgrad Med J* 1984; **62:** 581–4.
43. Keogh A. M., Billingham M. E., Schroeder J. S. Rapid histologic changes in endomyocardial biopsy specimens after myocarditis. *Br Heart J* 1990; **64:** 406–8.
44. Chow L. H., Radio S. J., Sears T. D., McManus B. M. Insensitivity of right ventricular endomyocardial biopsy in the diagnosis of myocarditis. *J Am Coll Cardiol* 1989; **14:** 915–20.
45. Baandrup U., Florio R. A., Olsen E. G. J. Do endomyocardial biopsies represent the morphology of the rest of the myocardium? *Eur Heart J* 1982; **3:** 171–8.
46. Billingham M. E. Acute myocarditis: Is sampling error a contraindication for diagnostic biopsies? Editorial Comment. *J Am Coll Cardiol* 1989; **14:** 921–2.

4

Clinical spectrum of viral heart disease

P. Richardson and H. Why

Introduction

Myocarditis is defined as inflammation of the myocardium and may be due to multiple causes. These include both infectious and noninfectious agents. Injury to the myocardial cell can result directly not only from an infectious organism but also from an immune response triggered by a previous infection, often viral. Other mechanisms include allergies and responses to a systemic autoimmune disorder as well as a variety of physical agents. The diagnosis of suspected viral heart disease therefore involves the exclusion of the numerous conditions summarized in Table 4.1.

The clinical presentation of the patient with suspected viral heart disease is extremely variable. It depends upon the degree of involvement of the myocardium; in some patients virtually no impairment of heart function is found, whilst in others there may be severe heart failure with dilated, poorly contracting ventricles. In the latter situation the differential diagnosis includes dilated cardiomyopathy which is associated typically with dilatation of all cardiac chambers and significant impairment of systolic function. Adopting the classification of the International Society and Federation of Cardiology/World Health Organization (ISFC/WHO) Task Force,[1] dilated cardiomyopathy is disease of heart muscle of unknown cause or association. This definition implies that conditions such as valvular heart disease, endstage coronary heart disease and hypertensive heart disease have all been excluded. It is increasingly recognized, however, that some cases of dilated cardiomyopathy may represent the endstage of a preceding viral illness.

The current interest in viral heart muscle disease has been accelerated by two factors. Firstly, the advent of a safe method of percutaneous catheter endomyocardial biopsy[2,3] which has provided the clinician with a means by which to classify the various grades of myocarditis. In spite of this there is still considerable clinical diagnostic difficulty since human myocarditis does not present as an easily recognizable clinical syndrome because the presentation may include sudden death, paroxysmal arrhythmias, episodic cardiac failure or relentless progression to endstage heart failure. The second factor was the development of enteroviral group-specific cDNA probes[4,5] enabling detection of virus nucleic acid in small endomyocardial tissue samples. Not only has this observation strengthened the pathogenetic link between myocarditis and dilated cardiomyopathy, but it has also provided some evidence that the presence of virus may have prognostic implications.[6]

Table 4.1   Differential diagnosis of viral myocarditis.

Infection
  Viral (mainly enteroviral)
  Bacterial
  Rickettsial
  Protozoal – Chagas/Lyme disease
  Metazoal

Metabolic
  Endocrine: with catechol excess/thyrotoxic
  Electrolytic disturbances
  Nutritional deficiencies

Immune mediated
  Postvaccinal
  Serum sickness
  Urticarial
  Transplant rejection
  Peripartum

Toxic
  Alcohol
  Drugs
  Heavy metals
  Poisons
  Anaesthetics

Connective tissue disease
  Rheumatoid arthritis
  Systemic lupus erythromatosus
  Churg–Strauss syndrome
  Polymyositis

Granulomatous
  Sarcoid

Physical agents
  Cold/heat extremes
  Ionizing radiation
  Electric shock

Incidence

The true incidence of viral heart disease in the general population is unknown. It is probable that approximately 5% of a virus-infected population may experience some degree of cardiac involvement[7,8] and that this percentage rises during epidemics[9,10] or during outbreaks within institutions. Seasonal variations in virus infection may correspond with outbreaks of myopericarditis. There is, furthermore, an increased incidence of coxsackie B virus heart disease in neonates[11,12] as well as late childhood and adolescence. It has also been suggested that there is an increased risk in pregnancy and during the peripartum period. In spite of this, infections associated with cardiovascular symptoms and signs probably constitute less than 1% of recorded infections in the experience of the WHO.[13] However, the number of patients with cardiovascular sequelae is considerably higher when only coxsackie B virus-infected individuals are concerned (3.99%).

In dilated cardiomyopathy approximately 100 patients per million of the population are detected annually in the USA and approximately 9000 deaths annually are ascribable to dilated cardiomyopathy (DCM).[14] In 1978 the incidence of dilated cardiomyopathy was reported by Torp[15] to be of the order of 10 per 100 000 persons and a similar incidence has been recorded in the UK.[16] There appears to be an increasing frequency of diagnosis and, indeed, since 1970 three times more patients are now diagnosed. This may represent not only an increase in physician awareness, but also an improvement of both noninvasive and invasive cardiological investigations. In the latter context endomyocardial biopsy and the advent of cardiac transplantation have further promoted interest in diagnosis.

The spectrum of myocarditis and dilated cardiomyopathy

The realization that myocarditis and dilated cardiomyopathy may represent two ends of a spectrum of disease affecting the myocardium is not new. It has been recognized since the early descriptions of Fiedler in 1899[17] that inflammation may affect the myocardium with development of a clinical syndrome which includes fever, shortness of breath, vomiting, convulsions and even loss of consciousness. The autopsy findings described an acute interstitial myocarditis, but at that stage the viral origin of the inflammatory process was unknown. The diagnosis of myocarditis remained a widely accepted clinical entity but some of these were a case of mistaken diagnosis. Early clinical analyses clearly recognized the importance of myocarditis in the pathogenesis of heart muscle disease but failed to recognize the role of viral infection.[18] Evidence of viral involvement is more recent, particularly the implication of the coxsackie B virus.[19] Lerner has proposed a biphasic model of pathogenesis based upon a mouse model, with an early infectious phase associated with active virus replication and a second, immune-mediated phase. In humans the first phase lasts approximately 1 week followed by the later immune-mediated or hypersensitivity phase in which antibody develops and which results in the development of clinical symptoms which correlate with significant myocardial damage. In spite of the very considerable body of evidence both with regard to the virological aspects and the immune mechanisms involved in the pathogenesis of dilated cardiomyopathy, Lerner's original concept is still credible.

Clinical studies

Substantiation of a definite link between acute myocarditis and the subsequent development of dilated cardiomyopathy was initially based on clinical studies. These included the observation in 22 patients with proven coxsackie viral myocarditis that recovery might occur within a few weeks to several months. In five patients, however, persistent signs of heart failure as well as electrocardiographic abnormalities were noted.[20] In a similar series of 42 adults with coxsackie B virus-induced myopericarditis, 82% made a complete clinical recovery, although 12 patients took 3 months or longer to recover. Seven patients had one or more recurrences of their cardiac illness which was fatal in two cases. In six patients electrocardiographic abnormalities persisted for 6 months to 6 years and three patients had residual cardiomegaly, indistinguishable from dilated cardiomyopathy.[21] Kawai[22] suggested the infection immune theory as a cause of dilated cardiomyopathy when he found statistically significant differences in the antibody titres of coxsackie B and *Herpes simplex* viruses in patients compared with normal controls.

A series of patients of particular interest were reported by Levi *et al.*[23] who identified 22 with coxsackievirus-induced heart disease. The viral aetiology was based on a fourfold or greater rise in the neutralizing antibody titre, or by isolation of a coxsackievirus. They found that 33% of these patients, examined 4–5 years after the acute illness, still had impairment of myocardial function. In three patients the changes were consistent with a dilated cardiomyopathy.[23] Following their initial report, the same authors were able to follow up a similarly defined group of 42 patients after a 15-year period.[24] Ten patients died, three with myocarditis and the remainder with a cardiomyopathy.

Earlier studies, demonstrating the relationship between myocarditis and dilated cardiomyopathy, were based on virological rather than histological criteria, the cardiac diagnosis being made on clinical grounds. A study which overcame such limitations and reactivated interest in the role of coxsackie B viruses in the pathogenesis of dilated cardiomyopathy was reported by Cambridge *et al.*[25] who studied 50 patients for evidence of previous coxsackie B virus infection, comparing them with age- and sex-matched controls who were admitted to hospital for investigation of other cardiac diseases.[25] High neutralizing antibodies to coxsackie B virus (>1024) occurred significantly more frequently among patients with dilated cardiomyopathy, particularly among those with a short history, many of whom were febrile at the onset of their illness. Eighteen patients in this series had cardiac biopsies but none showed evidence of myocarditis. This included 12 patients in whom a viral aetiology was implicated. It was not possible to culture virus from any of the endomyocardial biopsy samples, and subsequent studies have also confirmed this finding.[26,27]

Biopsy-proven myocarditis

There is a lack of long-term prospective studies in patients with biopsy-proven myocarditis. Indeed, Goodwin suggested this approach in his 'Prospects and Predictions for the Cardiomyopathies 1974'.[28] In order to investigate the natural history of patients with biopsy-proven acute myocarditis serial clinical, echocardiographic, haemodynamic and histological studies were performed over a 4–5 year period with the purpose of documenting a progression to dilated cardiomyopathy. Twenty-three patients with biopsy-proven acute myocarditis (ACM) were studied at initial presentation and at 2, 6 and 12–24 months. The late follow-up of the survivors included radionuclide assessment of left ventricular function during exercise. It was found initially that left ventricular ejection fraction (EF) was severely impaired in 81% of patients (EF $31 \pm 4.4\%$). After 6–8 months of follow-up two groups emerged. Group 1 had normal ejection fractions (EF $62 \pm 1.9\%$, $n=9$) and group 2 had impaired left ventricular function (EF $29 \pm 4.47\%$, $n=8$). These groups were significantly different. On long-term follow-up group 1 patients remained clinically normal, but had an abnormal response to exercise. In group 2, with impaired ventricular function, the histological criteria for dilated cardiomyopathy were found in seven patients. It was concluded that characteristic clinical features of dilated cardiomyopathy had developed in 12 patients (52%), four of whom died. Assessment of left ventricular function approximately 6 months after acute myocarditis helped to predict outcome with a progression to dilated cardiomyopathy documented in 50% of cases.[29] In view of the experience in this study and subsequent clinical observations it is apparent that the natural history of acute myocarditis may be summarized in diagramatic form (Fig. 4.1).

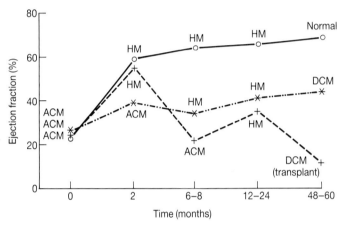

Fig. 4.1 Stylized diagram to illustrate the natural history of acute myocarditis. Three patients present identically with biopsy-proven acute myocarditis (ACM). The ventricular function of patient one (———) improves rapidly such that near normality is reached after 2 months, associated with the histological features of healing myocarditis (HM). These persist for up to 2 years before the histology becomes indistinguishable from normal. Patient two (– – –) also improves to the healing phase rapidly but relapses to acute myocarditis, improves once more and then progresses to the histological features of healed myocarditis/dilated cardiomyopathy (DCM) requiring cardiac transplantation. Patient three (·······) has an unresolved acute myocarditis at 2 months, and then progresses slowly through the healing phase to the clinical and histological features of dilated cardiomyopathy with continued impairment of left ventricular function.

Clinical presentation

The clinical spectrum of presentation of viral heart disease is variable and will depend upon the stage at which cardiac involvement is recognized. In approximately 30% of our patients there is a history of some form of 'viral illness'. This may include fever, upper respiratory tract infection, malaise or myalgia and occasionally a gastrointestinal upset. The symptom complex may include dyspnoea due to cardiac failure, chest pain relating to pericarditis, pulmonary infarction or infection or palpitation related to arrhythmias (e.g. sinus tachycardia, atrial fibrillation either sustained or paroxysmal, ventricular extrasystoles or even ventricular tachycardia). Sudden death may be due to ventricular tachycardia or ventricular fibrillation. The formation of thrombus within any of the cardiac chambers may result in embolization to either pulmonary or systemic circulations. The frequency with which the various presentations listed above occur in patients who have been classified as a result of endomyocardial biopsy into either having acute myocarditis or healing myocarditis is seen in Table 4.2 which also summarizes the degree of disability classified according to the New York Heart Association (functional class) – grading I–IV and symptoms at presentation. Table 4.3 uses a similar classification but the patients are divided according to whether enterovirus was detected in their myocardium at the time of presentation or not. It will be seen that, apart from an increased frequency of arrhythmias, there is no correlation between the presence of virus and the presenting features of the disease.

The differential diagnosis has to consider all the possible agencies responsible for myocarditis as listed in Table 4.1. In clinical practice, however, the most frequently encountered diagnoses include silent coronary artery disease, hypertensive heart disease and alcohol-induced heart muscle disease. A history of alcohol excess should be specifically enquired for and documented with regard to the type of alcohol, its quantity and duration. Heart muscle disease is most frequently encountered in those drinking in excess of 80 g

Table 4.2   Clinical and historical variables of 153 consecutive patients with suspected inflammatory heart muscle disease classified according to endomyocardial biopsy histology.

		Acute myocarditis (%) $n = 11$	Healing myocarditis (%) $n = 44$	Dilated cardiomyopathy (%) $n = 98$
NYHA class:	I	<5	3	11
	II	20	39	21
	III	20	32	41
	IV	>55	26	27
History of viral illness		55	32	20
History of excessive alcohol		<5	13	24
Chest pain		38	17	33
Documented arrhythmias		44	43	34
Clinical cardiac failure		67	62	62

Table 4.3   Clinical and historical variables of 153 serial patients with suspected inflammatory heart muscle disease according to the presence or absence of enterovirus RNA in endomyocardial biopsy tissue by cDNA hybridization probe.

		Enterovirus positive (%) $n = 47$	Enterovirus negative (%) $n = 106$
NYHA class:	I	2	10
	II	30	25
	III	35	38
	IV	33	27
History of viral illness		18	25
History of excessive alcohol		13	20
Chest pain		26	33
Documented arrhythmias*		58	25
Clinical cardiac failure		60	62

*$P < 0.001$, all other values $P = $ NS.

alcohol a day with an exposure of more than 10 years.[30] It is not clear whether alcohol can predispose to viral illness and, in eight patients where alcohol was thought to be the major pathogenic mechanism, three were found to have enterovirus RNA in their myocardium.

Clinical signs

The findings in the cardiovascular system include arrhythmias. Examination of the pulse may reveal a sinus tachycardia, atrial fibrillation or ventricular ectopic activity. In those patients with marked impairment of ventricular function there may be a degree of hypotension with a systolic pressure of less than 100 mmHg indicating poor systolic and left ventricular function. The heart is frequently enlarged and is associated with the presence of a gallop rhythm with easily audible third and fourth heart sounds. Some degree of functional mitral and tricuspid regurgitation may also be present. In those with pericardial involvement, a pericardial friction rub may be detectable. Signs of biventricular failure may be present with the most severe cases revealing signs of pleural effusion, sacral and peripheral oedema, as well as hepatomegaly with ascites. Although embolic complications only occur in approximately 25% of patients during the natural history of the disease, there may be signs of recent embolization to the peripheral vasculature. Cerebral embolization may give rise to neurological sequelae. Lyme borreliosis should always be considered as a possible cause for the combination neurological abnormalities and myocarditis.[31]

Clinical investigation

The clinical diagnosis of myocarditis is suggested by a history of a previous viral-like illness, electrocardiographic changes, a change in heart size on the chest X-ray and, in addition, a rise, preferably fourfold, in the appropriate viral antibody titres. In addition, the echocardiogram is now available as a noninvasive means of determining whether suspected viral disease has affected the myocardium and pericardium. The invasive approach to diagnosis includes assessment of the coronary arterial anatomy by selective coronary arteriography, measurement of the intracardiac pressures and, finally, confirmation of the suspected diagnosis of inflammation of the myocardium from tissue obtained by endomyocardial biopsy.

Electrocardiogram and arrhythmias

Whilst in many patients the involvement of the myocardium and atrium by the inflammatory process is diffuse, in some it may be focal. It will readily be appreciated that a small single lesion involving the conducting system may have serious consequences.[32] In the majority of patients the electrocardiographic abnormalities are in the main transient, and are more common than the clinical manifestations of myocardial involvement. The most common abnormalities are ST segment and T wave changes, atrioventricular arrhythmias, atrioventricular and intraventricular conduction defects; rarely, typical Q wave formation may be seen.[33] Life-threatening arrhythmias have been described not only in varicella[34] but also in coxsackie B3 myocarditis.[35] Figure 4.2 illustrates two electrocardiograms taken from a 16-year-old male

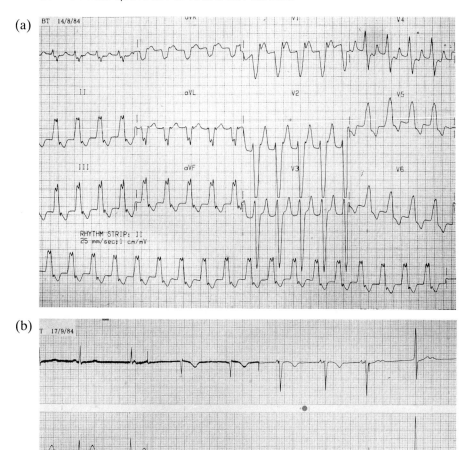

Fig. 4.2   Electrocardiograms of a 16-year-old male who presented with severe left ventricular failure due to myocarditis. Histology revealed healing myocarditis and the patient was not treated with immunosuppression. (a) Nodal tachycardia with left bundle branch block. (b) Sinus rhythm with T wave inversion in lead aVL and biphasic T waves in V_{2-4}. The voltage criteria for left ventricular hypertrophy are fulfilled.

presenting with biopsy-proven healing myocarditis and associated cardiac failure.

The spectrum of electrocardiographic changes in acute viral myocarditis or myopericarditis have been well described by Kitaura and Morita.[36] Eleven patients were followed up from 1.5 to 13 years. Ten of these patients underwent myocardial biopsy. The electrocardiographic changes in the acute stage were as follows: ST elevation in five patients, ventricular tachycardia in one, first degree A–V block in one, second degree A–V block in a further patient and third degree A–V block in four patients. ST elevation at presentation was associated with a normal electrocardiogram and long-term follow-up. However, those patients with third degree A–V block had the worst prognosis. Atrial fibrillation, when present, was frequently long-standing. In a further study of 20 patients with biopsy-proven myocarditis followed for 10 years the electrocardiogram returned to normal in only two patients. The remainder showed persistent changes including intraventricular conduction disturbance. Three patients required permanent pacemakers. In this series three of the patients progressed from myocarditis to dilated cardiomyopathy.[37]

The use of 24-hour Holter monitoring will clearly give better documentation of arrhythmias since those not only of atrial but also of ventricular origin are often paroxysmal. In patients with unsuspected arrhythmia their postmyocarditic origin may be confirmed by obtaining their endomyocardial biopsies. In a series of 65 patients who had been resuscitated from sudden death, had ventricular tachycardia resistant to standard anti-arrhythmic therapy or had high-grade ventricular arrhythmias (Lown class greater than or equal to IV B) with or without syncope, 17 patients had none of the usual causes identified. Twelve of these 17 patients underwent right ventricular biopsy and in six of them clinically unsuspected lymphocytic myocarditis was diagnosed[38]. Strain *et al.*[39] studied 18 patients with ventricular tachycardia or fibrillation in whom no structural heart disease was apparent. None of those patients was found to have significant coronary arterial lesions or impairment of left ventricular function at cardiac catheterization. Right ventricular biopsy, however, revealed histological abnormalities in 16 of 18 patients (89%); whilst nine patients (50%) had histological changes of nonspecific cardiomyopathy, three (17%) had subacute inflammatory myocarditis diagnosed.

X-ray examination
Routine chest X-rays are mandatory; indeed many patients are first identified because of unexplained cardiomegaly. In the acute phase of presentation there may be additional changes in the lung fields relating to the presence of cardiac failure. Since pericardial effusion is frequently associated with myopericarditis, the apparent cardiomegaly may not always be related to underlying myocardial dysfunction and echocardiography is diagnostic in such situations. Change in heart size may occur quite rapidly relating to spontaneous improvement of ventricular function. Figure 4.3 illustrates this comparing a series of four chest radiographs from the same patient whose electrocardiograms are illustrated in Fig. 4.2.

Echocardiography
Echocardiography has provided a simple noninvasive means of visualizing not only the myocardium but also the pericardium in patients with suspected cardiomyopathy or myocarditis. The assessment may include M-mode echo which allows measurement of the left ventricular dimensions and exclusion of underlying valvular heart disease. The technique is limited since definition

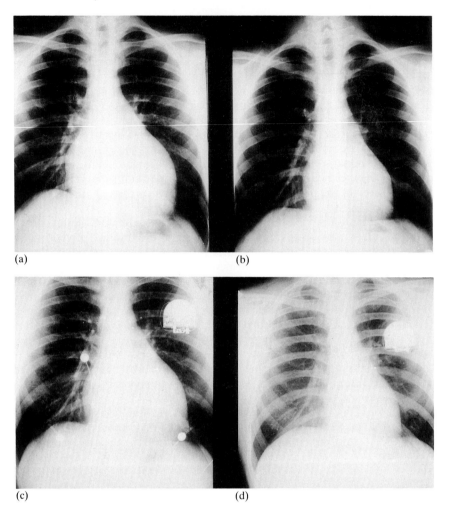

Fig. 4.3 Serial chest X-rays from a 16-year-old male with healing myocarditis on endomyocardial biopsy whose electrocardiograms are shown in Fig. 4.2. No pericardial effusion was demonstrated on an echocardiogram at any stage. (a) X-ray at the time of initial investigation. (b) Spontaneous improvement over a 2-week period. (c) Following the insertion of a permanent pacemaker for complete heart block 1 month later. (d) Three months after presentation with spontaneous reduction in heart size.

of the anatomy of the coronary arterial tree cannot be achieved. Recent developments in two-dimensional sector echo and Doppler as well as colour flow imaging have, however, added to diagnostic sophistication. Specific heart muscle disease, particularly amyloid can usually be differentiated and atrial myxomas excluded. Confirmation of the suspected diagnosis of amyloid heart disease requires endomyocardial biopsy.

In view of the sophistication of the diagnostic information now achieved by echocardiography, this investigation is performed prior to any invasive studies. Furthermore, it has been found that echocardiography is invaluable in the serial assessment of a patient's ventricular function, allowing more detailed assessment of its deterioration or recovery.

Typical findings in the patient with suspected myocarditis are those of a globally dilated left ventricular cavity with an overall reduction of systolic contraction. The left ventricular dimensions are markedly increased in both systole and diastole. These typical findings are usually present in those patients with diffuse myocardial involvement. In those, however, with more focal disease the finding may be that of segmental wall motion abnormalities with relatively minor dilatation of left ventricular cavity size. In the occasional patient there may be a localized ventricular aneurysm. These changes may be very similar to those seen in coronary artery disease and therefore arteriography is mandatory to be certain of the origin of the focal disease. Additional evidence regarding the presence of intracavity thrombus can also be obtained by echocardiography. This may on occasions be present in the form of a discrete pedunculated lesion, but most frequently as thrombus adherent to the intracavity wall related to the areas of maximal hypokinesia (Fig. 4.4).

In addition, echocardiography is a sensitive means of detecting and assessing the presence of a pericardial effusion. This is very frequently found in association with myocarditis. The combination of sector imaging and mitral inflow Doppler studies may allow the detection of haemodynamic compromise and cardiac tamponade. In addition, some degree of pericardial

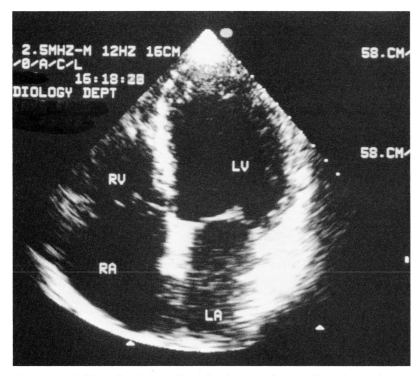

Fig. 4.4 Apical four chamber two-dimensional echocardiogram of a patient with acute myocarditis showing dilation of all cardiac chambers, particularly the left ventricle. Intracavity thrombus is seen at the apex of the left ventricle.

thickening can occasionally be seen. The differential diagnosis of possible infiltration of the pericardium by a tumour such as lymphoma or metastatic carcinoma is a rare finding.

Radionuclide techniques

Radionuclide techniques can be used in the detection of myocarditis. The initial application of radionuclide scanning was in experimental viral myoperi-carditis where the possibility of detecting myocardial inflammation using tech-nitium-99m pyrophosphate uptake was demonstrated.[40] Subsequently, gallium-67 imaging has been used to predict myocarditis which was then correlated to biopsy findings in patients with suspected dilated cardiomyo-pathy.[41] Indium-111 monoclonal antimyosin antibody imaging has shown some promise in the diagnosis of acute myocarditis in patients with suspected dilated cardiomyopathy.[42,43] Initial studies using this technique have shown a specificity of 58% and a sensitivity of 100%. The detection of monoclonal antimyosin antibody in patients with dilated cardiomyopathy and myocarditis indicates the possibility of an ongoing process of active myocyte damage. These changes have not as yet been correlated with the myocardial histology nor with the detection of underlying enterovirus RNA sequences. Gated radionuclide ventriculography can be used to assess left ventricular function and provide serial assessment of the ejection fraction in patients being followed up after an initial diagnosis of acute myocarditis. The technique, being noninvasive, like echocardiography may also be used to assess diastolic function in the ventricle.

Invasive investigation

In order to achieve complete diagnostic classification of a patient with sus-pected myocarditis, it is always appropriate to visualize the coronary anatomy by selective coronary arteriography. As already stated, some patients with myocarditis may have focal disease producing segmental changes in ven-tricular wall motion and even areas of aneurysmal dilation. However, it is not only in those with focal abnormalities, but occasionally in those with globally dilated left ventricles which are poorly contracting that silent cor-onary artery disease can be present.[44]

The haemodynamic findings in biopsy-proven acute myocarditis were studied in a group of 17 patients. At presentation the mean left ventricular ejection fraction was $31.5 \pm 35.6\%$. This was associated with a left ventricular end-diastolic pressure of 20.5 ± 2.9 mmHg, a systemic systolic blood pressure of 105.3 ± 4.4 mmHg, a pulmonary artery systolic pressure of 38.0 ± 4.8 mmHg and a mean pulmonary artery pressure of 26.5 ± 5.4 mmHg.[45] Nine of these patients were followed up after 2 months of immunosuppressive therapy. The left ventricular ejection fraction rose from 26 to 49%, and the cardiac index from 2.7 to 3.9 l/min/m.[2] The left ventricular end-diastolic pressure fell from 26.4 to 15.2 mmHg and pulmonary artery systolic pressure from 40 to 27 mmHg.

Endomyocardial biopsy

The technique of endomyocardial biopsy pioneered by Sakakibara and Konno[2] has been modified with the development of a percutaneous method of introduction using the long sheath and an adapted biopsy forceps.[46] The main value of endomyocardial biopsy has been the ability to confirm suspected myocarditis by histopathological evaluation. Three phases may be seen and these will depend upon the stage in the natural history of the illness when the tissue is obtained.[47] Myocarditis is defined as an inflammatory cell infiltrate of the myocardium with necrosis and/or degeneration of adjacent myocytes, not typical of ischaemic damage associated with coronary artery disease. In the acute phase the chief histological features include widening of the interstitium with inflammatory cells being in intimate contact with the adjacent myocardial fibres which show extensive fraying. In the healing (resolving) phase, whilst inflammatory cells are still evident, they are no longer in contact with the adjacent myocardial fibres and evidence of myocyte necrosis is no longer present. In the healed (resolved) phase there is an increase in the interstitial fibrous tissue with few inflammatory cells present and some degree of myocardial fibre hypertrophy. This stage is indistinguishable from dilated cardiomyopathy. The above classification is widely adopted and now constitutes the so-called Dallas criteria classification (see Chapter 3).[48] This classification was defined for the purposes of assessing the histological response to treatment. The histological distribution of our last 153 patients with suspected inflammatory heart muscle disease is shown in Fig. 4.5.

In spite of the controversy surrounding the frequency with which myocarditis is diagnosed on histological examination, the Dallas criteria must remain the 'gold standard' for making the diagnosis. The sensitivity of biopsy is clearly limited by the often focal nature of the inflammation. The incidence of myocarditis has varied widely from 3 to 63% in different studies.[49,50] In the analysis of a large series of patients, our own experience is that myocarditis is present in approximately 4.5%.[51] Whilst we are being quoted as having found an 80% incidence of myocarditis in one of our studies, this was in fact a very highly selected population of patients who were found to have typical acute myocarditis on histopathological criteria, deemed to be suitable for consideration of immunosuppression.[52]

Whilst there is a variable incidence of myocarditis in any population investi-

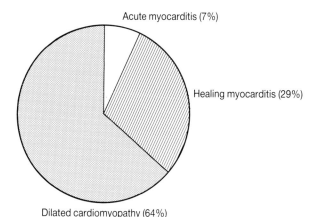

Fig. 4.5 Graphical representation of the spread of histological diagnoses of 153 consecutive patients with suspected inflammatory heart muscle disease over the past 3 years.

gated by myocardial biopsy, it is undoubtedly of value to the clinician to be able to determine whether his or her patient has the histological findings of dilated cardiomyopathy, i.e. the findings are consistent with a healed phase of myocarditis, or that they have some degree of myocarditis. Even those patients with acute myocarditis at the time of diagnosis with considerable impairment of ventricular function (ejection fraction <30%) may spontaneously improve within the next 6 months. Those patients who have the appearances of a healing or resolving myocarditis without myocyte necrosis may similarly improve.[29] Furthermore, serial endomyocardial biopsy may provide the opportunity to document the progression from acute to healed myocarditis. This can occur spontaneously and is not dependent upon the use of immunosuppressive therapy. The role of immunosuppression will be discussed separately in the section on treatment.

As well as affording the opportunity to diagnose typical lymphocytic myocarditis, endomyocardial biopsy will also provide the clinician with the opportunity to diagnose and exclude the rarer forms of heart muscle disease, for example giant cell myocarditis.[53] The apparent importance of diagnosing this form, compared with lymphocytic myocarditis, is that the prognosis is definitely worse. It was found that 20% of patients with giant cell myocarditis were alive or had not undergone cardiac transplantation at follow-up compared with 70% of those with lymphocytic myocarditis. Moreover, the follow-up period of those patients with lymphocytic myocarditis was 50% longer. Giant cell myocarditis was more likely to be associated with ventricular arrhythmias and, in many, a permanent pacemaker was indicated. There was a gradual decline in left ventricular function with time. A further condition which can also be diagnosed by endomyocardial biopsy and which indeed has been suggested as being related to giant cell myocarditis is sarcoidosis. The latter condition can be differentiated from giant cell myocarditis[54] but from the clinical point of view it is well recognized that cardiac sarcoidosis may respond to immunosuppressive therapy[55] and thus has a different natural history and prognosis.

Rarer forms of myocardial pathology occasionally present in a manner which may mimic myocarditis. One of these is amyloid heart disease. This is readily diagnosed by endomyocardial biopsy. It is known to have an extremely poor prognosis and is unresponsive to any form of medical treatment. Heart transplantation may be indicated. There is considerable controversy concerning the entity of arrhythmogenic right ventricular dysplasia. In a proportion of these patients who have predominantly right ventricular myocardial involvement with extensive fatty deposition, there are some in whom the histological changes of myocarditis may be found at the time of endomyocardial biopsy.[56–58]

Endomyocardial disease, which is usually seen in the tropics as endomyocardial fibrosis, has three stages which are pathologically well documented.[59] In the UK it is a very rare form of inflammatory heart muscle disease but, nevertheless, it needs to be differentiated from lymphocytic myocarditis. The first phase is an inflammatory phase in which eosinophilic infiltration occurs in the myocardium with appearances which may be similar to those of myocarditis. The eosinophils in this condition have been shown to have a characteristic degranulated appearance. This relates to the release of cationic proteins from the granules which have been shown by Spry *et al.*[60] to be cytotoxic.

The degranulated eosinophils are not only seen in the myocardium in some patients but also in the peripheral blood. Furthermore, the cationic protein levels can be measured in serum. The importance of recognizing this condition in its early myocarditic stage is that it can be treated with immunosuppressive therapy.[61]

The role of endomyocardial biopsy in the diagnosis and management of patients with myocarditis and their treatment with immunosuppressive therapy will be dealt with separately under the treatment section.

Virological diagnosis (see Chapter 9)

Whilst many viruses have been implicated in the pathogenesis of myocarditis and dilated cardiomyopathy,[62] the most frequently encountered group are the enteroviruses of which the coxsackie B viruses are the most frequently encountered. In determining whether a diagnosis of viral heart disease can be made by the clinician there are orders of magnitude of association which need to be fulfilled to reach this diagnosis. The criteria for the implication of a virus in myocarditis have been laid down by Lerner and Wilson.[63] However, in view of the ubiquitous nature of the enteroviruses it is possible that isolation of a virus or demonstration of an antibody response may be a coincidental finding.

Attempts to detect antigens to coxsackie B1–5 viruses by immunofluorescence in cardiac tissue have also been reported. Although Burch et al.[64] claimed to have identified coxsackie B viral antigens in the myocardium and endocardium of patients with myocarditis and valvulitis, these findings have not been confirmed independently. Employing radio labelled antigens, neither we[26] nor Takatsu et al.[27] were able to demonstrate coxsackie B virus antigen in cardiac biopsies from patients with heart muscle disease.

In practice routine viral serology together with coxsackie B neutralizing antibody tests may be helpful. However, a fourfold rise in neutralizing antibody titre in paired sera may be diagnostic.[9] An elevated titre of coxsackie-specific IgM may also indicate a recent infection. More recently in the study of 86 patients with dilated cardiomyopathy, the enterovirus-specific IgM response was investigated. Twenty-eight patients (33%) were shown to have persisting evidence of enterovirus infection compared with only 12% in a population of asymptomatic blood donors.[65]

The development of cDNA technology has made it possible to detect evidence of enterovirus infection in tissue from patients in all endomyocardial stages of myocarditis and dilated cardiomyopathy.[4] Employing slot blot hybridization, enteroviral RNA was detected in 43% of patients with myocarditis, either acute or healing, compared with 41% of patients with dilated cardiomyopathy and 5% of healthy controls (Table 4.4). Employing *in situ* hybridization, Kandolf et al.[5] demonstrated viral RNA not only in parts of the myocardium with histological evidence of acute myocarditis but also in apparently normal areas of myocardium from the same patient. In a further study replicating enterovirus RNA was found to be present in 23 of 95 patients with clinically diagnosed myocarditis, including 10 of 33 patients with dilated cardiomyopathy of recent onset. All the 53 patients comprising a pathological control group with other specific heart muscle disease not consistent with a primary viral aetiology (e.g. ischaemic injury, hypertrophic cardiomyopathy

Table 4.4 Incidence of enterovirus RNA in myocardial biopsy tissue from patients with myocarditis and dilated cardiomyopathy compared with control tissue from patients with specific heart muscle diseases ($n = 193$ patients).

	Myocarditis	Dilated cardiomyopathy	Controls
RNA +ve	23 (43%)	40 (41%)	2 (5%)
RNA −ve	31	57	40
Total	54	97	42

and metabolic cardiomyopathy) were negative when their myocardial tissue was examined by *in situ* hybridization.[66]

In addition to demonstrating enterovirus RNA in myocarditis it has also been possible to detect virus sequences in 30% of tissue samples taken from explanted hearts in patients undergoing cardiac transplantation for endstage dilated cardiomyopathy. This differed significantly from those with endstage coronary heart disease in whom enterovirus was detected in only 5%.[67] Virus RNA has also been demonstrable using *in situ* hybridization in 4 of 19 patients undergoing heart transplantation.[66] These studies clearly show that virus may be present in spite of the absence of inflammatory response on histopathological evaluation. The virus persists in a defective mutant form. This is the result of an aberration of viral RNA synthesis in a nonproductive replication cycle.[6]

Implications of virus persistence

The recognition that patients with a clinical diagnosis of myocarditis or dilated cardiomyopathy have a poor prognosis led to the investigation of patients with suspected heart muscle disease to determine whether there was an association between enterovirus infection and survival. One hundred and twenty-three patients with all grades of myocarditis or dilated cardiomyopathy were investigated to enable clinical and histological classification. Virus was detected in endomyocardial biopsy tissue using the hybridization probe in 41 patients. It was found that detection of persisting enteroviral RNA was the single most powerful predictor of survival.[6]

The polymerase chain reaction (PCR) gene amplification technique is sensitive and specific and can be applied to the diagnosis of viral disease in small tissue samples where low copy numbers of the viral genome may be present. Applying this technique 48 patients with clinically suspected myocarditis or dilated cardiomyopathy were investigated.[68] Five of the patients investigated had positive enteroviral signals by PCR, in two cases myocarditis was present histologically, whereas the remaining three had changes consistent with dilated cardiomyopathy. Whilst the PCR technique would appear to be a sensitive means of detecting enterovirus in myocardial biopsy tissue, there have been somewhat conflicting results from different centres. The technique has not been rigorously compared with the now more widely used molecular hybridization probes. Thus at the present time, although the hybridization probes are largely research tools, they probably provide the clinician with the most reliable way of diagnosing suspected viral heart disease. The development of a reliable PCR technique will, in the long-term, represent a major technological advance.

Treatment (see Chapter 11)

The treatment of viral heart disease relates predominantly to those patients who have important sequelae from the viral infection. As already stated the majority of patients may well improve spontaneously. At the present time no specific antiviral therapy is available, although Ribavirin has been used in an animal model with some success[69] and preliminary studies with interferon-α have been shown to inhibit virus replication and reduce the inflammatory response of the myocardium.[70] Since there is much evidence that heart muscle damage is caused by immune-mediated mechanisms, even if they are virus triggered, considerable interest has focussed on the use of various forms of immunosuppression in experimental murine coxsackie B3 myocarditis employing cyclosporin, prednisone and monoclonal antibodies, T helper and cytolytic suppressor T lymphocytes.[71] In a similar manner the effects of tumour necrosis factor, interleukin-2 and anti-interleukin-2 receptor antibodies were studied[72] (see Chapter 5, part II). The authors, however, were unable to demonstrate any consistent benefit using these types of treatment.

The relationship between virus infection and myocarditis is now well established. However, as described earlier, the model for the development of myocarditis and subsequently dilated cardiomyopathy is biphasic as described by Lerner.[19] In this model the period during which the virus undergoes active replication lasts probably no more than 10–14 days in the human. Subsequently, however, the virus may persist in a defective mutant form without an inflammatory response in the myocardium.[6,67] During the second phase innumerable antibodies have been identified which include cytolytic or cytotoxic anti-sarcolemmal or anti-myolemmal antibodies.[73] Further immune mechanisms which have been implicated include antibodies to the adrenergic β-receptor.[74] The sarcolemma may also act as an antigen[75] and the cardiac proteins can result in circulating heart-reactive antibodies in patients with myocarditis or cardiomyopathy.[76] While some evidence has been identified to indicate that the anti-myolemmal antibody system may have a prognostic implication[77] none of these systems have provided a precise basis for specific therapy (see Chapter 7).

The similarity of the histological features seen in heart transplant rejection to those seen in myocarditis provided the basis for the concept that immunosuppressive therapy might be beneficial in the treatment of this condition.[78] In that study 10 patients with congestive heart failure were investigated by biopsy and treated with immunosuppression (either prednisone alone, or prednisone in combination with azathioprine). Serial invasive and noninvasive assessment of cardiac performance was made, and 9 of the 10 patients had one or more follow-up myocardial biopsies. Four patients showed a dramatic improvement associated with immunosuppressive therapy. A further patient also showed improvement and four had stabilization of previously progressive heart failure. In the six patients who underwent a second myocardial biopsy following treatment, the inflammatory infiltrate had been eliminated. After discontinuation of therapy, signs and symptoms of myocarditis recurred in two patients.

Against the background of the Stanford experience, 9 of 12 patients who presented with congestive cardiac failure following a viral-like illness and who had acute myocarditis on endomyocardial biopsy were treated with immunosuppressive therapy (prednisolone and azathioprine in seven and prednisolone alone in two.[52] Following 2 months of treatment, seven patients showed clinical and haemodynamic improvement (ejection fraction rose from 27 to 46% and the left ventricular end-diastolic filling pressure fell from 26 to 16 mmHg). In these patients there was histological improvement to a healed pattern, although in two patients a healing pattern with persistent activity was seen. However, at 6 months only four patients had maintained improvement. One had relapsed after stopping treatment, improving again on reinstatement of therapy. Two patients developed severe interstitial myocardial fibrosis and gradually deteriorated. It was suggested that multicentre controlled trials would be necessary to assess fully the role of immunosuppressive treatment in this condition. There have been many small clinical studies of immunosuppressive therapy in active myocarditis and these are summarized by O'Connell.[79]

Against the background of the variable results of immunosuppressive therapy, a multicentre myocarditis treatment trial was sponsored by the National Institutes of Health which randomly assigned therapy to patients with active myocarditis according to the Dallas criteria.[48] This study has incorporated 23 centres in the USA, Canada and Japan and is coordinated by the University of Utah. Patients with unexplained congestive heart failure and an ejection fraction of <45% were randomized to receive either conventional therapy for congestive heart failure or conventional therapy plus prednisolone and cyclosporin for 6 months. The patients were then followed up for a further 6 months on conventional anti-failure therapy before final assessment of ejection fraction and exercise testing at 1 year. The results of this trial are not yet published, but preliminary analysis of the data indicates that there does not appear to be a significant difference with regard to outcome between those receiving conventional anti-failure therapy and those treated with immunosuppression. Improvement in ejection fraction appeared to occur in both groups and perhaps as importantly, no patient deteriorated as a result of receiving immunosuppressive therapy. Unfortunately the results appear to bear some similarity to the findings of the long-term follow-up study of acute myocarditis reported by Quigley *et al.*[29] who reported that two groups of patients emerged, those with severely impaired ejection fractions and those who were apparently normal. It is possible that a subset of patients exists in whom ventricular function does not recover and where an immune-mediated process could be responsible for the continued impaired ventricular function. The other alternative is that there is persistence of defective mutant virus which is impairing the cellular basis of myocardial contractile function. The detailed studies which are available to the myocarditis trial investigators may provide insight into the pathogenetic mechanisms. However, at the present time there does not appear to be any rational basis for immunosuppressive therapy in patients with either biopsy-proven myocarditis or dilated cardiomyopathy based on the current data. The clinician may, however, have to consider immunosuppression when faced with a patient with active myocyte necrosis on biopsy and a deteriorating clinical pattern.

The clinical complications of myocarditis include cardiac failure, arrhythmias and the development of dilated cardiomyopathy. The conventional treatment of these include diuretic therapy, digitalis where appropriate, ACE inhibitors, vasodilator therapy, anti-arrhythmics and inotropic support if required. The patients in the group requiring inotropic agents are likely to be candidates for heart transplantation. There is evidence that those patients who deteriorate rapidly with acute myocarditis are more likely to have a greater number of rejection episodes when they undergo transplantation (O'Connell, personal communication).

Acknowledgements

The authors gratefully acknowledge the contributions made by Dr E. G. J. Olsen, MD, FRCPath, Consultant Pathologist, Royal Brompton and National Heart Hospital with respect to the histological studies, and by Dr L. C. Archard, PhD, Senior Lecturer in Biochemistry, Charing Cross and Westminster Medical School with respect to the molecular virological studies.

References

1. Report of the International Society and Federation of Cardiology/World Health Organisation. Task force on the definition and classification of cardiomyopathies. *Br Heart J* 1980; **44:** 672–3.
2. Sakakibara S., Konno S. Endomyocardial biopsy. *Jpn Heart J* 1962; **3:** 537–43.
3. Richardson P. J. King's endomyocardial bioptome. *Lancet* 1974; **i:** 660–1.
4. Bowles N. E., Richardson P. J., Olsen E. G. J., Archard L. C. Detection of coxsackie B virus-specific RNA sequences in myocardial biopsy samples from patients with myocarditis and dilated cardiomyopathy. *Lancet* 1986; **ii:** 1120–3.
5. Kandolf R., Ameis D., Krischner P. *et al. In situ* detection of enteroviral genomes in myocardial cells by nucleic acid hybridization – an approach to the diagnosis of viral heart disease. *Proc Natl Acad Sci (USA)* 1987; **84:** 6272–6.
6. Archard L. C., Bowles N. E., Cunningham L. *et al.* Molecular probes for the detection of persisting enterovirus infection of human heart and their prognostic value. *Eur Heart J* 1991; **12** (suppl D): 56–9.
7. Gore I., Saphir D. Myocarditis: a classification of 1402 cases. *Am Heart J* 1947; **34:** 827–30.
8. Woodruff J. F. Viral myocarditis. *Am J Pathol* 1980; **101:** 427–78.
9. Grist N. R., Bell E. J. A six year study of coxsackievirus B infections in heart disease. *J Hyg (Cambs)* 1974; **73:** 165–72.
10. Helin M., Savola J., Lapinleimu K. Cardiac manifestations during a coxsackie B5 epidemic. *Br Med J* 1968; **iii:** 97–9.
11. Kirbrick S., Bernirscke K. Acute aseptic myocarditis and meningo-encephalitis in the newborn child infected with coxsackievirus group B type 3. *N Engl J Med* 1956; **255:** 883–9.
12. Kaplan M. H. Coxsackievirus infection in children under 3 months of age. In: Bendinelli M., Friedman H. eds. *Coxsackieviruses: a general update.* New York: Plenum Press, 1988: 241–52.
13. Grist N. R., Reid D. General pathogenicity and epidemiology. Coxsackieviruses: a general update. In: Bendinelli M., Friedman H. eds. *Coxsackieviruses: a general update.* New York: Plenum Press, 1988: 221–40.
14. Gillum R. F. Idiopathic cardiomyopathy in the United States, 1970–1982. *Am Heart J* 1986; **111:** 752–5.
15. Torp A. Incidence of congestive cardiomyopathy. *Postgrad Med J* 1978; **54:** 435–9.

16. Williams D. G., Olsen E. G. J. Prevalence of overt dilated cardiomyopathy in two regions of England. *Br Heart J* 1985; **54:** 153–5.
17. Jarco S. Fiedler on acute interstitial myocarditis. I. *Am J Cardiol* 1973; **32:** 221–3; II. *Am J Cardiol* 1973; **32:** 616–18.
18. Saphir O. Myocaditis: A general review with an analysis of 240 cases. *Arch Pathol* 1941; **32:** 1000–51.
19. Lerner A. M. Coxsackievirus myocardiopathy. *J Infect Dis* 1969; **120:** 496–9.
20. Saini G., Krompotic E., Slotki S. J. Adult heart disease due to coxsackievirus B infection. *Medicine* 1968; **47:** 133.
21. Smith W. G. Coxsackie B myopericarditis in adults. *Am Heart J* 1970; **80:** 34.
22. Kawai C. Idiopathic cardiomyopathy. A study on the infectious immune theory as a cause of the disease. *Jpn Circ J* 1971; **35:** 765.
23. Levi G. F., Proto C., Quadri A., Ratti S. Coxsackievirus heart disease and cardiomyopathy. *Am Heart J* 1977; **93:** 419–21.
24. Levi G. F., Scalvini S., Volterrani M. *et al*. Coxsackievirus heart disease: 15 years after. *Eur Heart J* 1988; **9** (suppl J): 1303–7.
25. Cambridge G., MacArthur C. G. C., Waterston A. P. *et al*. Antibodies to coxsackie B viruses in congestive cardiomyopathy. *Br Heart J* 1979; **41:** 692–6.
26. Morgan-Capner P., Richardson P. J., McSorley C. *et al*. Virus investigations in heart muscle Disease. In: Bolte H.-D. ed. *Viral Heart Disease*. Berlin: Springer-Verlag, 1984: 99–115.
27. Takatsu T., Kitamura Y., Morita H. *et al*. Viral myocarditis and cardiomyopathy. In: Sekiguchi M., Olsen E. G. J. eds. *Cardiomyopathy – clinical, pathological and theoretical aspects*. Tokyo: University of Tokyo Press, 1988: 341–63.
28. Goodwin J. F. Prospects and prediction for the cardiomyopathies. *Circulation* 1974: **50:** 210–19.
29. Quigley P. J., Richardson P. J., Meany B. T. *et al*. Long-term follow up of acute myocarditis: Correlation of ventricular function and outcome. *Eur Heart J* 1987; **8** (suppl J): 39–42.
30. Richardson P. J., Wodak A. D., Atkinson L. *et al*. Relation between alcohol intake, myocardial enzyme activity, and myocardial function in dilated cardiomyopathy: Evidence for the concept of alcohol induced heart muscle disease. *Br Heart J* 1986; **56:** 165–70.
31. Klein J., Stanek G., Bittner R. *et al*. Lyme borreliosis as a cause of myocarditis and heart muscle disease. *Eur Heart J* 1991; **12** (suppl D): 73–5.
32. James T. N., Schlant R. C., Marshall T. K. Randomly distributed focal myocardial lesions causing destruction of the His bundle or a narrow origin left bundle branch. *Circulation* 1978; **57:** 816.
33. Reyes M. P., Lerner A. M. Coxsackie myocarditis – with special reference to acute and clinical effects. *Prog Cardiovasc Dis* 1985; **27:** 373.
34. Woolf P. K., Chung T. S., Stewart J. *et al*. Life threatening dysrhythmias in varicella myocarditis. *Clin Paed* 1987; **26:** 480–2.
35. Sareli P., Schramroth C. L., Passias J., Schramroth L. Torsade de pointes due to coxsackie B3 myocarditis. *Clin Cardiol* 1987; **10:** 361–2.
36. Kitaura Y., Morita H. Secondary myocardial disease, virus myocarditis and cardiomyopathy. *Jpn Circ J* 1979; **43:** 1017–31.
37. Sekiguchi M., Hiroe M., Kaneko M., Kusakase K. Natural history of 20 patients with biopsy proven acute mycarditis – 10 year follow up. *Circulation* 1985; **72** (suppl 3): 109.
38. Vignola P., Kazutara A., Pauls S. *et al*. Lymphocytic myocarditis presenting as unexplained ventricular tachycardia: Diagnosis with endomyocardial biopsy and response to immunosuppression. *J Am Coll Cardiol* 1984; **4:** 812–19.
39. Strain J., Grose R., Factor S., Fisher J. Results of endomyocardial biopsy in patients with spontaneous ventricular tachycardia without apparent structural disease. *Circulation* 1983; **68:** 1171–81.

40. Matsumori A., Kadoja K., Kawai C. Technium 99m – pyrophosphate uptake in experimental viral perimyocarditis. Sequential study of myocardial uptake and pathologic correlates. *Circulation* 1980; **61:** 802–7.
41. O'Connell J. B., Henlan R. E., Robinson J. A. *et al.* Gallium-67 imaging in patients with dilated cardiomyopathy and biopsy proven myocarditis. *Circulation* 1984; **70:** 58–62.
42. Yasuda T. S., Palacios I. F., Dec W. *et al.* Indium-111 monoclonal antimyosin antibody imaging in the diagnosis of acute myocarditis. *Circulation* 1987; **76:** 306–11.
43. Rezkella S., Khoner R. A., Khaw B. A. *et al.* Detection of experimental myocarditis by monoclonal antimyosin antibody FAB fragments. *Am Heart J* 1989; **117:** 391–5.
44. Raftery E. B., Banks D. C., Oram S. Occlusive disease of the coronary arteries presenting as pacing congestive cardiomyopathy. *Lancet* 1969; **ii:** 1147–50.
45. Richardson P. J., Daly K., Gishen P. Haemodynamic findings in biopsy proven myocarditis. In: Bolte H.-D. ed. *Viral Heart Disease.* Berlin: Springer-Verlag, 1984: 165–72.
46. Richardson P. J. Endomyocardial biopsy: technique and evaluation of a new disposable forceps and catheter sheath system. In Bolte H.-D. ed. *Viral Heart Disease.* Berlin: Springer-Verlag, 1983: 173–6.
47. Olsen E. G. J., Meany B. T., Richardson P. J. Role of biopsy in the diagnosis and follow up of myocarditis – a critical review. In Schultheiss H.-P. ed. *New Concepts in Viral Heart Disease.* Berlin: Springer-Verlag, 1988: 285–94.
48. Aretz H. T., Billingham M. E., Edwards W. D. *et al.* Myocarditis: a histopathologic definition and classification. *Am J Cardiovasc Pathol* 1986; **1:** 3–14.
49. Zee Cheng C. S., Tsai C. C., Palmer D. C. *et al.* High incidence of myocarditis diagnosed by endomyocardial biopsy in patients with idiopathic congestive cardiomyopathy. *J Am Coll Cardiol* 1984; **3:** 63–70.
50. Dec G. W., Palacios I. F., Fallon J. T. *et al.* Active myocarditis in the spectrum of acute dilated cardiomyopathies – clinical features, histologic correlates and clinical outcome. *N Engl J Med* 1985; **312:** 885–90.
51. Baandrup U., Florio B. A., Rehalin M. *et al.* Critical analysis of endomyocardial biopsies from patients with suspected cardiomyopathy II. Comparison of histology and clinical/haemodynamic information. *Br Heart J* 1981; **45:** 487–93.
52. Daly K., Richardson P. J., Olsen E. G. J. *et al.* Acute myocarditis: role of histological and virological examination in the diagnosis and assessment of immunosuppressive treatment. *Br Heart J* 1984; **51:** 30–5.
53. Davidoff R., Palacios E., Southern J. *et al.* Giant cell and lymphocytic myocarditis – comparison of clinical factors and long term outcome. *Circulation* 1991; **83:** 953–61.
54. Johanssen A. Isolated myocarditis versus myocardial sarcoidosis. *Acta Pathol Microbiol Scand* 1967; **67:** 15–26.
55. Lorell B., Alderman E. L., Mason J. W. Cardiac sarcoidosis: diagnosis with endomyocardial biopsy and treatment with corticosteroids. *Am J Cardiol* 1978; **42:** 143–6.
56. Marcus F., Fontaine G., Guiraudon G. *et al.* Right ventricular dysplasia: a report of 24 adult cases. *Circulation* 1982; **65:** 384–98.
57. Hisaoka T., Kawai S., Ohi H. *et al.* Two cases of chronic myocarditis mimicking arrhythmogenic right ventricular dysplasia. *Heart and Vessels* 1990; (suppl 5): 51–4.
58. Thiene G., Corrado D., Nava A. *et al.* Right ventricular cardiomyopathy: is there evidence of an inflammatory aetiology. *Eur Heart J* 1991; **12** (suppl D): 22–5.
59. Davis J., Spry C. J. F., Vijayaraghavan G., De Souza J. A. A comparison of the clinical and cardiological features of endomyocardial disease in temperate and tropical regions. *Postgrad Med J* 1983; **59:** 179–83.

60. Spry C., Tai P.-C., Davis J. The cardiotoxicity of eosinophils. *Postgrad Med J* 1983; **59:** 147–51.
61. Spry C. J. F. Eosinophils and endomyocardial fibrosis: a review of clinical and experimental studies 1980–1986. In: Kawai C., Abelmann W. H. eds. *Pathogenesis of Myocarditis and Cardiomyopathy.* Tokyo: University of Tokyo Press, 1987: 293–310.
62. Lansdown A. B. G. Viral infection and diseases of the heart. In Melnick J. L. ed. *Progress in Medical Virology.* Basel: Karger, 1978: 70–113.
63. Lerner A. M., Wilson F. M. Virus myocardiopathy. *Prog Med Virol* 1973; **15:** 63–91.
64. Burch G. E., Sun S. C., Colcolough H. L. *et al.* Coxsackie B viral myocarditis and valvulitis identified in routine autopsy specimens by immunofluorescent techniques. *Am Heart J* 1967; **74:** 13.
65. Muir P., Tilley A., English T. A. M. *et al.* Chronic relapsing pericarditis and dilated cardiomyopathy; serological evidence of persistent enterovirus infection. *Lancet* 1989; **i:** 804–7.
66. Kandolf R., Canu A., Klinger K. *et al.* Molecular studies in enteroviral heart diseases. In: Brinton M. A., Henry F. X. eds. *New Aspects of Positive-strand RNA Viruses.* Washington: American Society for Microbiology, 1990: 340–8.
67. Bowles N. E., Rose M. L., Taylor P. *et al.* End-stage dilated cardiomyopathy: persistence of enterovirus RNA in myocardium at cardiac transplantation and lack of immune response. *Circulation* 1989; **80:** 1128–36.
68. Jin O., Sole M. J., Butany J. W. *et al.* Detection of enterovirus RNA in myocardial biopsies from patients with myocarditis and cardiomyopathy using gene amplification by polymerase chain reaction. *Circulation* 1990; **82:** 8–16.
69. Matsumori A., Wang H., Abelman W. H., Crumpacker C. S. Treatment of viral myocarditis with ribavirin in an animal preparation. *Circulation* 1985; **71:** 834–9.
70. Matsumori A., Kawai C., Crumpacker C. S., Abelmann W. H. The use of an animal model for preventive and therapeutic trials of viral myocarditis. In: Kawai C., Abelmann W. H. eds. *Pathogenesis of Myocarditis and Cardiomyopathy.* Tokyo: University of Tokyo Press, 1987: 37–47.
71. Herzum M., Huber S. A., Weller R. *et al.* Treatment of experimental immune coxsackie B3 myocarditis. *Br Heart J* 1991; **12** (suppl D): 200–2.
72. Matsumori A., Yamada T., Kawai C. Immunomodulatory therapy in viral myocarditis: effect of tumour necrosis factor, interleukin 2 and anti-interleukin 2 receptor antibody in an animal model. *Eur Heart J* 1991; **12** (suppl D): 203–5.
73. Maisch B. Immunologic regulation and effects on function in perimyocarditis, postmyocarditic heart muscle disease. In: Jacob R. ed. *Controversial Issues in Cardiac Pathophysiology. Basic Res Cardiol* 1986; **81** (suppl 1): 217–41.
74. Limas C. J., Limas C. Betareceptor autoantibodies in idiopathic dilated cardiomyopathy. In: Schultheiss H. P. ed. *New Concepts in Viral Heart Disease.* Berlin: Springer-Verlag, 1988: 217–24.
75. Maisch B. The sarcolemma as antigen in secondary immunopathogenesis of myopericarditis. *Eur Heart J* 1987; **8** (suppl J): 155–6.
76. Neuman D. A., Burer L. C., Baughman K. L. *et al.* Circulating heart-reactive antibodies in patients with myocarditis or cardiomyopathy. *J Am Coll Cardiol* 1990; **16:** 839–46.
77. Maisch B., Outzen H., Roth D. *et al.* Prognostic determinates in conventionally treated myocarditis and perimyocarditis – focus on antimyolemmal antibodies. *Eur Heart J* 1991; **12** (suppl D): 81–7.
78. Mason J. W., Billingham M. E., Ricci D. R. Treatment of acute inflammatory myocarditis assisted by endomyocardial biopsy. *Am J Cardiol* 1980; **45:** 1037–44.

79. O'Connell J. B. Immunosuppressive therapy in active myocarditis. In: Baroldi G., Camerini F., Goodwin J. F. eds. *Advances in Cardiomyopathies*. Berlin: Springer-Verlag, 1990: 325–30.

5

Experimental studies

Part I

Animal models: immunological aspects

S. A. Huber

Introduction

Viruses comprise a remarkable and unique 'life' form: the ultimate obligate intracellular parasite. Although the evolutionary source of viruses remains obscure, these entities have developed a diverse range of shapes, sizes and replicative cycles. Every 'higher' organism from bacteria to human beings is susceptible to virus infection. Interestingly, while most infections in humans have a viraemic phase (when virus enters the circulation either as free particles or as passengers in blood cells such as monocytes) and are therefore spread throughout the body, disease due to the infection is usually limited to selected organs or cell types. For example, rabies viruses causes disease of the central nervous system (CNS); hepatitis virus causes disease of the liver; and rhinovirus causes upper respiratory infections. Thus, certain viruses have a predilection for causing certain diseases.

To date, viruses have been most closely associated with three types of clinical cardiovascular disease. These are myocarditis, dilated cardiomyopathy and atherosclerosis. Details of the clinical diseases and evidence for a specific viral aetiology are discussed in other chapters and are therefore only briefly alluded to here. This chapter is primarily directed towards describing animal models of these clinical diseases and what these can tell us about pathogenesis. Clinical studies determining how viruses induce particular diseases are inherently limited, firstly, because any precipitating infections may have occurred months or years prior to the onset of symptoms, thus obscuring important cause and effect relationships. Secondly, the genetic, environmental and physiological characteristics of the individual as well as the type and genetics of the initiating infectious agent may affect the incidence, severity and pathogenesis of the disease process. Thirdly, detailed sequential studies are difficult to carry out because of the limitations in tissue availability and patient follow-up. Many different viruses or even genetic variants of the same virus may trigger processes, resulting ultimately in the same disease. However, the intervening pathways leading from infection to tissue injury may be remarkably different for each virus or for each patient. Animal models allow the investigator to limit variables and delve in depth into the complex cellular and molecular events whereby viruses alter cells directly and stimulate host responses. These host responses may simultaneously be beneficial and detrimental to the individual in that they control the virus infection but may also (1) change the virus increasing or decreasing its pathogenicity and (2) cause substantial immune-mediated tissue damage. The major weakness of animal models is determining whether a particular model truly reflects the clinical disease as a whole or a specific subset of patients with that disease. Where a clinical disease results from multifactorial mechanisms, animal models restricted to studying only selected variables may give either misleading or confusing conclusions on pathogenesis.

Characteristics of picornavirus and herpesvirus replication

The major animal models of virus-induced heart disease primarily use either picornaviruses or herpesviruses. A basic understanding of the viruses and their replication cycles is necessary to evaluate the pathogenic mechanisms in the various diseases.

Picornavirus (see also Chapters 1, 2 and 9)

Picornaviruses are small, nonenveloped viruses containing a single RNA strand with positive sense (i.e. the genome RNA can be directly translated into viral proteins). The genome comprises 30% of the molecular mass of the virus particle and is enclosed within an icosahedral protein capsid. The capsid is comprised of 60 promoters, each containing a single copy of the four structural proteins VP1 to VP4.[1-3] The topography of the capsid has been elucidated by X-ray crystallography and shows that the surface of the virion is irregular with elevated 'peaks' and 'grooves' or 'pits'. Proteins VP1, VP2 and VP3 are primarily involved in producing the outward topography of the capsid. Protein VP4 is an internal capsid protein and is located beneath the other three virus proteins. The role of VP4 is not absolutely clear, but it probably plays a dual role in stabilizing the interaction/tertiary structure of the other capsid proteins and facilitating in the interaction between the capsid and genome.

The basic picornavirus replication cycle can be divided into (1) virus attachment to the cell membrane, (2) virus penetration into the cytoplasm, (3) uncoating of the genome, (4) replication, (5) assembly of progeny virions, and (6) release of progeny virions into the extracellular space (Fig. 5.1a). Virus attachment occurs through binding specific membrane components (called virus receptors) primarily to the groove regions of the viral capsid.[3-6] The virus receptor is often cited as a major (but not exclusive) factor controlling both species specificity and tissue tropism of infection.[7-9] Many picornaviruses including polioviruses, coxsackieviruses, rhinoviruses and echoviruses are primarily primate pathogens while cardioviruses and aphthoviruses (foot-and-mouth disease virus) are picornavirus pathogens of mice and cloven-footed animals, respectively.[7] Even within a susceptible species,

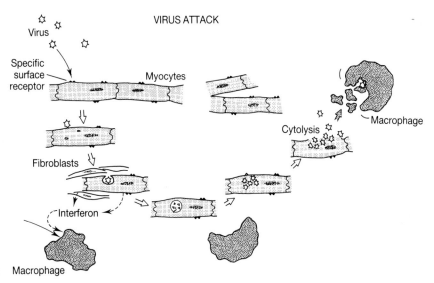

Fig. 5.1 (a) *Virus replication cycle*. Virus attaches to specific receptors on myocytes, is internalized into lysosomes and the viral protein capsid is enzymatically degraded to release the viral RNA into the cytoplasm. Virus RNA is translated and transcribed in the cytoplasm to produce new progeny virions. The progeny are released by lysis of the infected cell. Infection stimulates the release of interferon-α interferon-β which increases resistance of surrounding cells to infection and activates both macrophage and natural killer cells.

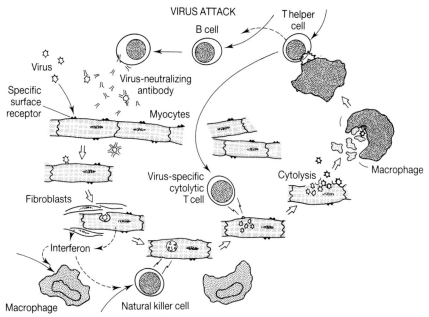

Fig. 5.1 (b) *Host defense mechanisms*. Activated macrophage phagocytize cellular debris and virus and present viral antigens to T and B lymphocytes stimulating both cellular and humoral virus-specific immunity. Virus-specific antibodies bind to virus preventing attachment to uninfected myocytes (limits spread of infection). Virus-specific T and natural killer cells lyse infected cells before completion of virus replication cycle to limit virus production.

VIRUS ATTACK

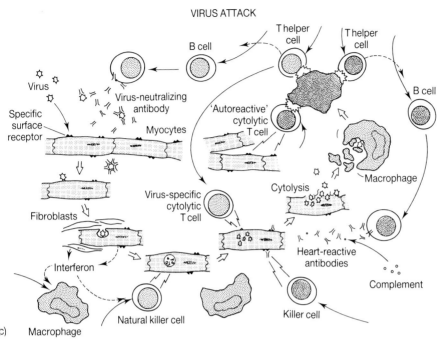

Fig. 5.1 (c) *Autoimmunity in viral heart disease.* Activated macrophage may stimulate autoimmunity by (1) presenting virus antigens which cross-react with host cell molecules (antigenic mimicry) or (2) presenting cellular antigens engulfed during phagocytosis of virus. Both cellular and humoral autoimmunity occurs. Autoimmune cytolytic T cells directly lyse myocytes. Heart reactive autoantibodies may lyse myocytes. Heart reactive autoantibodies may lyse myocytes through complement-dependent or antibody-dependent cell-mediated cytotoxicity (ADCC) mechanisms.

however, viruses may have distinct tropisms for certain tissues. Well-known examples of tissue tropism include poliovirus infection of the anterior horn cells of the spinal cord and rhinovirus infection of the epithelial cells of the nasopharynx. Evidence that the virus receptor may contribute directly to both species and tissue tropism comes from studies in which tropism can be (1) altered by changing receptor utilization of the virus and (2) circumvented by exposing usually nonsusceptible cells to infectious RNA. In this manner, poliovirus replication can occur even in nonprimate cells (e.g. chick embryos).

The receptor for the major family of rhinoviruses has been identified as ICAM-1, an adhesion molecule belonging to the immunoglobulin superfamily and an important element in immune responses.[5,6] A distinct immunoglobulin superfamily member has additionally been identified as the poliovirus receptor.[4] Most likely other molecules belonging to this family act as receptors for different picornaviruses. Evidence from this laboratory (N. Van Houten, unpublished observations) indicates that murine ICAM-1 is not the receptor for coxsackie B3 virus (CVB3), although another immunoglobulin superfamily member may be. Immunoglobulin superfamily members include not only a wide-range of cell–cell adhesion molecules but also the major histocompatibility complex (MHC) antigens, T cell receptor (TcR) molecules, and T cell accessory molecules (CD4 and CD8, etc.). There are certain inherent advantages for viruses to use members of this immunologically important family for their receptors. Firstly, the natural host response to infection involves induction of virus-specific immunity designed to eliminate the virus. Part of the immune response releases certain cytokines (interferon-γ, interleukin-1 and tumor necrosis factor) which enhance expression of many immunoglobulin superfamily proteins on cells. Thus, tissue cells which normally lack these proteins can be induced into *de novo* synthesis of them during virus immune responses, while cells which express only moderate or minimal levels of immunoglobulin superfamily members may increase expression many fold.[10–12] Undoubtedly, the biological relevance of increased expression of these molecules is to enhance the antigenicity of virally infected tissues and allow more efficient elimination of the infectious agent.[13] However, this process simultaneously creates more receptors for the virus suggesting that any infectious virions remaining in a tissue are likely to find a susceptible host cell. A second possible advantage for the virus in using immunoglobulin superfamily members as receptors is the presence of these molecules on immunoreactive cells. Selective infection of these lymphoid cells may either alter or disable the virus–immune response. Coxsackie B3 virus and encephalomyocarditis (EMC) virus clearly infect macrophages and may also infect at least some T lymphocytes[14] (S. A. Huber, unpublished observations).

Secondly, virus must be internalized into the cell through a process called viropexy. Attachment of the virus to the plasma membrane is clearly not adequate to allow infection of the cell. Schultz and Crowell[15] showed that a nonfusing myogenic cell line could express receptors for coxsackievirus group A and consequently bind these viruses, although internalization of the virus did not occur. Other fusible myogenic lines permitted virus entry and supported virus replication. This observation implies that characteristics of membrane fluidity or cytoskeletal elements must participate in internalization of the virus. Receptor-mediated endocytosis of picornaviruses involves clustering and cross-linking of at least five receptor molecules into clathrin-coated pits and invagination of the receptor–virus complexes into vesicles within the cytoplasm.[16,17] This process would require fluidity of the membrane to allow appropriate positioning of the receptors and involvement of the cytoskeletal elements in the internalization of the virus. Once inside the cell, the virus-containing vesicles fuse with other intracellular vesicles such as lysosomes to form endosomes. Uncoating of many picornaviruses requires low pH within the vesicles, suggesting enzyme directed degradation of the protein capsid and release of the viral RNA.

Once the viral RNA has successfully entered the cytoplasm, translation of the genome begins. Poly(C) tracts at the 5′ noncoding region of the viral RNA direct internal entry of ribosomes onto the RNA.[18,19] The picornavirus RNA encodes a single polyprotein which, subsequent to translation, is enzymatically processed to yield the four capsid proteins as well as several noncapsid proteins. Once translation has occurred, a virally encoded polymerase allows the infecting viral RNA to act additionally as a template for the production of more viral RNA. Complementary (negative strand) RNA is produced from the infecting (positive strand) viral RNA using the viral polymerase.[7] These negative strand RNAs are subsequently transcribed into additional positive strand viral RNAs which can either be inserted into progeny virions or used to continue the virus replication cycle. One interesting characteristic of picornaviruses is their ability to shut down host protein and RNA synthesis. The mechanism is not clearly understood but appears to involve the gradual dissociation of host mRNA–polysome complexes to be replaced by larger complexes involving the viral RNA.[20] The tertiary structure of the 5' noncoding region of the virus genome may be responsible for the preferential translation of virus RNA in the cell. Engineered alterations in the poly(C) tract of the virus can have dramatic effects on polysome attachment and viral replication.[18,19] Importantly, the efficacy of host protein shutdown can vary between virus variants, and this characteristic may play a role in the virulence of the infection.[21]

Assembly of the progeny virion capsids occurs within the cytoplasm. A provirion particle lacking the viral genome is initially constructed. Next, the viral RNA becomes associated with the procapsid and a proteolytic step seals the genome into the capsid, forming the mature virus particle.[7] Release of the progeny virions usually occurs with lysis of the infected cell. Cytopathic effects of picornavirus infections are increased plasma membrane permeability, leakage of the cytoplasm and disintegration of the cell.[22] Cell death may result from interference with normal cellular metabolism, but a more probable explanation is that a virus-encoded toxic factor is produced which ultimately lyses the cell. Whether the release of progeny virions always requires cell lysis is not clear. Long-term, chronically infected cell cultures have been established which release infectious CVB3 over many months or years.[23] This might be accomplished by low-grade lytic infections of a small number of cells at any particular time in the culture. Replication of the remaining cells would constantly replace lysed cells and provide new host cells for the progeny virus. Alternatively, picornaviruses may be released without cell lysis. Possibly, progeny virions might enter the endosome network and be released from the intact cell. Observations by several investigators indicate that some primary cell cultures such as myocytes, can be infected with CVB3 and even release virus into the medium over a period of several days without apparent cytopathic effect to the cells[24] (C. Gauntt, personal communication). Furthermore, continued culture of the infected cells ultimately results in cessation of infectious virus production while the myocytes continue to appear quite healthy. Similar transient infections occurring *in vivo* may have little detrimental effect on cardiac function. A related question is whether the picornavirus is completely eliminated from cells capable of surviving infection. The above studies defined transient infection by measuring infectious virus produced by infected myocytes and by demonstrating that such production is curtailed with time. However, several investigators detect persistent viral genomic material in myocardial cells *in vivo* in the absence of infectious virus.[25,26] Furthermore, while cells producing functional progeny virus show a predominance of positive strand viral RNA in the cytoplasm, the persistently infected cells show equal concentrations of both positive and negative strand RNA.[26,27] This could imply that the persistent infection is not designed to produce viable progeny virus. The infection may be maintained at the RNA level, i.e. replication of RNA may be occurring with either defective or minimal virus protein synthesis. The persistent infection might not cause cell lysis under these conditions but could perhaps detrimentally affect host protein and RNA synthesis. Whether certain host cells can be persistently infected while remaining basically viable and functional may be crucial to understanding the pathogenesis of viral heart disease.

Herpesvirus (see Chapter 1)

The herpesvirus family contains herpes simplex 1 (HSV-1), herpes simplex 2 (HSV-2), Epstein–Barr virus (EBV), cytomegalovirus (CMV) and human herpesvirus 6 (HHV-6). They are enveloped DNA viruses and are comprised of four major architectural components: the core, capsid, tegument and envelope. The core contains the linear double-stranded DNA genome with a size of approximately 10^8 D. The replication cycle of the herpesvirus involves adsorption of the viruses to the cell's plasma membrane followed by entry of the virus into the cytoplasm.[28] The receptors for most herpesviruses are not known, although EBV can use the CD8 molecule on T lymphocytes as a functional receptor.[29] This suggests that the herpesviruses, like picornaviruses and the human immunodeficiency virus (HIV), prefer immunoglobulin superfamily molecules for attachment sites. Viral entry into the cell may occur through one of two mechanisms. Either the virus is phagocytized into vesicles or the outer lipid membrane (envelope) of the virus fuses with the plasma membrane of the cell. In either case, disaggregation of the virus capsid occurs in the cytoplasm and the core (DNA–protein complex) is transported to the nucleus. The initial step in virus replication involves transcription of viral RNA for a set of immediate-early proteins which presumably include the virus-encoded DNA-dependent RNA polymerase (transcriptase) and other molecules needed for synthesis and processing of the initial proteins. There is a clear sequential and coordinated process of virus protein synthesis throughout the replication cycle. Furthermore, new RNA synthesis is required between synthesis of the different classes of viral proteins (immediate-early, intermediate and late). The need for new RNA synthesis probably reflects the post-transcriptional processing of the viral RNA which is required for translation of any particular set of viral proteins. Viral RNA in the nucleus is complementary to 40% of the viral DNA while RNA in the cytoplasm is complementary to only 12% of the genome. This indicates a significant reduction in RNA size between the time of transcription in the nucleus and translocation/translation of the viral RNA in the cytoplasm. The post-transcriptional processing of the viral RNA possibly depends upon specific enzymes produced during the different stages of the replication cycle.

Viral RNA is translated in the cytoplasm and the peptides frequently undergo post-translational modifications. These modifications can include either rapid or slow cleavage of a large polypeptide into two or more smaller, biologically active proteins, similar to the process seen during picornavirus replication. More frequently, however, the modifications involve alterations and/or additions of specific groups to the peptide backbone. These modifications include glycosylation, phosphorylation, amidation, acetylation, methylation and sulphation. All of the intermediate-early proteins appear to undergo phosphorylation while only some of the intermediate and late polypeptides are similarly treated. The phosphorylation of certain proteins may be essential for their translocation back into the nucleus where they participate in further RNA and DNA synthesis. Since both core and capsid assembly occur in the nucleus, DNA binding proteins and some structural (capsid) proteins must also be able to translocate into this organelle. Once the core and capsid have been assembled, the herpesvirus buds through the inner nuclear membrane where the maturing virus may pick up its envelope. Egress from the cell may be accomplished either by budding of the virus through the plasma membrane, entry into vacuoles and secretion of the virus through the plasma membrane or entry into the cell's vesicular system with direct connection into the extracellular space.

As with picornaviruses, herpesviruses can have serious detrimental effects on the infected cells. Cytopathic effects are commonly observed in susceptible cultured monolayers with foci of rounded and 'blebbed' cells. Infection efficiently inhibits cellular DNA, RNA and protein synthesis, and alterations in the plasma membrane are visible by electron microscopy. The most notable alterations evident by light microscopy are nuclear and cellular inclusion bodies. These are dense aggregates of membrane and granular materials which appear rich in virus-specific elements. Their appearance can be indicative of a herpesvirus infection, however, it is important to realize that not all infected cells develop inclusion bodies and not all of the herpesviruses are equally effective in inducing them.

Virus-induced heart disease

Myocarditis

Myocarditis is defined as an inflammatory infiltration of the muscles of the heart with accompanying myocardial cell damage in a pattern not resembling ischaemic heart injury.[29] That is, ischaemia and other forms of trauma which result in muscle necrosis can stimulate inflammatory cell invasion of the dead tissue to aid healing. However, the inflammatory cell infiltrate is often not intimately associated with the necrotic areas. In contrast, myocyte necrosis in myocarditis predominately occurs only with direct physical contact of mononuclear cells with the myocytes. Adjacent cardiac cells or even distal portions of the same myofibre bundle may appear perfectly healthy.

Myocarditis has both an infectious and noninfectious aetiology. Hypersensitivity reactions to a wide range of therapeutic and illicit drugs will trigger cardiac inflammation.[30,31]Worldwide, *Trypanosoma cruzi*, the aetiological agent in Chagas' disease, has the highest incidence of myocarditis *per capita* of infected population.[32] Rheumatic heart disease, while decreasing in importance in the industrialized world, remains a serious form of bacterial inflammatory heart disease in many of the developing countries.[33] In the industrialized nations, Lyme disease caused by a spirochaete infection is being reported with increasing frequency and is the predominant source of bacterial myocarditis.[34] Viral infections are most often implicated in myocarditis in the USA and Europe, when an aetiological agent can be identified.[35] Although virtually any virus may be capable of inducing myocarditis, most studies agree that the picornavirus family predominates.

Murine models of viral myocarditis give useful insights into the complex interactions between the virus and host and into the processes leading to tissue injury. Three viruses are most often studied these being CVB3 and EMC virus and murine CMV. Since group B coxsackieviruses (CVB) are major aetiological agents in the clinical disease, using the same virus in the murine model might replicate the same pathogenic and immunogenic processes as well. Histologically, clinical and CVB murine myocarditis share many similarities.[36–49] The disease occurs in either acute (lasting days to weeks) or chronic (lasting months) forms. In each case, scattered foci are initially found throughout the ventricles. The lesions consist of necrotic myofibres with pyknotic or absent nuclei intimately associated with varying numbers of inflammatory cells. Lesions also occur around blood vessels and resemble periarteritis. As the disease progresses, the number of inflammatory cells decreases and the necrotic tissue is replaced by repair elements. Inflammatory cells are usually far more abundant in murine models of myocarditis than observed clinically and consist primarily of macrophage, lymphocytes and fibroblast-like cells. The components of the lymphocyte contingent change with the different stages of the disease. Natural killer (NK) cells arrive early (days 2–5) and may remain throughout the acute disease. Beginning at about day 5, CD4+ and CD8+ T cells are observed in a ratio of approximately 2:1. Later, the proportion of CD8+ cells increases. Plasmacytes and B lymphocytes are rare during acute myocarditis but are more numerous in chronic disease.

Generally, virus appears in the heart within hours of inoculation of the mice.[48,50,51] Concentrations increase rapidly, reaching peak titres between 3 and 7 days after infection (Fig. 5.2). Afterwards, the infectious virus is rapidly eliminated. Complete infectious virus eradication can take between 2 and 4 weeks depending upon the host. Genetically different strains of mice vary markedly in their ability to localize, replicate and rapidly eliminate CVB3 in the heart. Often, strains of mice showing the highest and most persistent cardiac virus titres also develop the more severe and chronic forms of myocarditis. Despite the direct correlation between infectivity and pathogenicity, inflammation and accompanying myocyte necrosis usually become evident at a time when infectious virus concentrations are decreasing in the heart. Chronic inflammation may persist in the myocardium for months after infectious virus can no longer be detected.[48,49] This kinetic discordance between virus titres and tissue injury provides the foundation for a growing schism of opinion between myocarditis investigators. Does tissue injury result from viral replication directly or does the ensuing inflammation cause the cardiac damage? At present, most investigators favour an immune pathogenesis hypothesis where infection acts primarily as the disease trigger (see Chapter 6).

Immunity clearly participates in virus elimination. Virus-specific antibody binds to the elevated regions of the virus capsid and interferes with virus–receptor binding (virus neutralization). IgM neutralizing antibody response is detected as early as 2 days after infection and IgG antibody is observed by day 6.[48,51,52] Neutralizing antibodies alone can passively prevent virus infection when adoptively transferred into recipient mice immediately before or after virus inoculation.[53] However, passive transfer of antibody at later times when virus is established in peripheral organs is largely ineffective. Giving infected mice cortisone, a drug which completely abrogates inflammation in the heart, increases cardiac viral titres 10^4- to 10^5-fold and causes extensive myocyte necrosis despite high virus neutralizing antibody titres in the serum.[54] This observation suggests that the neutralizing antibody response is more effective in the viraemic phase of the infection and may be primarily involved in preventing virus localization in target organs. Other immune factors are re-

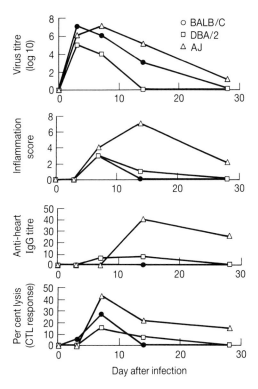

Fig. 5.2 *Comparison of coxsackie B3 virus (CVB3) infection and host responses in different inbred strains of mice.* Male, 6–8-week-old mice were inoculated with 6×10^4 plaque-forming units of virus intraperitoneally. Viral titres and inflammation in the heart, serum heart-reactive antibody titres and autoreactive cytolytic T lymphocyte responses were determined at various times after infection.

sponsible for clearance of established infections. Macrophage and NK cells probably control virus within organs.[38,54–59] Both cell types appear early in myocardial lesions and can kill CVB3-infected myocytes *in vitro* and *in vivo*. Selective elimination of either cell from infected animals significantly enhances cardiac injury and virus replication, while adoptive transfer of macrophage can accelerate virus clearance.

Although macrophages can directly eliminate, phagocytize and degrade virus, most probably, these cells and NK cells control infection through lysis of infected cells before completion of the virus replication cycle. Early interruption in the cycle would dramatically decrease progeny virion production which in turn, would result in fewer new cells becoming infected. Antibody should work coordinately with macrophage/NK cells by neutralizing free extracellular virus (limiting spread) while the cells halt new virus production. Antibody also clumps viruses together (antigen–antibody aggregates), then enhances phagocytosis by binding the virus–antibody aggregates to the macrophage Fc receptors. Adoptive transfer of suboptimal concentrations of macrophage and neutralizing antibody simultaneously augments protection compared to administration of the individual factors.[38,57]

Interferons may also participate in controlling infection. Interferons are pharmacologically potent molecules which act on uninfected cells.[60,61] They stimulate expression of selected genes in the nucleus and production of new classes of RNA and proteins. Three types of interferons are known. These are interferon-α (INF-α), interferon-β (INF-β) and interferon-γ (INF-γ). Interferon-α and INF-β are also known as type I or 'fibroblast' interferons while INF-γ is known as type II, 'immune' or 'lymphocyte' interferon. All three INFs are produced after infection. Interferon-α and INF-β are 25 to 35 kD glycoproteins. Interaction of these molecules with uninfected cells causes production of new proteins which apparently interact with the cell's ribosomes and prevent preferential translation of viral RNA. In the absence of this competitive advantage, virus protein synthesis is either slowed or stopped and progeny virion production is dramatically reduced. Interferon-α and INF-β are less likely to help already infected cells since the virus very rapidly interferes with host RNA and protein synthesis; the protective effect cannot, therefore, be induced. The very characteristic of viruses which aids in their shut down of host protein and RNA synthesis may be the factor stimulating INF production during infection. Poly(I)–poly(C) have been used for decades as potent INF stimulators. The poly(C) tract at the 5' noncoding region of the picornavirus RNA contains the important ribosome recognition structures allowing preferential attachment but may also be necessary for cytokine stimulation in infected cells. Interferon-γ was originally considered to have direct antiviral activity identical to INF-α and INF-β. It is now known, however, that INF-γ is capable of inducing INF-α and INF-β synthesis and the antiviral activity of INF-γ results from these other INFs.[62]

Picornavirus infections are highly susceptible to the effects of INF. Interferon-α and INF-β administered to CVB3-infected mice can reduce virus titres in the heart 100-fold or more, while administering anti-INF-α/β allows enhanced replication.[63–65] Variants of EMC virus have been selected primarily for their ability to induce INF. Encephalomyocarditis virus, the low INF inducer, is far more pathogenic to mice than EMC-B virus, the high INF inducer. As with neutralizing antibody and macrophage, INF may act synergistically with other antiviral effectors. Interferon contributes to NK cell activation and may also stimulate macrophage.

Interferon-γ has even more far-ranging effects since this INF enhances immunoglobulin superfamily protein expression on cells. Both clinical and murine studies demonstrate dramatic up-regulation of major histocompatibility complex (MHC) antigen expression on various cells in the heart during virus infection or myocarditis.[66,67] To date, each mammalian species has been shown to have at least two classes of MHC molecules. Class I MHC molecules consist of a polypeptide of approximately 44 kD which is associated with a molecule of β2-microglobulin.[68] The outer domains of the MHC molecule fold to give a deep groove in the protein. This groove contains the haplotype differences between distinct MHC molecules and is also the region which binds and presents antigens to T lymphocytes.[69] The class II MHC molecule has the same tertiary structure as the class I molecule but is comprised of two polypeptides (α and β chain). The external groove and haplotype differences are contributed by the 5' variable domains of both α and β chains. Class I and class II MHC mRNA leaves the nucleus and is translated by ribosomes on rough endoplasmic reticulum (ER). The MHC proteins progress through the Golgi where they are glycosylated and enter the endosome pathway for transport to the plasma membrane.

Evidence indicates that during translation and transport through the Golgi, the antigen-binding groove of the MHC molecules is blocked with another peptide termed the invariant chain (I-chain).[70,71] At some point in the endosomal pathway, however, the vesicles containing the MHC molecules fuse with lysosomes. The acid pH dissociates the I-chain and any viral peptides in the lysosomes (released during degradation of the virus capsid) may bind to the opened groove of the MHC and be transported to the cell surface.[13]

T lymphocytes are most often antigen specific and MHC restricted. That is, T lymphocytes have receptors (T cell receptor, TcR) on their cell surface which are specific for the tertiary structure made by the foreign antigen peptide and the MHC molecule.[72] CD4+ T cells generally react to peptides in class II MHC molecules while CD8+ T cells recognize peptides in class I MHC molecules. Major histocompatibility complex restriction means that only MHC molecules of the same type as the responding T lymphocyte can successfully 'present' the antigen. For example, CVB3-immune T lymphocytes from a DR3+ individual would respond to the viral antigens presented by DR3 MHC molecules but would not see CVB3 peptides presented by a different (DR4) MHC molecule. Part of the reason for this MHC restriction is that each MHC actually presents a different part of the virus.[73,74] The foreign peptides in the MHC groove are only about nine amino acids in length (the antigen epitope). Since the VP1 protein of CVB3 is approximately 35 kD, one can see that any particular T cell will recognize only a tiny portion of the whole virus protein. A DR3 MHC molecule may bind a completely different VP1 peptide than a DR4 molecule. The MHC locus is highly polymorphic and each individual inherits three class I and three class II molecules from each parent. Thus, few people show identical epitope recognition to any antigen. This level of genetic diversity actually acts as a survival mechanism for the species. Mutations in infectious organisms might prevent proper antigen processing and presentation of specific epitopes by a single MHC molecule. However, it is unlikely that any infectious agent would mutate all the epitopes associating with the six class I and six class II molecules coded within one individual or the more than 100 different MHC antigens within the species.

Distinct subsets of T lymphocytes have different effector functions. These include (1) T helper (Th) cells which, through the production of specific cytokines, direct the proliferation and activity of B lymphocytes, macrophage, delayed hypersensitivity, T cells and cytolytic T lymphocytes (CTL); (2) delayed hypersensitivity T cells (TDH) which cause the influx and aggregation of inflammatory cells within a site, increase capillary permeability and stimulate fibrosis; and (3) CTL, which directly lyse target cells. Basically, immunity can be divided into afferent and efferent responses. Afferent immunity involves clonal expansion of antigen-specific T cells while efferent immunity pertains more to the effector function of the lymphocytes. Stimulation of rapid T cell proliferation (clonal expansion) and differentiation into a highly efficient effector cell requires more than just the appropriate interaction between the lymphocyte's receptor and the antigen–MHC molecule complex.[75-77] Clonal T lymphocyte expansion is under autocrine control. The interaction of TcR–MHC–peptide stimulates interleukin-2 (IL-2, the lymphokine responsible for clonal T cell expansion) production and extracellular release by the T cell. This lymphokine must then bind to an IL-2 receptor on the T cell to stimulate cell division. However, unactivated T cells usually lack the appropriate IL-2 receptor on their cell surface. Induction of the IL-2 receptor depends upon a second signal from the antigen-presenting cell. Phagocytosis of the virus by a functional antigen-presenting cell (such as a macrophage) stimulates production of interleukin-1 (IL-1). This cytokine then acts on the T lymphocyte bound to the antigen-presenting cell through the TcR–MHC–peptide bridge to induce production of IL-2 receptors on the T cell. One may wonder why nature would have developed such a complex 'two-signal' system for T cell stimulation.

Immunity is an interesting mixture of both highly specific and completely nonspecific stimuli. For example, most cytokines/lymphokines act nonspecifically; the same lymphokine (IL-2) is used to expand clonally all Th cells irrespective of their antigen specificity. If this were the only signal required for T cell proliferation, a vigorous response to one antigen could result in sufficient IL-2 release to stimulate simultaneously clonal expansion of Th cells, to completely unrelated antigens. However, by requiring a second signal (IL-1 induction of IL-2 receptors), presumably the only Th cells which would express the IL-2 receptor would be those closely bound to the antigen-presenting cell through the TcR–MHC–peptide complex bridge. Thus, the TcR–MHC interaction confers the antigen specificity by keeping the antigen-presenting cell and antigen-specific T lymphocyte in close contact where concentrations of IL-1 are highest. T helper cells can be subdivided according to the type of secondary signal necessary for clonal expansion and the nature of the lymphokines they produce. T helper 1 (Th1) cells (producing IL-2 and INF-γ) use IL-1 as the secondary signal while T helper 2 (Th2) cells (producing interleukin-4 (IL-4), and interleukin-6, (IL-6)) use a different secondary signal (possibly adhesion molecules on cells such as endothelial cells can provide adequate secondary signal activity).

Understanding the two-signal hypothesis of T cell activation may be essential in viral immunity. Interferon-γ will induce MHC antigen expression on many tissues during infection, and these infected cells may process the viral epitopes and express them on their cell surface (Fig. 5.3). However, it is doubtful that an infected myocyte could act as a functional antigen-presenting cell to stimulate virus-specific (afferent) immunity since the myocyte is unlikely to produce the necessary secondary signal. Rather, enhanced MHC–virus peptide expression may primarily make infected myocytes targets for already differentiated effector cells (efferent immunity).

T lymphocytes play a major role in CVB3-induced murine myocarditis. Infection of T cell-depleted animals results in minimum cardiac inflammation and reduced myocyte necrosis compared to immunologically intact animals.[35,39,51,56] Viral titres in the hearts of T cell-deficient mice are equivalent to their immunocompetent counterparts and virus clearance occurs normally. This suggests that the T cell must contribute minimally to controlling the infection but could be important in causing tissue injury. Three major 'families' of responding T cells have been described, based largely on the nature of the antigens recognized[78] (see Fig. 5.4 for protocol used to isolate antigen-reactive T cell families). Virus-specific T lymphocytes (VSTL) react to viral epitopes on infected myocytes. In most mouse strains, VSTL appear

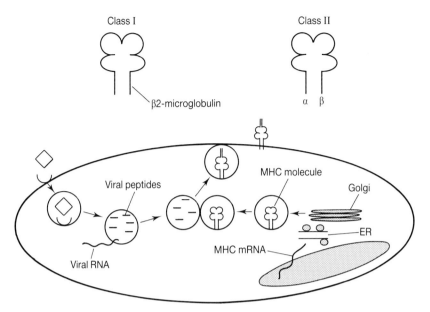

Fig. 5.3 *Viral antigen presentation.* Virus is engulfed into lysosomes and the protein capsid is enzymatically degraded to release the viral RNA. The viral peptides are transported to the cell surface in endosomal vessicles. Major histocompatibility complex (MHC) antigen mRNA is transcribed in the cell nucleus and translated on the endoplasmic reticulum (ER). The MHC proteins are subsequently glycosylated in the Golgi and transported to the plasma membrane through the endosome pathway. In the endosome, the viral peptides enter the MHC antigen groove.

to belong to the CD4+ subset. These cells have TDH and Th activity as well as some CTL function. Evidence in Balb/c mice suggests that the VSTL is responsible for the influx of inflammatory cells into the myocardium after infection.[79–81] Although these cells may not directly cause myocyte lysis during myocarditis, they may play an important role in pathogenesis through the lymphokines they release themselves or cause to be released by other inflammatory cells such as macrophages. Interleukin-1 and TNF inhibit β-adrenergic responsiveness of myocytes, and IL-1 also interferes with myocyte RNA and protein synthesis. Both effects could cause myocyte dysfunction without necessitating cell lysis.

A second population of T cells has been described which recognizes normal heart antigens.[79] These 'autoreactive' T cells (ATL) presumably represent an autoimmune response triggered by the virus infection. The autoantigens are many. Cardiac myosin and the mitochondrial antigens, adenine nucleotide translocator protein (ANT) and branched chain α-keto acid dehydrogenase (BCKD) are the major candidates for the relevant autoantigens in viral myocarditis.[79–85] Evidence that these three molecules are targetted depends upon demonstration that (1) both humoral and cellular autoimmune responses correlate with development of cardiac inflammation after infection; (2) only mouse strains which are susceptible to myocarditis after CVB3 infection develop these autoimmune responses; (3) immunization of mice with the iso-

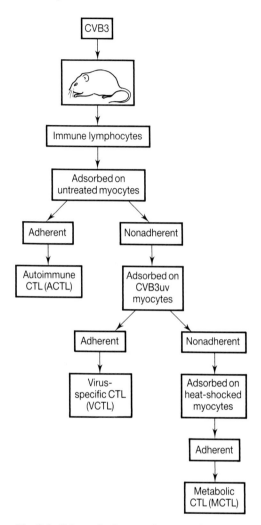

Fig. 5.4   Schematic diagram demonstrating three CTL families in coxsackie B3 virus-infected mice by selective immunoadsorption to myocyte monolayers.

lated self-proteins induces myocarditis independently of infection; and (4) adoptive transfer of autoimmune antibodies will produce cardiac disease in uninfected recipient animals. Other autoantigens may also be involved. These autoantigens include such molecules as fibronectin, laminin and vimentin (extracellular matrix and cytoskeleton components).[86]

Several mechanisms may be responsible for virus-induced autoimmunity and occur concurrently. The most likely mechanism involves antigenic mimicry between the virus and self-proteins (Table 5.1).[87] In this case, immune responses to the infectious agent also recognize normally expressed tissue antigens. Different CVB3 neutralizing antibodies react to cardiac myosin, ANT and vimentin, as well as to some as yet unidentified heart antigens.[88–90] Interestingly, at least one antibody made to the M protein of streptococcus

Table 5.1 Antigens implicated in coxsackie B3 virus (CVB3) induced myocarditis.

Antigen	Mimicry to CVB3 (Y,N,ND)	Induction of myocarditis in CFA (Y,N,ND)	Reference
1. Cardiac myosin	Y	Y	Neu *et al.*[84,85] Cunningham *et al.*,[88]
2. Extracellular matrix (fibronectin, laminin etc.)	Y	ND	Maisch *et al.*,[86] Cunningham *et al.*,[88]
3. Adenine nucleotide translocator (ANT) protein/calcium channel	Y	Y	Schultheiss *et al.*,[82,83] Schwimmbeck *et al.*,[89]
4. Heat shock proteins (60 kD hsp)	ND	ND	Huber *et al.*[78] (Huber unpublished observations)
5. Branched chain α-keto acid dehydrogenase (BCKD)	ND	ND	Herskowitz *et al.*[66]
6. CVB3 receptor molecule	ND	ND	Lyden *et al.*,[50] Weller *et al.*,[106] Van Houten *et al.*[107]

Y = Yes. ND = Not determined.

cross-reacts not only to heart but has strong CVB3-neutralizing activity. This shows that a bacterial epitope responsible for cardiac autoimmunity in rheumatic heart disease may be very similar to the viral epitope inducing autoimmunity in CVB3-induced myocarditis. A second mechanism for stimulating autoimmunity depends upon both the influx of inflammatory cells and on the aberrant expression of MHC molecules in the heart. The macrophages present in the inflammatory infiltrate could phagocytize cellular debris and stimulate self-antigen sensitive lymphocytes. This alone might not lead to pathogenic autoimmunity, however, if the myocytes do not express MHC antigens (CTL bind by TcR–MHC–peptide bridges to lyse target cells). Enhanced MHC expression in infected organs would make myocytes susceptible to autoimmune-mediated lysis. Aberrant MHC expression may be responsible for a number of autoimmune diseases including multiple sclerosis, post-infectious paralysis and insulin-dependent (type 1) diabetes mellitus.[91,92]

A third mechanism for CVB3-induced autoimmunity may be through anti-idiotypy.[93–96] When CVB3 is inoculated into mice, they respond as indicated above by both virus-specific humoral and cellular immunity. The specificity of the immune effectors is carried in the antigen-binding (variable) regions of the antibody and TcR. This constitutes the idiotype. Since each lymphocyte is predetermined to respond to only one antigen, and each individual can react to approximately 10^7 different antigens, the number of lymphocytes specific for any one antigen is limited. When the antigen is introduced into the host, however, rapid clonal expansion dramatically increases the number of antigen-specific (idiotypic) immune cells. The idiotype which was rare in the unstimulated state becomes more common after sensitization. The immune system had never become 'tolerant' (unresponsive) to the idiotype because there were too few antigen-specific cells initially. Now that the idiotype is abundant, it will act as a 'foreign' antigen itself, giving rise to an 'anti-idiotypic' response. This process, termed the network theory, can continue even further, much like the image of an object caught between two mirrors at opposite sides of a room.[97–99] Networking is a potent mechanism for immunoregulation. In fact, network theory has largely replaced the concept of specific immunoregulatory cells (suppressor T cells) as the mechanism for controlling immune responsiveness.

Idiotype–anti-idiotype responses have other uses as well. This is becoming a major thrust in vaccine development.[100,101] The variable region of a virus-neutralizing antibody is a three-dimensional 'negative image' of the part of the virus involved in receptor binding. Making an antibody to this variable region means the anti-idiotype has the tertiary structure of the original antigen (in this case, the virus). Thus, one could immunize individuals with the anti-idiotype and obtain fully functional virus-neutralizing antibodies. This has been successfully accomplished in a number of infectious disease models and is being developed for practical application. The advantage to immunization using anti-idiotype antibodies is that the antigen region essential to inducing good protective immunity is preserved but no virus is actually needed in the vaccine. The potential disadvantage is that the anti-idiotype is a faithful reproduction of the receptor-binding region of the virus, the anti-idiotype will also bind to the virus receptor on cells, thus inducing autoimmunity. As long as the anti-idiotypic response is transient, little tissue injury would accrue from this form of autoimmunity. If the anti-idiotypic response is large and persistent, clinical autoimmunity may occur.

Autoimmunity in CVB3 myocarditis partly results from anti-idiotypic responses to virus-specific immune effectors.[102,103] Anti-idiotypic antibodies have been demonstrated in CVB3-infected mice which react to virus-neutralizing antibodies. These anti-idiotypic antibodies bind to myocytes and inhibit both virus binding and infection of the cells. Adoptive transfer of anti-idiotypic antibodies into CVB3-infected mice protects the animals (abrogates myocarditis) and is incapable of causing myocarditis in uninfected recipients.[102,104] The anti-idiotypic humoral response, then, may bind to cells but apparently has only beneficial activity.

Autoimmunity to the CVB3 receptor on myocytes does occur, however, and can be highly pathogenic.[104–106] *In vitro*, various factors can modulate virus receptor expression on cultured myocytes. Susceptibility of the myocytes to autoimmune CTL-mediated lysis correlates directly with virus receptor expression. Furthermore, tissue cells lacking the cardiac CVB3 receptor are not lysed.[106] Finally, because of the high mutability of picornaviruses, variants of CVB3 can be selected which show different receptor binding characteristics.[106,107] Changing which cellular molecule binds virus or how virus interacts with its receptor can dramatically alter pathogenesis without inhibiting infection. How cellular autoimmunity to the virus receptor occurs *in vivo* is unclear. Anti-idiotypy such as observed in human immunity is unlikely. Most likely, myocytes dying from either virus or immune-mediated lysis fragment, and the debris will be cleared by macrophages. Virus receptors released in this manner may already be bound by virus. The virus may also attach virus-specific antibodies which allows the virus–receptor–antibody complex to be rapidly taken up by macrophage through Fc receptor-directed phagocytosis. Once in the macrophage, the virus receptor is enzymatically processed identically to virus capsid proteins and ultimately transported to the macrophage plasma membrane associated with MHC molecules, thereby stimulating autoimmunity.[108–110]

The third family of immune effector cells reacts to cellular neoantigens induced during the infection process.[78] These neoantigens are not virus epitopes and are not usually present on normal myocytes. Rather, the metabolic alterations in the cells caused by the infection induce new cellular proteins to be expressed at the plasma membrane. The nature of these neoantigens has been recently determined in this laboratory. They belong to the heat-shock protein (hsp) family.[111'–115] Cells exposed to a variety of stress conditions including heat shock, virus infection, interference with metabolic activity, exposure to oxygen free radicals and nutrient starvation stimulate the production of hsp. Heat shock proteins are usually grouped according to their molecular weight, are highly conserved between prokaryotic and eukaryotic cells, and appear to play essential roles in cell function and protein transport in both normal and stress conditions. Proteins in the 60, 70 and 90 kD families aid in assembling and disassembling protein complexes, and may interact with and correct improperly folded proteins. Those of the 90 kD family interact with steroid hormone receptors, cytoskeletal components and kinases. Those of the 70 kD family interact with DNA replication complexes and may facilitate the presentation of antigenic peptides to the immune system. Genes for two 70 kD proteins are located within the MHC locus. These 70 kD proteins anchor processed antigens to the cell surface in a manner which improves interaction between the MHC–peptide–TcR complex.

T lymphocytes recognize both self- and microbial hsp. Different infections may also induce identical hsp expression, provided the viruses interfere with cellular metabolism. Additionally, even noninfectious events in the heart might induce hsp expression. Thus, an individual experiencing multiple exposures to drugs, ischaemia or infectious agents might develop increasingly more aggressive hsp-specific immunity until this antigen-specific effector is the predominant cause of tissue injury. Preliminary studies from this laboratory indicate that mice given subcardiotoxic concentrations of adriamycin, then rested for 9 weeks, will develop twice as severe myocarditis when infected with CVB3 than age-matched animals not given the drug. Similarly, animals infected sequentially with two CVB belonging to different serotypes show significant augmentation of both cardiac inflammation and heart virus concentrations compared to animals infected with either virus separately.[111,112]

All the above autoimmune, virus-immune and hsp-immune responses can occur in the CVB3 myocarditis model either simultaneously or independently and contribute to pathogenesis.[116–123] In any particular individual, which specific responses are present probably depends upon both the genetic disposition of the host and the characteristics of the infecting virus (Table 5.2). Many host factors influence both the susceptibility to and severity of myocarditis. Some genetic strains of mice will develop myocarditis when infected while others show minimal or no cardiac injury. The MHC locus clearly controls susceptibility.[46,117] Interestingly, different myocarditic viruses (CVB3 versus EMC virus) and even different genetic variants of the same virus (CVB3 Woodruff strain versus CVB3 Lerner strain) may have distinct MHC associations. If many viruses cause clinical myocarditis, a clear MHC association may not be observed if each pathogenic infection is controlled by a different MHC allele.

Table 5.2   Factors influencing severity and incidence of experimental myocarditis.

Host factors

Major histocompatibility complex (MHC) (different MHC associations for each virus/virus variant)

Sex hormones, pregnancy (androgen ↑ oestrogens ↓ myocarditis)

Age (neonatal and post-puberty ↑ myocarditis)

Exercise (↑ myocarditis)

Prior exposure to other cardiotropic drugs, bacteria or viruses

Virus factors

Tropism (virus must infect heart)

Antigenic mimicry (autoimmunity induced to cross-reactive epitopes shared by virus and self-proteins)

Cytokine induction (viruses inducing ↑ or ↓ cytokine production can alter host immunity and either immune-mediated cardiac damage or virus clearance)

Virus replication (virus with either defective or highly efficient replicative cycles can affect disease by the concentration of infectious progeny virus released – high virus production could extend infection to more myocytes while low virus production could lead to rapid virus elimination

---

Age of the individual at infection also influences myocarditis.[57,118] Clinical myocarditis occurs predominantly in either the neonatal or postpuberty period. Children 1–9 years of age might be infected but show a lower incidence of viral heart disease compared to individuals in the susceptible age groups. The murine CVB model shows much the same pattern of disease. Many investigators report that suckling mice are highly susceptible to CVB myocarditis. It has also been shown that CVB3-induced myocarditis is limited in weanling mice (3 weeks old) of either sex. However, by sexual maturity (7–8 weeks old), male mice increase in myocarditis susceptibility dramatically while female age-matched animals continue to be relatively nonsusceptible. As the mice enter old age (40–48 weeks old), male susceptibility decreases while female susceptibility increases gradually. Thus, by this time, male and female mice are again equivalent in their myocarditis susceptibility.

The differences between male and female mice can be linked to sex-associated hormones. Androgens (testosterone and progesterone) enhance myocarditis susceptibility while oestrogens decrease susceptibility. Hormonal differences not only explain variations in susceptibility between males and females with age, but also why pregnant and postpartum females can develop as severe or more severe heart disease than males.[119,120] The age and sex association of murine myocarditis clearly resembles the clinical disease. Here, also, myocarditis predominates after sexual maturity and males are affected twice as often as females. Those females developing myocarditis, moreover, are either in the third trimester of pregnancy or postpartum when progesterone levels are elevated. The pattern of female susceptibility might alter in the future if (1) progesterone is the risk factor in pregnancy-associated clinical myocarditis and (2) use of progesterone-based contraceptives increases.

Animal studies also suggest that exercise is a substantial risk factor in both experimental and clinical viral myocarditis.[121–123] In a review published in 1980, Woodruff[35] reported several anecdotal cases of sudden unexpected death due to myocarditis occurring in physically active individuals. Experimental studies demonstrate that even moderate exercise such as swimming 30 min a day can convert mild viral myocarditis into severe forms of the disease with associated increases in mortality and cardiac necrosis. The mechanisms explaining dramatically enhanced myocarditis subsequent to exercise are incompletely understood. Both virus titres in hearts and immunity are enhanced in exercised animals, but T cell depletion of the exercised mice protects them from myocarditis. Presumably then, immunopathogenic rather than direct virus-mediated myocyte injury remains important in exercise-enhanced heart disease.

Finally, virus variants might be naturally 'selected' within an individual depending upon the humoral immunity present.[116,124] Picornaviruses are highly mutable with approximately one in a thousand viruses representing a distinct variant.[124] Antibodies arising in an individual during previous infections might selectively inactivate certain viruses while allowing replication of others. If the virus variants differ in their pathogenic potential, this selection process could influence disease severity. Thus, a CVB3 variant selected by its ability to infect and replicate in myocytes in the presence of an anti-virus receptor antibody largely retained its cardiotropism (ability to infect the heart) but was incapable of inducing myocarditis.[107]

Although much of the above discussion deals with viruses as inducers of immune-mediated myocarditis, viruses may also directly injure myocytes.[39,125] The amount of virus-mediated damage may differ depending upon the infectious agent used. Coxsackie B virus infection of cultured myocytes, endothelial cells or fibroblasts results only in transient infections.[23] These cells show no obvious cytopathic effect and will not release intracellular radio-isotope markers. Furthermore, both infected and uninfected myocytes beat with identical rates despite active virus production occurring in the infected cell cultures.[107] These observations imply CVB infections may not cause physiological dysfunction in infected myocytes. The pattern changes with EMC virus, however. This picornavirus causes complete lysis of myocyte cultures in 12 hours even with low concentrations of virus (one plaque forming unit virus per 10 myocytes). Myocytes cease beating within hours of EMC virus exposure. As one might expect, while T lymphocyte depletion of CVB-infected mice curtails myocardial necrosis, similar treatment of EMC virus-infected mice either has no effect or can enhance cardiac damage. Thus, EMC virus infection appears to be directly detrimental to myocardial cell physiology without involving immunological mediators.

Besides picornaviruses, CMV is the other major virus used in animal models of myocarditis.[126–128] Here also, the mouse is the preferred host, and susceptibility depends partly on MHC haplotype of the host. CMV apparently is incapable of infecting myocutes, but concentrate primarily in vascular endothelial cells.[128,129] As with CVB3, the endothelial cell may play an essential part in CMV tropism. CMV variants can be selected which show preferential infectivity for either lung or cardiac endothelial cells.[129] Thus, only certain variants of CMV may be cardiotropic and capable of inducing inflammatory heart disease. Since the endothelial cell is the primary target of CMV infection, it is not surprising that inflammation is generally restricted to perivascular spaces. Immunocompetent mice may develop only mild myocarditis and infectious virus is only transiently demonstrable in the heart.[127] Elimination of either all T lymphocytes or CD4+ cells results in increased virus concentrations and persistence, suggesting that CD4+ T cells are important in controlling virus infections. As with CVB3-infected mice, animals depleted of all T cells and infected with CMV develop minimal myocarditis. Thus, myocarditis is dependent on CD4+ T cell-mediated responses. The CD8+ T cell also influences CMV heart disease. This cell population apparently contains immunoregulation activity which prevents CD4+ cell-dependent cardiac injury. In the immunologically 'normal' individual, the immunoregulatory CD8+ cell prevents pathogenic CD4+ T cell responses without similarly affecting the CD4+ cell-dependent virus clearance. This suggests that the beneficial and detrimental CD4+ lymphocyte responses are not mediated by identical cells.

Dilated cardiomyopathy (See also Chapters 3 and 4)

Although myocarditis may resolve within weeks or months of onset, in some patients the disease becomes chronic with persistence of interstitial fibrosis often accompanied by inflammation, myocardial hypertrophy, chamber dilation and congestive heart failure (dilated cardiomyopathy). The incidence of dilated cardiomyopathy in the USA has been given as 10/100 000/year.[24] What percentage of these cases might result from prior myocarditis or viral infection of the heart is controversial. Long-term follow-up studies on myocarditis patients indicate that only approximately 25% develop chronic myocarditis and only 30% of all myocarditis patients show evidence of dilated cardiomyopathy.[23,130,131] Considering the paucity of well-documented myocarditis cases (usually those confirmed by histological evidence of inflammation in myocardial biopsy samples), one might be tempted to conclude that relatively few dilated cardiomyopathy patients had predisposing inflammatory or viral heart disease. However, most cases of myocarditis in the population are probably subclinical, and any symptoms may be nonspecific and mild. Thus, earlier episodes of myocarditis or viral infections of the heart might have gone unnoticed in dilated cardiomyopathy patients.

Despite the clinical evidence for viral infections in dilated cardiomyopathy, animal models of this disease are rare and inconsistent.[132] coxsackie B virus infections infrequently cause chamber dilation and wall thinning. The only notable exception is in exercised and CVB3-infected mice which will show dramatic heart weight gains and anatomical alterations similar to clinical dilated cardiomyopathy.[121] Possibly the increased or sustained workload and physiological stress on the remaining viable myofibres is required to convert CVB3 myocarditis into dilated cardiomyopathy. EMC virus infections will induce ventricular aneurysms, especially in the apical portion of the heart. Congestive heart failure and associated peripheral oedema will also occur in EMC virus-infected mice. The ability of EMC virus to induce these cardiac changes directly may largely reflect the more devastating effects of EMC virus infection on myocytes and the fact that generally a much greater proportion of the myocardium is involved in infections with this virus than in CVB infections.

Atherosclerosis (see also Chapter 8)

Atherosclerosis is a very common cardiovascular disease which primarily results in the narrowing or occlusion of the medium and large arteries. It is a leading cause of myocardial infarction and cerebrovascular insufficiencies. Early lesions presumably begin with the induction of focal proliferative lesions in the arterial wall, and accumulation of lipid-rich vacuoles containing high concentrations of cholesteryl esters (foam cells). Death of the foam cells and release of the intracellular contents leads to both accumulation of lipid in the extracellular space and fibrosis, with the deposition of collagen and elastin in the lesions. Herpesvirus genomic sequences and viral proteins can be demonstrated in aortic endothelial and smooth muscle cells.[133,134] Such infections may be an initiating event in atherosclerosis. Animal models provide the best evidence for a viral aetiology in this disease. The best model is found in chickens and uses Marek's disease virus, an avian herpesvirus.[135-137] These studies show that infection of birds on high cholesterol diets results in atherosclerotic plaques which appear very similar to those observed in humans. Infection of animals not on a high fat diet results in mild aortic lesions including proliferation of the smooth muscle cells within the intima, but little lipid accumulation. Uninfected birds fail to develop atherosclerotic plaques irrespective of diet. Viral antigens can be demonstrated at the sites of lesion development. *In vitro* studies indicate that the herpesvirus-infected smooth muscle cells accumulate more cholesterol and cholesteryl esters than uninfected cells. This suggests that virus infection may affect lipid transport control at the plasma membrane, or that damage to cytoplasmic vesicles causes aberrant accumulation of lipid. Herpesviruses are not the only viruses which might cause vascular injury. Coronary artery occlusion has been demonstrated in at least one patient with severe myocarditis.[138] Furthermore, mice placed on a high cholesterol diet and infected with CVB3 show nearly twice the cholesterol accumulation in both the myocardium and aorta as compared to uninfected animals on the same diet.[139]

References

1. Chen Z., Stauffacher C., Li Y. *et al*. Protein–RNA interactions in an icosahedral virus at 3.0 A resolution. *Science* 1989; **245**: 154–6.
2. Jackson R. J., A detailed kinetic analysis of the *in vitro* synthesis and processing of encephalomyocarditis virus products. *Virology* 1986; **149**: 114–21.
3. Luo M., Vriend G., Kamer G. *et al*. The atomic structure of Mengo virus at 3.0 A resolution. *Science* 1987; **235**: 182–3.
4. Mendelsohn C. L., Wimmer E., Racaniello V. R. Cellular receptor for poliovirus: molecular cloning, nucleotide sequence, and expression of a new member of the immunoglobulin superfamily. *Cell* 1989; **56**: 855–63.
5. Staunton D. E., Merluzzi V. J., Rothlein R. *et al*. A cell adhesion molecule, ICAM-1, is the major surface receptor for rhinoviruses. *Cell* 1989; **56**: 849–56.
6. White J. M., Littman D. R. Viral receptors of the immunoglobulin superfamily. *Cell* 1989; **56**: 725–30.
7. Raeckert R. Picornaviruses and their replication. In: Fields B. ed. *Virology*. New York: Raven Press, 1985: 705–38.
8. Smith H. Host and tissue specificities in virus infections of animals. In: Poste G. ed. *Virus Infection and the Cell Surface*. Amsterdam: Elsevier/North-Holland Publishing Co., 1977: 1–46.
9. Crowell R. L. Comparative generic characteristics of picornavirus–receptor interactions. In: Beers R., Bassett E. eds. *Cell Membrane Receptors for Viruses, Antigens, and Antibodies, Polypeptide Hormones, and Small Molecules*. New York: Raven Press, 1976: 179–202.

10. Bottazzo G. F., Dean B. M., McNally J. M. *et al. In situ* characterization of autoimmune phenomena and expression of HLA molecules in the pancreas in diabetes insulitis. *N Engl J Med* 1985; **313:** 353–5.
11. Mazza P. T., Ter Meulen V., Fontana A. Hyperinducibility of Ia antigen on asrocytes correlates with strain-specific susceptibility to experimental autoimmune encephalitis. *Proc Natl Acad Sci (USA)* 1987; **84:** 4219–28.
12. Todd I., Pujol-Borrell R., Hammond L. *et al.* Interferon gamma induces HLA-DR expression by thyroid epithelium. *Clin Exp Immunol* 1985; **61:** 265–73.
13. Germain R. N. Immunology: the ins and outs of antigen processing and presentation [news]. *Nature* 1986; **322:** 687–9.
14. Duke G. M., Osorio J. E., Palmenberg A. C. Attenuation of Mengo virus through genetic engineering of the 5′ noncoding poly(C) tract. *Nature* 1990; **343:** 474–6.
15. Schultz M., Crowell R. L. Eclipse of coxsackievirus infectivity: the restrictive event for a nonfusing myogenic cell line. *J Gen Virol* 1983; **64:** 1725–32.
16. Madshus I., Sandvig K., Olsnes S., van Deurs B. Effect of reduced endocytosis induced by hypotonic shock and potassium depletion on the infection of HEp-2 cells by picornaviruses. *J Cell Physiol* 1987; **131:** 14–22.
17. Zeichhardt H., Wetz K., Willingman P., Habermehl K. Entry of poliovirus type 1 and mouse Elberfeld virus into HEp-2 cells: receptor mediated endocytosis and endosomal or lysosomal uncoating. *J Gen Virol* 1985; **66:** 483–92.
18. Jang S. K., Krausslick H.-G., Nicklin M. J. H. *et al.* A segment of the 5′ nontranslated region of encephalomyocarditis virus RNA directs internal entry of ribosomes during *in vitro* translation. *J Virol* 1988; **62:** 2636–43.
19. Simoes E. A., Sarnow P. An RNA hairpin at the extreme 5′ end of the poliovirus RNA genome modulates viral translation in human cells. *J Virol* 1991; **65:** 913–21.
20. Baltimore D. The replication of picornaviruses. In: Levy H. B. ed. *Biochemistry of Viruses*. New York: Marcel Dekker, Inc., 1969: 101–76.
21. Jen G., Thach R. E. Inhibition of host translation in encephalomyocarditis virus-infected L cells: a novel mechanism. *J Virol* 1982; **43:** 250–61.
22. Schnurr D. P., Schmidt N. J. Persistent infection of mouse fibroblasts with coxsackievirus. *Arch Virol* 1984; **81:** 91–101.
23. Huber S. A., Job L. P., Woodruff J. F. Lysis of infected myofibers by coxsackievirus B3 immune T lymphocytes. *Am J Pathol* 1980; **98:** 681–94.
24. Bowles N. E., Richardson P. J., Olsen E. G. J., Archard L. C. Detection of coxsackie B virus-specific RNA sequences in myocardial biopsy samples from patients with myocarditis and dilated cardiomyopathy. *Lancet* 1986; **i:** 1120–2.
25. Foulis A. K., Farguharson M. A., Cameron S. D. *et al.* A search for the presence of the enteroviral capsid protein VP1. *Diabetologica* 1990; **33:** 290–8.
26. Jin O., Sole M. J., Butany J. W. *et al.* Detection of enterovirus RNA in myocardial biopsies. *Circulation* 1990; **82:** 8–16.
27. Roizman B. The herpesviruses. In: Nayak D. P. ed. *The Molecular Biology of Animal Viruses*. New York: Marcel Dekker, Inc., 1978: 769–848.
28. Sauvageau G., Stocco R., Kasparian S., Menezes J. Epstein–Barr virus receptor expression on human CD8+ (cytolytic/suppressor) T lymphocytes. *J Gen Virol* 1990; **71:** 379–86.
29. Aretz H. T., Billingham M. E., Edwards D. Myocarditis – a histopathologic definition and classification. *Am J Cardiovasc Pathol* 1987; **1:** 3–14.
30. Billingham M. E. Morphologic changes in drug-induced heart disease. In: Bristow M. R. ed. *Drug-induced Heart Disease*. Amsterdam: Elsevier, 1980: 21–30.
31. Laposata E. A. Cocaine-induced heart disease: mechanisms and pathology. *J Thorac Imaging* 1991; **6:** 68–75.
32. Public Health Laboratory Service Report. Memorandum. *Br Med J* 1967; **4:** 575–7.

33. Elk Holy A., Rotta J., Wannamaker L. W. *et al.* Recent advances in rheumatic fever control and future prospects: a World Health Organization memorandum. *Bull WHO* 1978; **56**: 887–912.
34. Steere A. C., Grodzicki R. L., Kornblatt A. N. *et al.* The spriochetal etiology Lyme disease. *N Engl J Med* 1983; **308**: 733–40.
35. Woodruff J. F. Viral myocarditis. *Am J Pathol* 1980; **101**: 425–83.
36. Godman G. C., Bunting H., Melnick J. L. The histopathology of coxsackievirus infection in mice. I. Morphologic observations with four different viral types. *Am J Pathol* 1952; **28**: 223–57.
37. Grodums E. I., Dempster G. Myocarditis in experimental coxsackie B3 infection. *Can J Microbiol* 1959; **5**: 605–15.
38. Grodums E. I., Dempster G. The pathogenesis of coxsackie group B viruses in experimental infection. *Can J Microbiol* 1962; **8**: 105–13.
39. Kishimoto C., Abelmann W. H. *In vivo* significance of T cells in the development of coxsackievirus B3 myocarditis in mice. Immature but antigen specific T cells aggravate cardiac injury. *Circ Res* 1990; **67**: 589–98.
40. Herskowitz A., Wolfgram L. J., Rose N. R., Beisel K. W. Coxsackievirus B3 murine myocarditis: a pathologic spectrum of myocarditis in genetically defined inbred strains. *J Am Coll Cardiol* 1987; **9**: 1311–19.
41. Hirschman S. Z., Hammer G. S. Coxsackievirus myopericarditis: a microbiological and clinical review. *Am J Cardiol* 1974; **34**: 224–32.
42. Kilbourne E. D., Wilson C. B., Perrier D. The induction of gross myocardial lesions by coxsackie (pleurodynia) virus and cortisone. *J Clin Invest* 1956; **35**: 362–70.
43. Marboe C. C., Knowles O. M., Weiss M. B. *et al.* Characterization of the inflammatory infiltrate in human myocarditis – an endomyocardial biopsy study. In: Bolte H.-D. ed. *Viral Heart Disease*. Berlin: Springer-Verlag, 1984: 74–86.
44. Olsen E. G. J. Histomorphological relations between myocarditis and dilated cardiomyopathy. In: Bolte H.-D. ed. *Viral Heart Disease*. Berlin: Springer-Verlag, 1984: 5–12.
45. Rabin E. R., Hassan S. A., Jensen A. B., Melnick J. L. Coxsackievirus B3 myocarditis in mice: an electron microscope, immunofluorescent and virus-assay study. *Am J Pathol* 1964; **44**: 775–97.
46. Rose N. R., Neumann D. A., Herskowitz A. Genetics of susceptibility to viral myocarditis in mice. *Pathol Immunopathol Res* 1988; **7**: 266–78.
47. Fohlman J., Friman G., Ilback N.-G. *et al.* A qualitative and quantitative method for *in situ* characterization of the inflammatory response in experimental myocarditis. *Acta Pathologica microbiologica et Immunologic Scandinavica* 1990; **98**: 559–67.
48. Lodge P. A., Herzum M., Olszewski J., Huber S. A. Coxsackievirus B-3 myocarditis: acute and chronic forms of the disease caused by different immunopathogenic mechanisms. *Am J Pathol* 1987; **128**: 455–63.
49. Leslie K. O., Schwarz J., Simpson K., Huber S. A. Progressive interstitial collagen deposition in coxsackievirus B3-induced murine myocarditis. *Am J Pathol* 1990; **136**: 683–93.
50. Lyden D. C., Olszewski J., Feran M. *et al.* Coxsackievirus B-3 induced myocarditis. Effect of sex steroids on viremia and infectivity of cardiocyte. *Am J Pathol* 1987; **126**: 432–8.
51. Huber S. A., Job L. P. Cellular immune mechanisms in coxsackievirus group B type 3 induced myocarditis in Balb/c mice. *Adv Exp Med Biol* 1983; **161**: 491–508.
52. Huber S. A., Lodge P. A., Job L. P. The role of virus and immune mediated cardiocyte injury in coxsackievuris B3-induced myocarditis. In: Bolte H.-D. ed. *Viral Heart Disease*. Berlin: Springer-Verlag, 1984: 64–73.
53. Rager-Zisman B., Allison A. C. Effects of immunosuppression on coxsackievirus B-3 infection in mice and passive protection by circulating antibody. *Can J Microbiol* 1973; **5**: 605–512.

54. Woodruff J. F. Lack of correlation between neutralizing antibody production and suppression of coxsackievirus B-3 replication in target organs: evidence for involvement of mononuclear inflammatory cells in defense. *J Immunol* 1979; **123:** 31–6.
55. Godeny E. K., Gauntt C. J. *In situ* immune autoradiographic infection of cells in heart tissues of mice with coxsackievirus B3-induced myocarditis. *Am J Pathol* 1987; **129:** 267–76.
56. Woodruff J. F, Woodruff J. J. Involvement of T lymphocytes in the pathogenesis of coxsackievirus B3 heart disease. *J Immunol* 1974; **113:** 1726–34.
57. Grodums E. I., Dempster G. The age factor in experimental coxsackie B3 infection. *Can J Microbiol* 1959; **5:** 595–603.
58. Godeny E. K., Gauntt C. J. Involvement of natural killer cells in coxsackievirus B3 induced murine myocarditis. *J Immunol* 1986; **137:** 1695–1702.
59. Godeny E. M., Gauntt C. J. Murine natural killer cells limit coxsackievirus B3 replication. *J Immunol* 1987; **139:** 913–18.
60. Levy H. B., Riley F. L., Buckler C. E. Interferon. In: Nayak D. P. ed. *The Molecular Biology of Animal Viruses.* New York: Marcel Dekker, Inc., 1978: 41–62.
61. Knop J. Immunologic effects of interferon. *J Invest Dermatol* 1990; **95:** 725–45.
62. Balkwill F. R. Interferons: from molecular biology to man. *Microbiol Sci* 1986; **3:** 212–33.
63. Gaines K. L., Kayes S. G., Wilson G. L. Factors affecting the infection of the D variant of encephalomyocarditis in the B cells of C57 B1/6J mice. *Diabetologia* 1987; **30:** 419–26.
64. Kandolf R., Canu A., Hofschneider P. H. Coxsackie B3 virus can replicate in cultured human fetal heart cells and is inhibited by interferon. *J Mol Cell Cardiol* 1987; **17:** 167–75.
65. Wilson G. L., Bellomo S. C., Craighead J. E. Effect of interferon on encephalomyocarditis virus infection of cultured mouse pancreatic beta cells. *Diabetologia* 1983; **24:** 38–45.
66. Herskowitz A., Ahmed-Ansari A., Neumann D. A. *et al.* Induction of major histocompatibility complex antigens within the myocardium of patients with active myocarditis. *J Am Coll Cardiol* 1990; **15:** 624–32.
67. Seko Y., Tsuchimochi H., Nakamura T. *et al.* Expression of major histocompatibility complex I antigen in murine ventricular myocytes infected with coxsackievirus B3. *Circ Res* 1990; **67:** 360–7.
68. Nathenson S. G., Geliebter J., Pfaffenbach G. M., Zeff R. A. Murine major histocompatibility complex class I mutants: molecular analysis and structure–function implications. *Ann Rev Immunol* 1986; **4:** 471–502.
69. Falk K., Rotzochke O., Stevanovic S. *et al.* Allele-specific motifs revealed by sequencing of self-peptides eluted from MHC molecules. *Nature* 1991; **351:** 290–6.
70. Cresswell P., Blum J. S., Kelner N., Marks M. S. Biosynthesis and processing of class Ii histocompatibility antigens. *CRC Crit Rev Immunol* 1987; **7:** 31–53.
71. Alexander J., Payne J. A., Murray R. *et al.* Differential transport requirements of HLA and H-2 class I glycoproteins. *Immunogenetics* 1989; **29:** 380–8.
72. Haskins K., Kappler J., Marrack P. The major histocompatibility complex restricted antigen receptor on T cells. *Ann Rev Immunol* 1984; **2:** 51–66.
73. DeLise C., Berzofsky J. A. T cell antigenic sites tend to be amphipathic structures. *Proc Natl Acad Sci (USA)* 1985; **82:** 7048–52.
74. Sette A., Buus S., Appella E., Smith J. A. *et al.* Prediction of major histocompatibility complex binding regions of protein antigens by sequence pattern analysis. *Proc Natl Acad Sci (USA)* 1989; **86:** 3296–300.
75. Finberg R., Benacerraf B. Induction, control and consequences of virus specific cytolytic T cells. *Immunol Rev* 1981; **58:** 157–80.

76. Mossmann T. R., Coffman R. L. Th1 and Th2 cells: different patterns of lymphokine secretion lead to different functional properties. *Ann Rev Immunol* 1989; **7:** 145–73.

77. Unanue E. R. Antigen-presenting function of the macrophage. *Ann Rev Immunol* 1984; **2:** 395–428.

78. Huber S. A., Heintz N., Tracy R. Coxsackievirus B-3 induced myocarditis: virus and actinomycin D treatment of myocytes induces novel antigens recognized by cytolytic T lymphocytes. *J Immunol* 1988; **141:** 3214–19.

79. Huber S. A., Lodge P. A. Coxsackievirus B-3 myocarditis in Balb/c mice. Evidence for autoimmunity to myocyte antigens. *Am J Pathol* 1984; **116:** 21–9.

80. Estrin M., Huber S. A. Coxsackievirus B3-induced myocarditis: autoimmunity is L3T4+ T helper cell and IL-2 independent in Balb/c mice. *Am J Pathol* 1987; **127:** 335–41.

81. Estrin M., Smith C., Huber S. Coxsackievirus B-3 myocarditis T cell autoimmunity to heart antigens is resistant to Cyclosporin A treatment. *Am J Pathol* 1986; **125:** 18–25.

82. Schultheiss H.-P., Schulze K., Kuhl U. *et al.* The ADP/ATP carrier as a mitochondrial auto-antigen – facts and perspectives. *Ann NY Acad Sci* 1987; **448:** 44–68.

83. Schultheiss H.-P., Ulrich G., Janda I. *et al.* Antibody-mediated enhancement of calcium permeability in cardiac myocytes. *J Exp Med* 1988; **168:** 2105–20.

84. Neu N., Beisel K. W., Traystman M. D. *et al.* Autoantibodies specific for the cardiac myosin isoform are found in mice susceptible to coxsackievirus B3 induced myocarditis. *J Immunol* 1987; **138:** 2488–92.

85. Neu N., Rose N. R., Beisel K. W. *et al.* Cardiac myosin induces myocarditis in genetically predisposed mice. *J Immunol* 1987; **139:** 3630–6.

86. Maisch B., Wedeking U., Kochsiek K. Quantitative assessment of antilaminin antibodies in myocarditis and perimyocarditis. *Eur Heart J* 1987; **8** (suppl J): 233–6.

87. Oldstone M. B. A. Molecular mimicry and autoimmune disease. *Cell* 1987; **50:** 819.

88. Cunningham M. W., Antone S. M., Gulizia J. M. *et al.* Cytotoxic and viral neutralizing antibodies cross-react with streptococcal, M protein, enteroviruses, and human cardiac myosin. *Proc Natl Acad Sci (USA)* 1992; **89:** 1320–4.

89. Schwimmbeck H.-P., Schultheiss H.-P., Strauer B. G., Oldstone M. B. A. Antigenic determinants shared between myosin and cardiotropic virus: significance for virus-induced heart disease. *VIIIth International Congress of Virology*, Berlin, 1990.

90. Sadigursky M., Acosta A. M., Santos-Buch C. A. Muscle sarcoplasmic reticulum antigen shared by a *Tyrpanosoma cruzi* clone. *Am J Trop Med Hyg* 1982; **31:** 934–43.

91. Friedman A., Frankel G., Lorch Y., Steinman L. Monoclonal anti-IA antibody reverses chronic paralysis and demyelination in TMEV infected mice: critical importance of timing of treatment. *J Virol* 1987; **61:** 898–903.

92. Rodriguez M., Lafuse W. P., Leibowitz J. L., Davis C. S. Partial suppression of Theiler's virus induced demyelination with *in vivo* anti-IA monoclonal antibody. *Neurology* 1986; **36:** 964–1000.

93. Cooke A., Lydyard P. M., Roitt I. M. Autoimmunity and idiotypes. *Lancet* 1984; **ii:** 723–5.

94. Erlanger B. F., Cleveland W. L., Wasserman N. H. *et al.* Auto-anti-idiotypy: a basis for autommunity and a strategy for anti-receptor antibodies. *Immunol Rev* 1986; **94:** 23–48.

95. Marriott S. J., Roeder D. J., Consigli R. A. Anti-idiotypic antibodies to a polyomavirus monoclonal antibody recognize cell surface components of mouse kidney cells and prevent polyomavirus infection. *J Virol* 1987; **61:** 2747–52.

96. Kauffman R. S., Fields B. N. Pathogenesis of viral infections. In: Fields B. ed. *Virology*. New York: Raven Press, 1985: 153–87.

97. Herzenberg L. A., Tokuhisa T., Hayakawa K. Epitope specific regulation. *Ann Rev Immunol* 1983; **1:** 609–32.

98. Pereira P., Bandeira A., Coutinho A., Marcos M. A. V-region connectivity in T-cell repertoires. *Ann Rev Immunol* 1989; **7:** 209–49.

99. Jerne N. K. Idiotypic networks and other preconceived ideas. *Immunol Rev* 1984; **79:** 5–24.

100. Poltz P. H. Autoantibodies are anti-idiotype antibodies to antiviral antibodies. *Lancet* 1983; **ii:** 824–6.

101. Bruck C., Co M. S., Slaoui M. *et al.* Nucleic acid sequence of an internal image-bearing monoclonal anti-idiotype and its comparison to the sequence of the external antigen. *Proc Natl Acad Sci (USA)* 1986; **83:** 6578–82.

102. Paque R. E., Miller R. Autoanti-idiotypes exhibit mimicry of myocyte antigens in virus-induced myocarditis. *J Virol* 1991; **65:** 16–22.

103. Weremeichik H., Moraska A., Herzum M. *et al.* Naturally occurring anti-idiotypic antibodies – mechanisms for autoimmunity and immunoregulation. *Eur Heart J* 1991; **12:** 154–7.

104. Huber S. A., Simpson K., Weller A., Herzum M. Immunopathogenic mechanisms in experimental myocarditis. In: Schultheiss H.-P. ed. *New Concepts in Viral Heart Disease*. Berlin: Springer-Verlag, 1988: 179–87.

105. Huber S. A., Lodge P. A., Herzum M. *et al.* The role of T lymphocytes in the pathogenesis of coxsackievirus B3 myocarditis. In: Kawai C. C., Abelmann W. eds. *Pathogenesis of Myocarditis and Cardiomyopathy*. Tokyo: University of Tokyo Press, 1987: 9–22.

106. Weller A. H., Simpson K., Herzum M. *et al.* Coxsackievirus B3-induced myocarditis: virus receptor antibodies modulate myocarditis. *J. Immunol* 1989; **143:** 1843–50.

107. Van Houten N., Bouchard P. E., Moraska A., Huber S. A. Selection of an attenuated coxsackievirus B3 variant using a monoclonal antibody reactive to myocyte antigen. *J. Virol* 1991; **65:** 1286–90.

108. Takeichi N., Kuzumaki N., Kodama T. *et al.* Runting syndrome in rats inoculated with Friend virus. *Cancer Res* 1972; **32:** 445–51.

109. Eaton M. D. Autoimmunity induced by syngeneic splenocyte membranes carrying irreversibly absorbed paramyxovirus. *Infect Immun* 1980; **27:** 855–62.

110. Eaton M. D., Almquist S. J. P. Autoimmunity induced by injection of virus modified cell membrane antigens in syngeneic mice. *Infect Immun* 1977; **15:** 322–8.

111. Young R. A. Stress proteins and immunity. *Ann Rev Immunol* 1990; **8:** 401–20.

112. Born W., Happ M. P., Dallas A. *et al.* Recognition of heat shock proteins and γ-δ cell function. *Immunol Today* 1990; **11:** 40–7.

113. Linquist S., Craig E. A. The heat shock proteins. *Ann Rev Genet* 1988; **22:** 631–7.

114. Cheng M. Y., Harti F. U., Martin J. *et al.* Mitochondrial heat shock protein hsp60 is essential for assembly of protein imported into yeast mitochondria. *Nature* 1989; **337:** 620–5.

115. Sargent C. A., Dunham I., Trowsdale J., Cambell R. D. Human major histocompatibility complex contains genes for the major heat shock protein HSP70. *Proc Natl Acad Sci (USA)* 1989; **86:** 1968–72.

116. Beck M. A., Chapman N. M., McManus B. M. *et al.* Secondary enterovirus infection in the murine model of myocarditis. *Am J Pathol* 1990; **136:** 669–81.

117. Buie C., Lodge P., Herzum M., Huber S. A. Genetics of coxsackievirus B3 and encephalomyocarditis virus-induced myocarditis in mice. *Eur Heart J* 1987; **8:** 399–402.

118. Lyden D., Olszewski J., Huber S. Variation in susceptibility of Balb/c mice to

coxsackievirus group B type 3-induced myocarditis with age. *Cell Immunol* 1987; **105:** 332–9.

119. Huber S. A., Job L. P., Auld K. R. Influence of sex hormones on coxsackie B3 virus infection in Balb/c mice. *Cell Immunol* 1982; **67:** 173–89.

120. Lyden D. C., Huber S. A. Aggravation of coxsackievirus group B type 3-induced myocarditis and increase in cellular immunity to myocyte antigens in pregnant Balb/c mice and animals treated with progesterone. *Cell Immunol* 1984; **87:** 462–72.

121. Reyes M. P., Lerner A. M. Coxsackievirus myocarditis with special reference to acute and chronic effects. *Prog Cardiovasc Dis* 1985; **27:** 373–94.

122. Lerner A. M., Wilson F. M. Virus myocardiopathy. *Prog Med Virol* 1973; **15:** 63–91.

123. Cabinian A. E., Kiel R. J., Smith F. *et al.* Modification of exercise-aggravated coxsackievirus B3 murine myocarditis by T lymphocyte suppression in an inbred model. *J Lab Clin Med* 1990; **115:** 454–62.

124. Prabhaker B. S., Srinivasappa J., Ray V. Selection of coxsackievirus B4 variants with monoclonal antibodies results in attenuation. *J Gen Virol* 1987; **68:** 865–9.

125. Melnick J. Enteroviruses: polioviruses, coxsackieviruses, echoviruses and newer enteroviruses. In: Fields B. ed. *Virology*. New York: Raven Press, 1985: 739–94.

126. Lawson C. M., O'Donoghue H., Bartholomaeus W. N., Reed W. D. Genetic control of mouse cytomegalovirus-induced myocarditis. *Immunology* 1990; **69:** 20–6.

127. Leung W. C. T., Hato J., Hashimoto K. Murine cytomegalovirus infection model in Balb/c mice – pericarditis with myocarditis involvement during virus infection. *Tokai J Exp Clin Med* 1986; **11:** 303–11.

128. Craighead J. E., Martin W. B., Huber S. A. Role of CD4+ (helper) T cells in the pathogenesis of murine cytomegalovirus myocarditis. *Lab Invest* 1992; **66:** 755–61.

129. Lodge P. A., Haisch C. E., Huber S. A. *et al.* Biological differences in endothelial cells depending upon origin of derivation. *Transplant Proc* 1991; **23:** 216–18.

130. Kline I. K., Saphir O. Chronic pernicious myocarditis. *Am Heart J* 1960; **59:** 681–97.

131. Fenoglio J. J. Jr., Ursell P. C.. Kellogg C. F. *et al.* Diagnosis and classification of myocarditis by endomyocardial biopsy. *N Engl J Med* 1983; **308:** 12–18.

132. Matsumori A., Kawai C., Crumpacker C. S., Abelmann W. H. The use of animal models for prevention and therapeutic trials of viral myocarditis. In: Kawai C., Abelmann W. H. eds. *Pathogenesis of Myocarditis and Cardiomyopathy*. Tokyo: University of Tokyo Press, 1987: 37–47.

133. Melnick J. L., Petrie B. L., Dreesman G. R. *et al.* Cytomegalovirus antigen within human anterial smooth muscle cells. *Lancet* 1983; **ii:** 644–7.

134. Hendrix M. G. R., Dormans P. H. J., Kilslaar P. *et al.* The presence of cytomegalovirus nucleic acids in arterial walls of atherosclerotic and nonatherosclerotic patients. *Am J Pathol* 1989; **134:** 1151–7.

135. Fabricant C. G., Fabricant J., Litrenta M. M., Minick C. R. Virus-induced atherosclerosis. *J Exp Med* 1978; **148:** 335–40.

136. Fabricant C. G., Fabricant J., Minick C. R., Litrenta M. M. Herpesvirus-induced atherosclerosis in chickens. *Fed Proc* 1963; **42:** 2476–9.

137. Hajjar D. P., Fabricant C. G., Minick C. R., Fabricant J. Virus induced atherosclerosis: herpesvirus infection alters aortic cholesterol metabolism and accumulation. *Am J Pathol* 1986; **122:** 62–70.

138. Morgan J. M., Gray H. H., Pillai R. G. Coronary arterial occlusion and myocardial infarction in acute myocarditis. *Int J Cardiol* 1990; **26:** 226–9.

139. Ilback N. G., Mohammed A., Fohlman J., Friman G. Cardiovascular lipid accumulation with coxsackie B virus infection in mice. *Am J Pathol* 1990; **136:** 159–67.

Part II

Animal models: pathological findings and therapeutic considerations

A. Matsumori

Introduction

A wide range of viruses may be implicated in infections associated with myocarditis. RNA viruses predominate and, among these, the picornaviruses are the most commonly identified agents. Clinically, viral myocarditis may present in a wide variety of ways, ranging from a total lack of clinical manifestations to sudden, unexpected death, which is not uncommon and may be caused by a fatal arrhythmia, high-degree atrioventricular block or circulatory collapse. In addition to the broad spectrum of clinical features associated with acute viral myocarditis, possible complications and late sequelae may give cause for concern. A subacute or even chronic myocarditis may lead to progressive myocardial failure and death.[1,2] However, the relative infrequency of cases of acute viral myocarditis together with the difficulty of obtaining appropriate clinical material, makes it difficult to study the pathogenesis of myocarditis in humans. Experimental models have therefore been used to study various aspects of the pathogenesis of viral myocarditis.

An animal model has been developed using encephalomyocarditis (EMC) virus which causes congestive heart failure in the acute and subacute stages of infection.[3] Dilation and hypertrophy, as seen in dilated cardiomyopathy, developed in the chronic stage of infection.[4] Animal models of coxsackievirus B1 and B4 myocarditis have also been studied in mice and hamsters[5,6] as well as the natural history and pathogenesis of viral myocarditis. Diagnostic methods and therapeutic and preventive interventions in these models have also been studied.[7–13]

Animal models of congestive heart failure and dilated cardiomyopathy

Encephalomyocarditis (EMC) virus is a picornavirus biologically similar to coxsackievirus. The virus was first isolated in 1945 from primates which experienced sudden death. A severe myocarditis developed in inbred Balb/c mice inoculated with the myocardiotropic variant of EMC virus. In our laboratory myocardial lesions appeared earlier and were more extensive than those detected in myocarditis induced by coxsackieviruses. The mortality rate was highest on the 4th day and then decreased gradually, only to increase again between days 11 and 14. Mice dying between days 8 and 14 had evidence of a pleural effusion, ascites, and congestion of the lungs and liver, the cause of death being congestive heart failure. The cavity dimensions of the right ventricle (RV) and left ventricle (LV) were significantly greater than those among noninfected controls. The thickness of the walls of the ventricles being decreased in this stage (Fig. 5.5).[3]

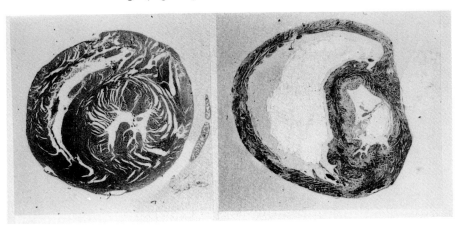

Control   14 Days after virus inoculation

Fig. 5.5 Balb/c mouse. Fourteen days after encephalomyocarditis (EMC) virus inoculation: dilation of ventricular cavities and decreased wall thickness are evident. Haematoxylin and eosin stain. Left: control. Right: 14 days after virus inoculation. × 10. Reproduced with permission of American Heart Association from Matsumori and Kawai.[3]

Microscopic features

The earliest microscopic changes following inoculation with EMC virus in mice is an increase in the eosinophilic staining of myocardial cells. Damaged myocardial fibres frequently appear fragmented, swollen and intensely eosinophilic. Cross-striations are not evident. Focal areas of basophilia are occasionally observed. Nuclei of the affected fibres frequently appear pyknotic or undergo karyorrhexis. Inflammatory cells are either sparse or have yet to appear (Fig. 5.6a). Later, fine haematoxylinophilic granules are seen in some of the necrotic fibres. These granules gradually enlarge, and some coalesce to fill the necrotic cytoplasmic segments. Stains for calcium are positive. Necrosis and dysplastic mineralization are limited to individually affected cells. This is most evident in hearts with the greatest injury. At this stage some cellular infiltration is apparent (Fig. 5.6b). At a later stage, the inflammatory cellular response predominates. This infiltrate consists of histiocytes, lymphocytes, plasma cells and a few polymorphonucler leukocytes (Fig. 5.6c). During the final stages interstitial mononuclear cell infiltrates gradually disappear, to be replaced by fibrosis (Fig. 5.6d). In relatively few instances, small foci composed of a few necrotic fibres appear to have been removed without mineralization and are replaced by fibrous scars. Myocardial fibrosis persists long after virus inoculation.

DBA/2 mice inoculated with EMC virus also developed a severe myocarditis and died of congestive heart failure in the acute stage. Surviving mice

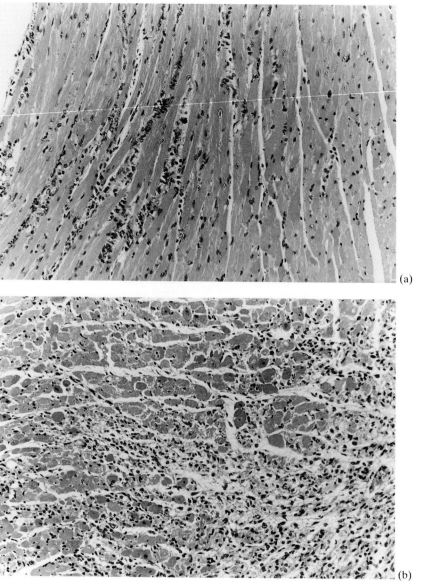

Fig. 5.6 Photomicrographs of the heart of mice inoculated with encephalomyocarditis virus. (a) On day 5 focal myocytolysis is present. (b) On day 7 necrosis of myocardial cell and cellular infiltration are evident.

developed dilation and hypertrophy similar to changes observed in patients with dilated cardiomyopathy.[4] The heart weight was not significantly greater in infected mice than among controls on days 4–5, but was significantly greater by day 90. The heart weight to body weight ratio was greater in infected mice and the cavity dimension of the LV was significantly greater in infected mice. The wall thickness of the RV, the interventricular septum and the LV, al-

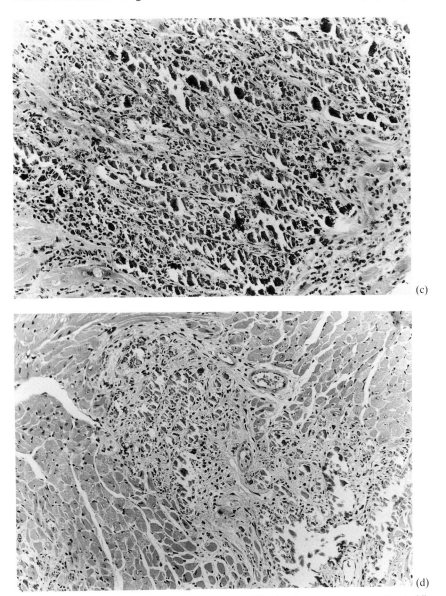

Fig. 5.6 (c) On day 14 cellular infiltration and calcification become more prominent. (d) On day 28 myocardial fibrosis is evident but cellular infiltration decreases. Haematoxylin and eosin stain. × 180. Reproduced with permission of American Heart Association from Matsumori *et al.*[35]

though decreased in the acute stage, increased during the chronic phase to a comparable thickness with age-matched control mice. Histological changes were similar to those seen in Balb/c mice in the acute stage although more prominent myocardial calcification occurred in DBA/2 mice. By day 30, cellular infiltration had decreased, but myocardial calcification persisted; myocardial fibrosis was evident at this stage. By day 90, the heart showed dilation and hypertrophy[4] (Fig. 5.7); myocardial fibrosis being prominent and hypertrophy of myocardial cells evident. Although myocardial calcification persisted, there was no mononuclear cell infiltration. Congestion of the lungs was noted at this stage. These findings suggest that dilated cardiomyopathy may develop as early as 3 months after infection with EMC virus. Dilation and hypertrophy of the heart persisted long after inoculation with EMC virus in DBA/2 as well as in C3H/He mice.[14] Myocardial lesions were also seen in the atria from the acute to the chronic stage. EMC virus was isolated from the hearts and EMC virus antigen was detected in the myocardium up to the second week of infection (Fig. 5.8), but neither was found thereafter. Genetic

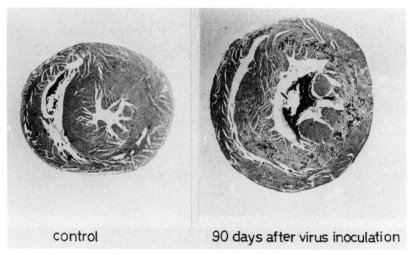

Fig. 5.7   DBA/2 mouse. Ninety days after encephalomyocarditis virus inoculation: dilation and hypertrophy are evident. Left: control. Right: 90 days after virus inoculation. × 8. Reproduced with permission of the American Heart Association from Matsumori and Kawai.[3]

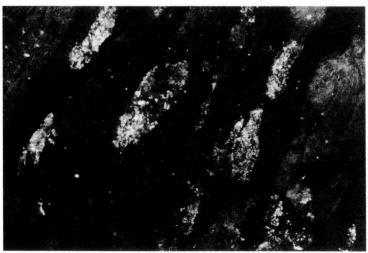

Fig. 5.8   Seven days after encephalomyocarditis virus inoculation. Virus antigen is seen in myocardial cells. Indirect immunofluorescence. × 500.

factors may play a role in susceptibility to infection and severity of the disease, and even in the differences in character of the pathological lesions. In EMC virus infections differences were found in the frequency of myocarditis in inbred strains of A/J, Balb/c, C3H/He, C57BL/6 and DBA/2 mice. Severe myocarditis was induced in Balb/c, C3H/He and DBA/2 mice inoculated with EMC virus, but A/J and C57BL/6 mice did not show cardiac abnormalities. Myocardial calcification was most severe in C3H/He mice, but there was little calcification in Balb/c mice. The reasons for these differences are not known, but genetic factors may play an important role in the pathogenesis.[14] The development of cardiac dilation and hypertrophy is dependent not on myocardial calcification, but on the severity of lesions, which, although extensive, permit animals to survive.

Mural thrombus in viral myocarditis

Mural thrombus formation, especially in the atria, was found in these models in the acute to chronic stages. The earliest fresh thrombi were seen on day 7 in mice with severely affected atrial endocardia. Thrombi were found more frequently in mice with congestive heart failure or cardiac dilation. However, thrombosis was also found in hearts without marked dilation of the ventricular cavity.[15]

Although myocardial lesion of the ventricles were particularly severe, in proportion to the relative mass of the ventricular muscle, a few mural thrombi in the ventricles were found. Moreover, the left ventricles were significantly enlarged in mice with thrombosis, and a significantly high incidence of thrombosis was seen in mice with congestive heart failure. These results indicate that the endocardial lesion and the cardiac dilation are factors for thrombus formation in acute viral myocarditis and that the latter may be closely related to thrombus formation. It is noteworthy, however, that some mice with thrombosis did not show cardiac dilation.

Case reports of *antemortem* diagnosis of thromboembolism in acute viral myocarditis are rare, and its incidence is not known. It is important, however, to recognize that mural thrombi develop during the early stage of the disease. Obviously, patients with acute viral myocarditis associated with mural thrombi have an increased risk of peripheral embolism. The results of this study suggest that prophylaxis with anticoagulant therapy should be considered before cardiac dilation is evident.

Ventricular aneurysm complicating viral myocarditis

There have been only a few reports relating to virus-induced ventricular aneurysm. Left ventricular aneurysm has been reported following coxsackie B1 and B4 virus myocarditis in mice.[16] However, there has been no evidence that viruses produce right ventricular aneurysms. Aneurysms have been found in the right ventricle during the acute and chronic stages of severe EMC virus myocarditis (Fig. 5.9).[17]

The disease known as right ventricular dysplasia is a pathological condition which primarily affects the right ventricle. The right ventricular musculature

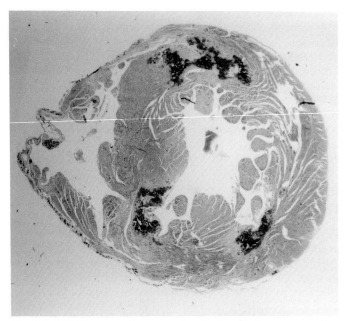

Fig. 5.9   DBA/2 mouse. Seven months after inoculation: transmural myocardial fibrosis and aneurysmal dilation of the right ventricle are noted. Haematoxylin and eosin stain. × 16. Reproduced with permission of Springer-Verlag from Matsumori and Kawai.[7]

is partially or totally absent and is replaced by fatty and fibrous tissue. If the dysplasia is extensive, the right ventricle is paper-thin and there is apposition of the endocardium to the epicardium. This condition has been described as Uhl's anomaly. Dysplasia may also involve the left ventricle and atria. Right ventricular aneurysm seen at the chronic stage following EMC virus myocarditis is similar to the changes in right ventricular dysplasia. Viral myocarditis may cause right ventricular aneurysms, albeit infrequently, and this suggests a pathogenic role of viral infection in right ventricular dysplasia or Uhl's anomaly. Although less frequent, ventricular aneurysms may also involve the left ventricle.

An animal model of chronic myocarditis: successive infection with coxsackievirus and encephalomyocarditis virus in mice

Acute myocarditis and subsequent myocardial fibrosis have been induced in C3H/He mice inoculated with coxsackie B3 virus, although myocardial lesions were less severe than those seen in EMC-induced virus myocarditis. As both coxsackie B3 virus and EMC viruses cause myocarditis in C3H/He mice, the effect of successive viral infections was investigated to see whether this caused additional myocardial damage and whether lesions similar to chronic myocarditis or dilated cardiomyopathy developed. Four-week-old C3H/He mice were first inoculated with coxsackie B3 virus (Nancy stain) intraperitoneally. Four weeks later, mice were infected with EMC virus. Mice which survived were sacrificed 2 weeks after the second infection, at the age of 10 weeks. Hearts of mice inoculated with coxsackie B3 virus alone showed myocardial calcification and fibrosis but little cellular infiltration. There was cellular infiltration and necrosis, but little fibrosis in the hearts of mice inoculated with EMC virus alone. However, in mice infected with both coxsackie B3 virus and EMC viruses, acute myocarditis with cellular infiltration and myocardial necrosis, and healed myocarditis with fibrosis and calcification occurred simultaneously.[18] These results suggest that successive virus infections may cause additional myocardial damage, infected mice developing lesions similar to those occurring in humans with chronic myocarditis or dilated cardiomyopathy.

Conduction disturbance and arrhythmias in viral myocarditis in mice with encephalomyocarditis virus

Various kinds of electrocardiographic abnormalities were detected in the mouse model. Significant numbers of mice developed various degrees of atrioventricular block associated with mononuclear cell infiltration: oedematous changes in the conduction cells were found in the conduction system of mice with complete A–V block. Serial electrocardiograms showed atrial and ventricular premature complexes (VPCs) in the acute stage and these ectopic complexes persisted in the chronic stage.[19] The presence of arrhythmias in surviving mice may suggest that some patients with arrhythmias, with no other clinical manifestations, have had a previous viral myocarditis.

Morphologic features and electric disturbances in experimental coxsackie B3 virus myocarditis in hamsters

Arrhythmias and conduction disturbance in coxsackie B1 virus myocarditis in hamsters

When 2-week-old Syrian golden hamsters were inoculated with coxsackie B1 virus which had been propagated seven times in hamster heart before experimental use, electrocardiogram (ECG) abnormalities and histological evidence of myocarditis were detected in 31 of 39 infected hamsters. Multiple abnormalities were recorded in four hamsters: three showed ST–T change followed by first-degree A–V block, complete A–V block and transient second-degree A–V block with supraventricular extrasystoles, respectively; one showed first-degree A–V block and left bundle branch block (LBBB) pattern simultaneously. Eighty per cent of the hamsters showed ST–T change either as the sole ECG abnormality or as the first of a number of other abnormalities. The ST was displaced in various ways. Usually, the T waves showed a transient flattening in most of the leads during the recovery phase which then gradually became normal. The occurrence of conduction disturbances on the ECG corresponded closely with the histological location of myocarditis: basal IVS was always injured by myocarditis in cases with A–V blocks. Complete A–V block was recorded on the third day.[20]

Ventricular aneurysms and ventricular arrhythmias complicating coxsackie B1 virus myocarditis of Syrian golden hamsters

Serial ECGs were recorded in hamsters surviving the acute and electrocardiographically proven myocarditis. In a mean 17.8-week follow-up period, chronic VPCs followed the acute ECG changes in three of the animals. In one hamster, an acute ECG abnormality, intraventricular conduction disturbance with flat T waves, and deviation of the electrical axis to the left were recorded on the 4th day. A few VPCs of uniform contour were detected for the first time in the hamster on day 63, and were recorded along with paired ventricular beats from day 70 until the death of the animal on day 217. Pathological examination of the heart disclosed thick fibrosis in the inner layers of the anterior wall of the left ventricle, and protrusion of that part of the ventricular wall. Thin fibrotic lesions were also found in both ventricles, particularly on the left of the interventricular septum. Ventricular premature complexes had two kinds of contour in the other two hamsters, each of which had two ventricular aneurysms. No VPC was recorded in the other seven hamsters, none having cardiac aneurysms. These results demonstrate a close relationship between chronic VPC of a uniform contour following coxsackie B1 virus myocarditis together with the formation of ventricular aneurysms in Syrian golden hamsters; hamsters surviving over an extended period despite having aneurysms.[6] Ventricular aneurysms following coxsackie B1 virus myocarditis in Syrian golden hamsters may perhaps provide an experimental model of human ventricular aneurysms of unknown aetiology.

Immunological probes in the pathogenesis and diagnosis of viral myocarditis

Lymphocyte subset in viral myocarditis

Lymphocyte subsets in the peripheral blood were measured by flow cytometry using monoclonal antibodies to T cells (Thy 1.2), helper-inducer T cells (Lyt 1), cytotoxic-suppressor T cells (Lyt 2) and B cells (goat anti-mouse IgG).

For immunocytochemical analysis, frozen sections of the myocardium were stained to detect T cell subsets by a labelled avidin–biotin technique; T cell subsets being expressed as a percentage of the inflammatory cells enumerated by methyl green counter staining. The percentage of Thy 1.2 cells increased on days 14 and 28. Lyt 1 cells decreased significantly on day 7. However, there was no change in Lyt 2 or B cells. Immunocytochemical study of the heart showed that a significant number of infiltrating cells were Thy 1.2 positive (10, 11 and 10% on days 7, 14 and 28, respectively), that Lyt 1 cells increased on day 14 (8%), but that Lyt 2 cells did not show any significant change and were present only in low numbers (Fig. 5.10). This study demon-

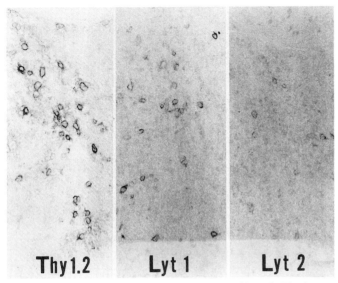

Fig. 5.10 Lymphocyte subset in the heart *in situ* (day 14). The frozen section was stained by the labelled avidin–biotin technique using monoclonal antibody against Thy 1.2 (T cells, left), Lyt 1 (helper-inducer T cells, middle) and Lyt 2 (cytotoxic-suppressor T cells, right). A significant number of infiltrating cells were Thy 1.2 positive cells and Lyt 1 cells predominate. × 220. Reproduced with permission of Springer-Verlag from Matsumori *et al.*[12]

strated that helper-inducer cells showed significant changes during the course of EMC virus myocarditis and suggests that these cells may be involved in the pathogenesis of this disease.[21]

Anti-heart antibody following encephalomyocarditis virus myocarditis (see also Chapter 6)

Patients with viral myocarditis as well as those with dilated cardiomyopathy have been reported to develop heart-reactive autoantibodies[22] and to have immunoglobulin deposits in their hearts.[23]

Anti-heart autoantibodies were found in the sera from DBA/2 mice infected with EMC virus.[24] Frozen sections of the hearts of uninfected mice were incubated with mouse sera and stained with anti-mouse IgG. Positive granular staining was first seen on day 4 and persisted to day 90; the titre was highest on day 21 (Fig. 5.11). The demonstration of anti-heart antibody in this model of viral myocarditis also suggests that this antibody may be involved in the pathogenesis of dilated cardiomyopathy.

In coxsackievirus B3 myocarditis, A. CA/SnJ and A. SW/SnJ mouse strains developed heart-specific autoantibodies as determined by indirect immunofluorescence. Western immunoblotting analyses demonstrated that antibodies to myosin were a prominent feature in the sera of strains which developed myocarditis.[25]

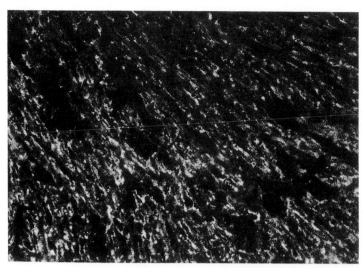

Fig. 5.11   Anti-heart antibody is seen in sera of DBA/2 mouse in encephalomyocarditis virus myocarditis. Indirect immunofluorescence. × 280.

Distribution of cardiac myosin isoenzymes as determined by selective monoclonal antibodies

It is known that gene expression for the ventricular myosin heavy chains which are composed of three myosin isoforms is developmentally regulated,[26] and that the myosin isoforms expressed in rats with pressure and volume overload states, and in cardiomyopathic hamsters, revert to the fetal and perinatal forms, presumably to mediate myocardial adaptation to the imposed cardiac load.[27,28]

Frozen sections of the hearts were stained with the monoclonal antibody specific for the myosin isoenzyme V_3 (R11D10). R11D10 did not stain myocytes of uninfected mice, whereas positive granular fluorescence was seen on the 5th day after infection. This persisted up to day 90, being most marked in myocytes near foci of myocardial fibrosis and calcification. Thus, the distribution of cardiac isoenzymes was altered following viral myocarditis.[29]

Antimyosin monoclonal antibody uptake in myocarditis

Recently, an antibody imaging technique was developed using antimyosin monoclonal antibodies which was found to be useful in the diagnosis of acute myocardial infarction,[30–32] myocarditis[31,33] and heart allograft rejection.[34] It has been demonstrated that the antimyosin monoclonal antibody was localized selectively in the heart from the acute to subacute stages of viral myocarditis.[35,36] When the myocardial uptake of [125]I- and ^{131}I-antimyosin monoclonal antibody Fab in experimental myocarditis was studied in Balb/c mice infected by EMC the highest ratio of ^{125}I-antimyosin appeared in the heart of infected mice on day 14. The uptake ratio for the heart increased significantly 3 days after virus inoculation and reached a maximum on day

14, when myocardial lesions were most extensive and prominent. The uptake ratio then decreased significantly, but still remained high compared with controls on day 28 when cellular infiltration had decreased and fibrosis was evident (Fig. 5.12). The scintigraphic images obtained with the ^{131}I-antimyosin monoclonal antibody clearly demonstrated that visualization of the heart in experimental myocarditis was possible 24 hours after administration of radiotracer, and localized activity was still observed in the 48-hour image. The pharmacokinetics of [131]In-antimyosin monoclonal antibody Fab were also investigated using the same model. Myocardial uptake 24 hours after intravenous injection of [131]In-antimyosin Fab increased significantly in EMC virus-infected mice 5, 7 and 14 days after virus inoculation, and correlated with myocardial cell necrosis. The *in vivo* kinetics study demonstrated that the heart-to-blood ratio reached a maximum 48 hours after the intravenous administration of [131]In-antimyosin Fab, which was considered to be the optimal time in [131]In-antimyosin Fab scintigraphy. High-performance liquid chromatographic analysis revealed the presence of antigen–antibody complexes in the blood of infected mice after injection of [131]In-antimyosin Fab; the antigen may perhaps be whole myosin. Antimyosin antibody imaging may therefore be useful in detecting and assessing myocardial injury in myocarditis.

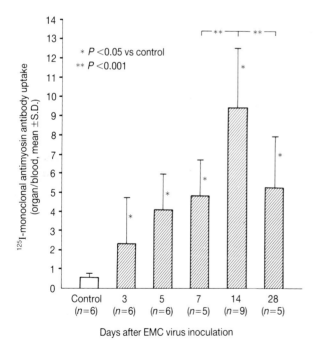

Fig. 5.12 Sequential study of myocardial uptake of ^{125}I-antimyosin monoclonal antibody Fab (ratio of percentage dose per gram for the heart to percentage dose per millilitre for blood). ^{125}I-antimyosin uptake ratio began to increase on day 3, reached a maximum on day 14, and remained elevated on day 28. Reproduced with permission of the American Heart Association from Matsumori *et al.*[35]

Atrial natriuretic polypeptide in viral myocarditis

Since atrial natriuretic polypeptide (ANP) has been isolated from the atria of mammalian species, much interest has been focussed on its implication in cardiovascular disease. Plasma ANP levels are increased in patients with congestive heart failure.[37] Although the atrial ANP level in cardiomyopathic hamsters was reported to be decreased[38] the ANP level in ventricles is increased in the hypertrophied heart caused by aortic ligation in rats, in cardiomyopathic hamsters with congestive heart failure,[38] and in patients with dilated cardiomyopathy.[39] These studies suggest that ANP plays a pathophysiological role in heart failure despite its function as a naturally occurring vasodilator and an endogenous diuretic. Increased synthesis and secretion of ANP have been reported in the ventricle and atrium in our model of EMC viral myocarditis.[40,41] Atrial natriuretic poly peptide-like immunoreactivity in the extracts was measured by a radioimmunoassay which recognizes the common C-terminal sequence of α-human ANP and α-rat ANP (α-rANP). The atrial ANP level decreased to 22% of that of the uninoculated age-matched mice on day 7, increased to a value 1.6 times higher than the control value on day 14, and returned to nearly the same value as that of the controls by day 28. The ventricles of the control mice contained approximately a 1000 times lower concentration of ANP than the atria. The ventricular ANP concentration of the infected mice was three times higher than the control value on day 7, increased to 21 times that of controls by day 14 and still remained nine times higher on day 28.

The plasma ANP level of the infected mice was also elevated: it was seven times higher on day 7, 20 times higher on day 14 and seven times higher than controls on day 28. Frozen sections were prepared from the atria and ventricles of the control and infected mice and indirect immunofluorescence and immunoperoxidase stains were performed. Anti-ANP antibody stained atrial myocytes but did not stain ventricular myocytes in normal hearts. Staining became more prominent in the atrial myocytes near the foci of myocardial lesions on day 7 and was more extensive on day 14. Positive staining was seen in the ventricular myocytes after day 7 (Fig. 5.13). Electron microscopy revealed an increased number of electron-dense granules in atrial myocytes 14 days after infection. Electron-dense granules were seen in the ventricles of inoculated mice on day 14, although such granules were not present in the ventricles of control mice.[12]

The most striking result in this study was a marked increase in the ventricular ANP level. Although the ventricular concentration and content of ANP were much lower than those of the atria even in the infected mice, it is noteworthy that the ventricular ANP level had increased to a value 21 times higher than that of controls, whereas the atrial ANP level showed only a two fold increase. This suggests that an increase in mechanical load during the development of heart failure gives rise to the re-expression of the ANP gene in ventricular myocytes, this being suppressed in the normal adult ventricle. In addition, since ANP staining was particularly marked in the areas surrounding lesions, local effects stimulating ANP synthesis may possibly be present. Further studies are necessary to elucidate the possible mechanism responsible for enhanced ANP synthesis in this model.

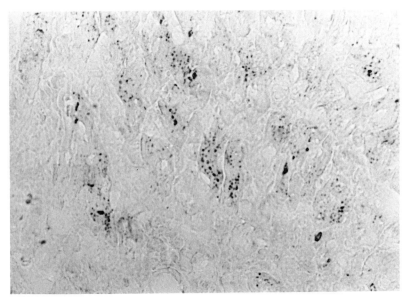

Fig. 5.13 Immunoperoxidase staining of the interventricular septum of a mouse by anti-atrial natriuretic polypeptide (ANP) antibody 14 days after encephalomyocarditis virus inoculation. Positive staining was seen in the ventricular myocytes near the foci of myocardial lesions after day 7 of infection. Anti-ANP antibody did not stain ventricular myocytes in normal hearts. × 360.

The viral genome in experimental myocarditis

In order to evaluate the aetiologic significance of enteroviruses in myocarditis and cardiomyopathy, especially the dilated type, several investigators have attempted to detect the viral genome in hearts using nucleic acid probes. Bowles et al.[42] claimed positive hybridization signals in 9 of 17 samples from patients with histological evidence of active or healing myocarditis or dilated cardiomyopathy with inflammatory changes. Studying the effect of persistent infection by coxsackie B3 virus in the myocardium of athymic mice, another group detected the viral genome in the myocardium of immunodeficient mice for up to 56 days post inoculation and suggested that the presence of the viral genome might possibly be related to the pathogenesis of dilated cardiomyopathy.[43] Other studies have used biotinylated cDNA probes to study human *post mortem* cardiac tissues by *in situ* hybridization[44] or radiolabelled probes for the *in situ* studies to investigate the natural course of EMC virus infection in mice.[45] The presence of viral genomes in the murine heart has been investigated in experimental coxsackievirus B3 myocarditis by Northern blotting. Four-week-old C3H/He mice were inoculated with coxsackie B3 virus. The ^{32}P-labelled cDNA probe was derived from the 5′ end sequence of the coxsackie B3 virus genome. Northern blot autoradiograms of heart RNA were positive for viral RNA up to day 7 and negative after day 10. No viral RNA was detected in the hearts of uninfected mice. Positive autoradiograms always had the strongest signal in the 7.4 kb region, corresponding to the size of the complete genome of the virus (Fig. 5.14). Hybridization signals were present

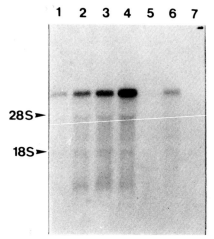

Fig. 5.14 Autoradiogram of Northern blot of total murine heart RNA from hearts infected with coxsackie B3 virus. Day 3 (lane 1), day 4 (lane 2), day 5 (lane 3), day 6 (lane 4), day 7 (lanes 5 and 6) and day 10 (lane 7). Reproduced with permission of the *Journal of Molecular Cell Cardiology* from Okada *et al.*[46]

prior to the appearance of histopathological changes.[46] Such studies may be useful in evaluating the effects of specific drugs on experimental viral myocarditis at the level of the viral genome.

The use of animal models in preventive and therapeutic interventions

Virus vaccine and passive immunization

Passive immunization with EMC hyperimmune rabbit serum given shortly after inoculation with EMC appears to protect mice from virus myocarditis.[47] A virus-specific formalin-inactivated vaccine also prevented the development of EMC-induced myocarditis. Neutralizing antibodies were demonstrated after two doses of vaccine. After subsequent challenge with the virus, all vaccinated mice survived without developing myocarditis, whereas all unvaccinated animals developed fatal disease.[47]

Encephalomyocarditis virus is periodically isolated in domestic swine,[48] captive wild animals or nonhuman primates.[49] Episodic outbreaks of EMC virus infection have been reported in swine manifesting a severe and often fatal myocarditis. Vaccination or passive immunization may be of value in preventing EMC virus infection in animals. Vaccination of animals before pregnancy completely inhibited myocardial virus replication and had a protective effect on EMC virus infection in offspring.[50] Consideration may be given in due course to the development of such vaccines against picornaviruses, particularly coxsackie B virus, which have a recognized role in myocarditis in humans.

The effect of interferon

Natural human interferon preparations do not show significant activity in mouse cells. However, a recombinant human leukocyte interferon subtype α D and hybrid interferon-α A/D were shown to have relatively high antiviral activity in murine cell cultures and also *in vivo*.[51] Because interferon has multiple immunological effects, it may contribute to the body's defence against various microbial assaults. However, interferon probably plays a significant role in the control of viral infections. This assumption has been supported by a number of studies which suggest that neutralization of interferon using specific antisera enhances the severity of viral infection.[52]

In an animal model of EMC virus myocarditis, it was demonstrated that human leukocyte interferon-α A/D given one day before or simultaneously with inoculation with EMC virus inhibited multiplication of virus in the heart and protected mice from developing myocarditis. Prevention was dependent on dosage and on the time of initiation of treatment. When treatment was started before or simultaneously with virus inoculation, interferon-α A/D in a dose of 10^7 units/kg day effectively reduced the inflammatory response and myocardial damage.[53]

Interferon-β inhibits replication of coxsackie B3 virus in cultured human heart cells.[54] and murine interferon-β reduces the number of coxsackie B3 virus-induced myocardial lesions in CD-1 mice but does not reduce viral infectivity in heart tissue.[55] Murine interferon-α/β has been shown to be effective against lethal infection of coxsackie A16 virus and enterovirus 71 in mice when administered simultaneously with or early after infection.[56] Using an animal model of coxsackievirus myocarditis, it has been shown that human leukocyte interferon-α A/D given 1 day before or simultaneously with inoculation with virus inhibited multiplication of virus in the heart and protected mice from developing coxsackie B3 virus myocarditis.[57]

Being a broad-spectrum antiviral agent interferon may be potentially useful in treating a disease such as viral myocarditis which may be caused by different viruses.

Effect of ribavirin on encephalomyocarditis virus myocarditis

Ribavirin (virazole, 1-β-D-ribofuranosyl-1,2,4-triazole-3-carboxamide) is a synthetic nucleoside analogue, structurally related to inosine and guanosine, and has a broad antiviral activity against RNA and DNA viruses. Clinically, its efficacy has been demonstrated in measles, influenza and respiratory syncytial virus infections.[58,59]

When administered subcutaneously at a dose of 100, 200 or 400 mg/kg immediately after EMC virus inoculation ribavirin-treated mice survived significantly longer that controls. The degree of inhibition of viral replication in the heart was influenced by drug dosage; 200 mg/kg ribavirin significantly inhibited viral replication. Cellular infiltration was significantly less marked in mice treated with 200 mg/kg ribavirin, and myocardial necrosis was significantly less severe in mice treated with 400 mg/kg compared with that in controls.[60] Ribavirin was also effective at a dose of 400 mg/kg beginning 1 day or 3 days after inoculation.

Effect of ribavirin on coxsackie B3 virus myocarditis

The effect of ribavirin on coxsackie B3 virus myocarditis has also been investigated. Four-week-old C3H/He mice were inoculated intraperitoneally with 3 × 10⁴ PFU of coxsackie B3 virus. Ribavirin was administered subcutaneously at a dose of 50, 100 or 200 mg/kg daily immediately after virus inoculation. All mice survived and were sacrificed on day 7. The myocardial virus titre on day 7 was significantly lower in mice treated with 100 mg/kg ribavirin compared with controls.

Histological examination of the myocardium showed less cellular infiltration and necrosis in mice treated with 100 or 200 mg/kg. Thus, ribavirin effectively inhibited myocardial virus replication and reduced the inflammatory response and myocardial damage in this experimental model of coxsackie B3 virus myocarditis. The minimal effective dose which induced an effect on coxsackievirus myocarditis was less than that for EMC virus myocarditis.[9]

Synergistic treatment with interferon and ribavirin

Although simultaneous administration of interferon-α A/D and ribavirin inhibited multiplication of EMC virus in the heart and protected mice from developing myocarditis, large amounts of these drugs were necessary to obtain beneficial effects. The side effects of these drugs are usually dose related, but synergistic combinations of drugs may allow effective treatment at lower drug concentrations. This strategy has been highly successful in the treatment of some bacterial diseases and cancers. Since the mode of action of interferon may differ from that of ribavirin, the possibility was investigated that recombinant interferon-α A/D might act synergistically with ribavirin. Plaque reduction assays in tissue cultures showed that ribavirin and interferon-α A/D inhibited EMC virus replication synergistically.[9] In our study, ribavirin, 100 mg/kg, or interferon, 10⁶ units/kg, alone did not inhibit EMC virus replication in the heart. When used together daily, 100 mg/kg ribavirin and 10⁶ units/kg interferon achieved a striking synergistic effect. There was enhanced survival and myocardial virus titre was also effectively reduced (Fig. 5.15). There was a significant reduction in the inflammatory response and in myocardial damage. Combined therapy achieved its effects at lower concentrations than when either preparation was used alone. It is possible that such a combination would reduce the frequency of undesirable side effects for either drug used at a higher concentration. The use of combinations of antivirals deserves further careful study for other serious viral infections.

The effect of tumour necrosis factor

Tumour necrosis factor (TNF) is a cytokine released mainly by activated macrophages.[61] Recently, *in vitro* antiviral effects against EMC virus in selected cell lines have been reported.[62] The mechanism by which TNF acts is still unknown, but it has been shown that interferon-β is a mediator of the antiviral effect of TNF.[63] Matsumori *et al.* investigated whether TNF has an antiviral effect *in vivo* in our model of EMC virus myocarditis.[13] The specific activity of recombinant human TNF (rhTNF) (Suntory Institute for Biochemical Research, Osaka, Japan) is about 4.8 × 10⁷ units/mg protein, based

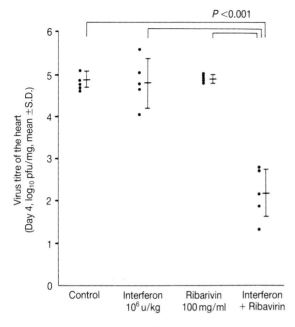

Fig. 5.15 Synergistic treatment of interferon-α A/D and ribavirin in encephalomyocarditis virus myocarditis. Interferon-α A/D 10^6 units/kg, or ribavirin, 100 mg/kg, did not inhibit encephalomyocarditis virus replication in the heart, but combined treatment had a striking effect.

on its cytotoxic activity in L929 cells. Recombinant human TNF (10 μg in 0.2 ml) was injected intravenously 1 day before EMC virus inoculation, and the same dose was injected daily intraperitoneally from the day of inoculation to day 4. Myocardial virus titres in mice treated with rhTNF were significantly higher than among controls. Myocardial necrosis and cellular infiltration were also significantly more severe among treated mice. Thus, although an antiviral effect of TNF against EMC virus infection has been reported *in vitro*, the reverse effect appears to occur *in vivo* emphasizing that the *in vitro* effect cannot always be extrapolated to the *in vivo* situation.

The effect of interleukin-2

Interleukin-2 (IL-2) is a lymphokine which is produced by activated T cells. Interleukin-2 plays an important role in the immune system, for example, inducing differentiation and proliferation of T cells and B cells, proliferation of natural killer cells and induction of antigen-specific killer cells. Interleukin-2 has also been reported to have an anti-viral effect[64,65] induced by activation of natural killer cells and cytotoxic T cells. The effect of recombinant human IL-2 (rIL-2, TGP-3, Takeda Chemical Industries Ltd, Osaka, Japan) was investigated in EMC virus myocarditis in mice. Recombinant human IL-2, 1×10^6 units in 0.1 ml, was administered intravenously beginning 1 day before virus inoculation thereafter being given daily but intraperitoneally at the same dose. The mice were killed on day 5. There was no significant difference in myocardial virus titre or histopathology between treated mice and controls. Thus, no protective effect was demonstrated with rIL-2 against EMC virus infection in mice.

The effect of anti-interleukin-2 receptor monoclonal antibody

Activated T cells express a variety of plasma membrane receptors which are absent from the surface of resting T cells, e.g. receptors for interleukin-2, insulin and transferrin. *De novo* acquisition of membrane receptors for IL-2 marks a critical event in the course of T cell activation. M7/20, a rat anti-mouse IL-2 receptor monoclonal antibody, blocks IL-2-mediated growth and inhibits binding of IL-2 to its cellular receptor.[66] Intraperitoneal injection with M7/20 at a dose of 5 µg/mouse/day for 10 days results in indefinite survival of murine cardiac allografts.[67]

The effect of immunosuppressive therapy was investigated with anti-IL-2 receptor antibody M7/20 in EMC virus myocarditis. Balb/c mice were inoculated with EMC virus and injected intraperitoneally daily with M7/20, 5 µg/mouse, for 14 days. There was no significant difference in mortality or cardiac histopathology between treated mice and controls. Thus, the suggestion is that therapy with anti-IL-2 receptor monoclonal antibody is unlikely to be beneficial.

Immunosuppressive agents

The effect of corticosteroids
Steroids have been shown to reverse *in vivo* rejection episodes by preventing the production of IL-2, thereby denying activated T cells an essential trophic factor. Steroids do not act directly on the IL-2-producing T cell, but they inhibit production of this lymphokine by preventing monocytes from releasing IL-1, thereby blocking IL-1-dependent release of IL-2 from antigen-activated T cells.

Kilbourne *et al.*[68] reported that a single injection of cortisone at an early stage of infection with coxsackie B3 virus increased both the severity of myocardial damage and the incidence of lethal disease in mice. In contrast, there have been many clinical reports of the successful use of these agents.[69,70] However, the influence of steroids on the different stages of viral myocarditis in an experimental model has not been studied.

The effects of prednisolone on acute EMC viral myocarditis have been studied.[71] BALB/c mice, 4 to 5 weeks old, were inoculated intraperitoneally with EMC virus. Prednisolone was administered intramuscularly, 10 mg/kg once a day, on days 4 to 13 to mice who were observed until day 23. The survival rate of mice treated with prednisolone was significantly lower than that of controls. Up to day 8 viral titres were similar to those of the controls but by day 10 they were considerably higher. The neutralizing titres of the prednisolone-treated group on days 8 and 10 were significantly lower than those of the controls. However, levels increased to the same as those among the controls by day 14. Prednisolone was also administered, 10 mg/kg/day, on days 8–17 and mice were observed until day 27. The survival rate of the prednisolone-treated group on day 27 was similar to that of the controls. Although the extent of myocardial necrosis on day 14 was slightly greater in the prednisolone-treated group in both experiments. There were no significant differences in the scores of myocardial necrosis and cellular infiltration between the prednisolone-treated and control groups on days 8, 10 and 14 in either experiment. This study suggests that although steroids may aggravate the course of acute viral myocarditis if administered if neutralizing antibody responses are poor but if given when the neutralizing antibody titres are high no deterrent effect is observed. Nevertheless, no beneficial effect of steroids was observed.

The effect of cyclosporin

Cyclosporin is a fungal metabolite with unique immunosuppressive properties which make it a particularly suitable agent for the therapy of autoimmune disorders characterized by a deficiency of T cell suppressor function. Cyclosporin blocks IL-2 release from activated helper T lymphocytes. The release of other lymphokines, such as interferon-γ, by activated T cells is also inhibited by cyclosporin, whereas the expression of IL-2 receptors and the responsiveness of activated T lymphocytes to lymphokines are not blocked. Coincident with the drug-induced inhibition of helper T cell function, cyclosporin spares, at least partly, the activation of suppressor T cells *in vitro* and *in vivo*. The effect of immunosuppressive therapy has been investigated with cyclosporin in EMC viral myocarditis.[72] Eight-week-old male DBA-2 mice were infected with EMC virus and randomized to a treatment or control group. Cyclosporin (25 mg/kg per day) was administered subcutaneously for 3 weeks, starting at 1 week after infection during viral replication. The mortality rate was significantly higher in mice treated with cyclosporin (Fig. 5.16). However, there was no apparent reduction in the score for gross myocardial lesions or myocardial hypertrophy as assessed by heart weight to body weight ratio, or in the extent of myocardial inflammation, necrosis or calcification on microscopic assessment. There was a tendency for the mice in the treatment group to have a more severe degree of inflammation. Cyclosporin was also administered for 3 weeks, starting 3 weeks after infection, i.e. *after* the period of viral replication. This resulted in a slightly but not significantly higher mortality in treated mice (Fig. 5.16). However, although there was no significant histological difference between treated and untreated mice cyclosporin-treated mice had significantly greater ratios for heart weight to body weight, lung weight to body weight and liver weight to body weight. This suggests that the mice may have more severe heart failure.

The effect of cyclosporin on the production of anti-heart autoantibodies has been further investigated in EMC virus-induced myocarditis.[73] Four-week-old BALB/c mice were infected with EMC virus and cyclosporin (25 mg/kg) was administered subcutaneously daily, starting on the fourth day after infection. On day 7, treated mice showed higher titres of anti-heart autoantibody than controls. However, histological lesions, lymphocyte subsets in the heart and in the peripheral blood, neutralizing antibody responses and virus concentrations in the heart showed no significant differences.

O'Connell *et al.*[74] studied the effect of intraperitoneally administered cyclosporin in the murine model of coxsackie B3 virus myocarditis. When com-

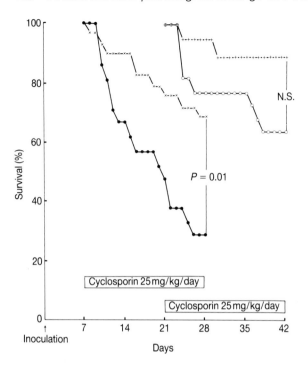

Fig. 5.16   The effect of cyclosporin on survival in encephalomyocarditis virus myocarditis. Mortality was significantly greater in the early treatment protocol (●–●). Later administration of cyclosporin did not show improvement of mortality (–). Control (x–x :+–+). Reproduced with permission of the American Heart Association from Monrad *et al.*[72]

pared with controls, mice given cyclosporin had a high mortality rate and a significantly reduced mononuclear infiltrate, but more cardiac necrosis. However, when cyclosporin was started a week after infection, the mortality rate was lower, although histological abnormalities were similar.

The effect of FK-506
The effect of FK-506, a macrolide antibiotic obtained from *Streptomyces tsukubaensis*, collected from the soil of the Tsukuba area in northern Japan has also been investigated.[75] A wide variety of pharmacological and immunological studies has shown that FK-506 has strong immunosuppressive activity against mixed lymphocyte reactions[75] and that it is a valuable drug for preventing graft rejection experimentally.[76] FK-506 suppresses T cell-mediated immunity, suppressing both IL-2 and IL-2 receptor expression on T cells.[75,77] Its immunosuppressive activity is up to 100 times greater than that of cyclosporin. However, FK-506 (0.5 or 1.0 mg/kg), given on the the same day as EMC virus inoculation, did not improve survival (Fig. 5.17) or myocardial lesions.

The implication of these studies with respect to inflammatory myocarditis in humans is that therapy with immunosuppressive agents such as corticosteroids, cyclosporin or FK-506, although potentially useful for myocarditis

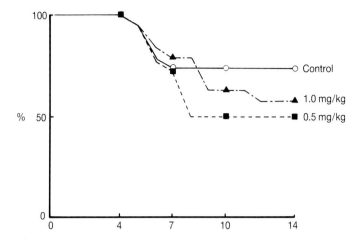

Fig. 5.17 Effect of FK-506 on survival in encephalomyocarditis virus myocarditis. FK-506 did not improve survival.

secondary to primary autoimmune disorders, is unlikely to be beneficial when the disease is the result of an acute picornavirus infection, at least during the early period of viral replication and shortly thereafter.

The effect of angiotensin converting enzyme inhibitor

Recently, it has been reported that captopril, an antihypertensive drug, which inhibits angiotensin coverting enzyme (ACE) activity, has anti-inflammatory properties and is effective in treating severe congestive heart failure (CHF).[78–80] The effect of captopril on EMC virus myocarditis has been studied in Balb/c mice. Captopril, 10, 30 or 100 mg/kg, was administered orally from day 4 to 14 after virus inoculation. Survival of mice treated with 100 mg/kg per day was significantly higher than in the placebo treatment group from days 12 to 14. The ratios of heart weight to body weight were significantly lower and histological examination showed less extensive myocardial necrosis, cellular infiltration and calcification in mice treated with 30 and 100 mg/kg compared with controls.[81]

Thus, captopril improved virus-induced myocardial injury, congestive heart failure and survival of mice dose dependently in an experimental model, even when treatment was started around the peak of virus replication. This study suggests that captopril may prove to be a promising new therapeutic agent for acute myocarditis.

Rezkalla *et al.*[82] also showed that captopril was beneficial in acute coxsackie B3 virus murine myocarditis. However, they found that the drug, although reducing heart weight and necrosis if started very early after infection, did not result in any improvement histologically if treatment was delayed.

Captopril dilates blood vessels by suppressing angiotensin II production and through a number of other mechanisms not related to conversion of angiotensin I to angiotensin II. The agent has also been shown to inhibit norepinephrine release from adrenergic nerve endings. It potentiates vasodilatory effects of kinins to block the breakdown of bradykinin. Bradykinin in turn stimulates the release of prostanoids and endothelium-derived relaxing factor.[83] Captopril has been proven to be effective for the treatment of congestive heart failure, and reduction of afterload and preload by these vasodilation effects is thought to underlie the beneficial effects of captopril. While there are no previous studies on congestive heart failure due to acute myocarditis, beneficial effects in our model of congestive heart failure may be partly explained by the above mechanisms. Captopril can scavenge free radicals because of its sulphydryl group.[84] It has been suggested that free radicals are involved in inducing an inflammatory response by activating a neutrophil chemotactic factor in plasma.[85] Thus, the action of captopril as a free radical scavenger may play an important role in improving myocardial injury during the acute to subacute stages of viral myocarditis.

The effect of β-adrenergic receptor blockers

Traditionally, congestive heart failure in patients has been considered to be a contraindication for the use of β-adrenergic receptor blockers. However, recent studies suggested that these agents can have beneficial effects and can improve survival in patients with dilated cardiomyopathy.[86–89] Although myocarditis may initiate dilated cardiomyopathy,[1,2] few studies have investigated the role of β-adrenergic blockers in viral myocarditis. To our knowledge, there has been only one published report[90] on the effects of β-adrenergic blockers on myocarditis. In that study, the effect of metoprolol on acute coxsackie B3 virus in a murine model of myocarditis was examined. There was an increase in mortality associated with severe pathological changes in the hearts of mice given metoprolol at 32.5 mg/kg per day. The adverse haemodynamic and immunological effects resulting from treatment with metoprolol were thought to induce these findings because the myocardial virus titre was increased. We have recently investigated the effect of carteolol on EMC viral myocarditis. Carteolol is a nonselective β-adrenergic blocker with moderate intrinsic sympathomimetic activity and little membrane stabilizing activity. It has about a 20- to 30-fold stronger β-adrenergic blocking effect per unit weight than propranolol. In our experimental model moderate doses of carteolol had no deleterious effect on survival, heart weight to body weight ratio, histopathological findings or myocardial virus titre in the acute and subacute stages. Thus, carteolol did not make viral myocarditis more severe in these mice. The difference between Rezkalla's study and our finding may reflect differences in the strain of mice used, the virus, or the β-blocker. In an experiment on chronic infection, DBA/2 mice were inoculated with EMC virus and then given carteolol, 1 or 10 mg/kg, or metoprolol, 30 mg/kg daily, starting on day 14; mice were killed on day 104. Heart weight to body weight ratio and histopathological scores were significantly lower in mice given carteolol than in infected controls. Furthermore, left ventricular cavity dimension, left ventricular wall thickness and myocardial fibre diameter of the left ventricle were significantly reduced in mice given carteolol compared with controls. Metoprolol did not cause any significant changes compared with the controls. This study suggests that carteolol may prevent development of myocardial lesions similar to those observed in dilated cardiomyopathy following myocarditis.[91]

Acknowledgments

This work was supported, in part, by a Research Grant from the Ministry of Health and Welfare, Grant-in-Aid for Scientific Research on Priority Areas and for General Scientific Research from the Ministry of Education, Science and Culture, Japan and Kanazawa Research Fund.

I thank Drs Tatsuo Hoshino, Nobuyoshi Tomioka, Chiharu Kishimoto, Yoshiki Matoba, Ikutaro Okada, Tomoko Ohkusa, Makoto Tominaga, Takehiko Yamada, Hiroshi Suzuki and Shingo Maruyama, Narito Morii and Scott E. Monrad for great contributions to the studies and Drs Chuichi Kawai, Clyde S. Crumpacker, Steven S. Tracy and Walter H. Abelmann for pertinent advice on the work.

References

1. Kawai C., Matsumori A., Kitaura Y., Takatsu T. Viruses and the heart: viral myocarditis and cardiomyopathy. *Prog Cardiol* 1978; **7:** 141–62.
2. Kawai C., Matsumori A., Fujiwara H. Myocarditis and dilated cardiomyopathy. *Ann Rev Med* 1987; **38:** 221–39.
3. Matsumori A., Kawai C. An experimental model for congestive heart failure following encephalomyocarditis virus myocarditis in mice. *Circulation* 1982; **65:** 1230–5.
4. Matsumori A., Kawai C. An animal model of congestive (dilated) cardiomyopathy: Dilatation and hypertrophy of the heart in the chronic stage in DBA/2 mice with myocarditis caused by encephalomyocarditis virus. *Circulation* 1982; **66:** 355–60.
5. Matsumori A., Kawai C. Coxsackievirus B3 perimyocarditis in BALB/c mice: experimental model of chronic perimyocarditis in the right ventricle. *J Pathol* 1980; **131:** 97–106.
6. Hoshino T., Matsumori A., Kawai C., Imai J. Ventricular aneurysms and ventricular arrhythmias complicating coxsackievirus B1 myocarditis of Syrian golden hamsters. *Cardiovasc Res* 1984; **18:** 24–9.
7. Matsumori A., Kawai C. Animal models of congestive heart failure and congestive (dilated) cardiomyopathy due to viral myocarditis in mice. In: Bolte H. D. ed. *Viral Heart Disease*. Berlin: Springer-Verlag, 1984: 35–56.
8. Matsumori A., Kawai C., Crumpacker C. S., Abelmann W. H. The use of animal models for preventive and therapeutic trials of viral myocarditis. In: Kawai C., Abelmann W. H., Matsumori A. eds. *Cardiomyopathy Uptake 1. Pathogenesis of myocarditis and cardiomyopathy*. Tokyo: University of Tokyo Press, 1987: 37–47.
9. Matsumori A., Okada I., Kawai C. *et al*. Animal models for therapeutic trials of viral myocarditis: effect of ribavirin and alpha interferon on coxsackievirus B3 and encephalomyocarditis virus myocarditis. In: Schultheiss H. P. ed. *New Concepts in Viral Heart Disease*. Berlin: Springer-Verlag, 1988: 377–84.
10. Matsumori A., Kawai C. Immunomodulating therapy in experimental myocarditis. In: Miescher P. A., Maisch B. eds. *Springer Seminars in Immunopathology: immunopathology of cardiac diseases*. Berlin: Springer-Verlag, 1989: 11, 77–88.
11. Matsumori A., Hoshino T., Kishimoto C., Kawai C. Morphological features and electric disturbances in experimental viral myocarditis. In: Olsen E. G. J., Sekiguchi M. eds. *Proceeding of the 2nd International Symposium on Cardiomyopathy and Myocarditis*. Tokyo: University of Tokyo Press, 1990: 217–22.
12. Matsumori A., Matoba Y., Tomioka N., Kawai C. Experimental viral myocarditis: immunopathogenetic aspects. In: Baroldi G., Camerini F., Goodwin J. F. eds. *Advances in Cardiomyopathies*. Berlin: Springer-Verlag, 1990: 181–9.

13. Matsumori A., Yamada T., Kawai C. Immunodulating therapy in viral myocarditis: effects of tumor necrosis factor, interleukin-2 and anti-interleukin-2 receptor antibody in an animal model. *Eur Heart J* 1991; **12** (suppl D): 203–5.
14. Matsumori A., Kawai C., Sawada S. Encephalomyocarditis virus myocarditis in inbred strains of mice: chronic stage. *Jpn Circ J* 1982; **46**: 1192–6.
15. Tomioka N., Kishimoto C., Matsumori A., Kawai C. Mural thrombus in experimental viral myocarditis in mice: relationship between thrombosis and congestive heart failure. *Cardiovasc Res* 1986; **20**: 665–71.
16. El-Khatib M. R., Chason J. L., Lerner A. M. Ventricular aneurysms complicating coxsackievirus group B, types 1 and 4 murine myocarditis. *Circulation* 1979; **59**: 412–16.
17. Matsumori A., Kishimoto C., Kawai C., Sawada S. Right ventricular aneurysms complicating encephalomyocarditis virus myocarditis in mice. *Jpn Circ J* 1983; **47**: 1322–4.
18. Okada I., Matsumori A., Tominaga M. *et al.* An animal model of chronic myocarditis: successive infection with coxsackievirus and encephalomyocarditis virus in mice. *Jpn Circ J* 1990; **54**: 788–9.
19. Kishimoto C., Matsumori A., Ohmae M. *et al.* Electrocardiographic findings in experimental myocarditis in DBA/2 mice: complete atrioventricular block in the acute stage, low voltage of the QRS complex in the subacute stage and arrhythmias in the chronic stage. *J Am Coll Cardiol* 1984; **3**: 1461–8.
20. Hoshino T., Matsumori A., Kawai C., Imai J. Electrocardiographic abnormalities in Syrian golden hamsters with coxsackievirus B_1 myocarditis. *Jpn Circ J* 1982; **46**: 1305–12.
21. Matsumori A., Tomioka N., Kawai C. Viral myocarditis: immunopathogenesis and the effect of immunosuppressive treatment in a murine model. *Jpn Circ J* 1989; **53**: 58–60.
22. Maisch B., Trostel-Soeder R., Stechemesser E. *et al.* Diagnostic relevance of human and cell-mediated immune reactions in patients with acute viral myocarditis. *Clin Exp Immunol* 1982; **48**: 533–45.
23. Bolte H. D., Schutheiss H. P. Variations in the susceptibility to coxsackievirus B_3-induced myocarditis among different strains of mice. *J Immunol* 1986; **136**: 1846–52.
24. Matsumori A., Thorp K., Crumpacker C. S., Abelmann W. H. Anti-heart antibody in an experimental model of viral myocarditis. *Circulation* 1984; **70 (II)**: 140.
25. Alvarez F. L., Neu N., Rose N. R. *et al.* Heart-specific autoantibodies induced by coxsackievirus B3: identification of heart autoantigens. *Clin Immunol Immunopathol* 1987; **43**: 129–39.
26. Lompre A. M., Nadal-Ginard B., Mahdavi V. Expression of the cardiac ventricular α- and β-myosin heavy chain genes is developmentally and hormonally regulated. *J Biol Chem* 1984; **259**: 6437–48.
27. Mercadier J. J., Lompre A. M., Wisnewsky C. *et al.* Myosin isoenzymatic change in several models of rat cardiac hypertrophy. *Circ Res* 1981; **49**: 525–32.
28. Wiegrand V., Stroh E., Henninges A. *et al.* Altered distribution of myosin isoenzymes in the cardiomyopathic Syrian hamster (BIO 8, 262). *Basic Res Cardiol* 1983; **78**: 665–70.
29. Matsumori A., Thorp K., Khaw B. A. *et al.* Distribution of cardiac myosin isoenzymes in the mouse with viral myocarditis as determined by selective monoclonal antibodies. *Circulation* 1984; **70 (II)**: 402.
30. Khaw B. A., Gold H. K., Yasuda T. *et al.* Scintigraphic quantification of myocarditial necrosis in patients after intravenous injection of myosin-specific antibody. *Circulation* 1986; **74**: 501–8.
31. Matsumori A., Yamada T., Tamaki N. *et al.*[111] In-monoclonal antimyosin antibody imaging: imaging of myocardial infarction and myocarditis. *Jpn Circ J* 1990; **54**: 333–8.

32. Matsumori A., Yamada T., Tamaki N. *et al.* Persistent uptake of indium-111 antimyosin monoclonal antibody in patients with myocardial infarction. *Am Heart J* 1990; **120**: 1026–30.

33. Yasuda T., Palacios I. F., Dec G. W. *et al.* Indium 111-monoclonal antimyosin antibody imaging in the diagnosis of acute myocarditis. *Circulation* 1987; **76**: 306–11.

34. Frist W., Yasuda T., Segall G. *et al.* Noninvasive detection of human cardiac transplant rejection with indium-111 antimyosin (Fab) imaging. *Circulation* 1987; **76** (suppl V): 81–5.

35. Matsumori A., Ohkusa T., Matoba Y. *et al.* Myocardial uptake of antimyosin monoclonal antibody in a murine model of viral myocarditis. *Circulation* 1989; **79**: 400–5.

36. Yamada T., Matsumori A., Watanabe Y. *et al.* Pharmacokinetics of indium-111-labeled antimyosin monoclonal antibody in murine experimental viral myocarditis. *J Am Coll Cardiol* 1990; **16**: 1280–6.

37. Burnett J. C., Kao P. C., Hu D. C. *et al.* Atrial natriuretic peptide elevation in congestive heart failure in man. *Science* 1986; **231**: 1145–7.

38. Ding J., Thibault G., Gutkowska J. *et al.* Cardiac and plasma atrial natriuretic factor in experimental congestive heart failure. *Endocrinology* 1987; **121**: 248–57.

39. Saito Y., Nakao K., Arai H. *et al.* Augmented expression of atrial natriuretic polypeptide gene in ventricle of human failing heart. *J Clin Invest* 1989; **83**: 298–305.

40. Matsumori A., Morii N., Tomioka N. *et al.* Atrial natriuretic polypeptide in experimental viral myocarditis: increased synthesis and secretion in the ventricle and atrium. *Circulation* 1987; **76** (suppl IV): 211.

41. Morii N., Nakao K., Matsumori A. *et al.* Increased synthesis and secretion of atrial natriuretic polypeptide during viral myocarditis. *J Cardiovasc Pharmacol* 1989; **13** (suppl 6): 5–8.

42. Bowles N. E., Richardson P. J., Olsen E. G. J., Archard L. G. Detection of coxsackie-B-virus specific RNA sequence in myocardial biopsy samples from patients with myocarditis and dilated cardiomyopathy. *Lancet* 1986; **ii**: 1120–2.

43. Kandolf R., Ameis D., Kirshner P. *et al. In situ* detection of enteroviral genomes in myocardial cells by nucleic acid hybridization: an approach to the diagnosis of viral heart disease. *Proc Natl Acad Sci (USA)* 1987; **84**: 6272–6.

44. Easton A. J., Eglin R. P. The detection of coxsackievirus RNA in cardiac tissue by *in situ* hybridization. *J Gen Virol* 1988; **69**: 285–91.

45. Cronin M. E., Love L. A., Miller F. W. *et al.* The natural history encephalomyocarditis virus-induced myositis and myocarditis in mice: viral persistence demonstrated by *in situ* hybridization. *J Exp Med* 1988; **168**: 1639–48.

46. Okada I., Matsumori A., Kawai C. *et al.* The viral genome in experimental murine coxsackievirus B3 myocarditis: a northern blotting analysis. *J Molec Cell Cardiol* 1990; **22**: 999–1008.

47. Matsumori A., Crumpacker C. S., Abelmann W. H., Kawai C. Virus vaccine and passive immunization for the prevention of viral myocarditis in mice. *Jpn Circ J* 1987; **51**: 1362–4.

48. Murnane T. G., Craighead J. E., Mondragon J., Shelekov A. Fatal disease of swine due to encephalomyocarditis virus. *Science* 1960; **131**: 498–9.

49. Helwig F. C., Schmidt E. D. H. A filter-passing agent producing interstitial myocarditis in anthropoid apes and small animals. *Science* 1945; **102**: 31–3.

50. Matsumori A., Crumpacker C. S., Abelmann W. H. Pathogenesis and preventive and therapeutic trials in an animal model of dilated cardiomyopathy induced by a virus. *Jpn Circ J* 1987; **51**: 661–4.

51. Weck P. K., Rinderknecht E., Estell D. A, Stebbing N. Antiviral activity of bacteria-derived human alpha interferons against encephalomyocarditis virus infection of mice. *Infection and Immunity* 1982; **35**: 660–5.

52. Gresser I., Tovey M. G., Bandu M.-T. *et al*. Role of interferon in the pathogenesis of virus diseases in mice as demonstrated by the use of anti-interferon serum. I. Rapid evolution of encephalomyocarditis virus infection. *J Exp Med* 1976; **144:** 1305–15.

53. Matsumori A., Crumpacker C. S, Abelmann W. H. Prevention of viral myocarditis with recombinant human leukocyte interferon-α A/D in a murine model. *J Am Coll Cardiol* 1987; **9:** 1320–5.

54. Kandolf R., Canu A., Hofschneider P. H. Coxsackie B3 virus can replicate in cultured human foetal heart cells and is inhibited by interferon. *J Molec Cell Cardiol* 1985; **17:** 167–81.

55. Lutton C. W, Gauntt C. J. Ameliorating effect of IFN-β and anti-IFN-β on coxsackievirus B3-induced myocarditis in mice. *J Interferon Res* 1985; **5:** 137–46.

56. Sasaki O., Karaki T., Imanishi J. Protective effect of interferon in infections with hand, foot and mouth disease virus in newborn mice. *J Infect Dis* 1986; **153:** 498–502.

57. Matsumori A., Tomioka N., Kawai C. Protective effect of recombinant alpha interferon on coxsackievirus B3 myocarditis in mice. *Am Heart J* 1988; **115:** 1229–32.

58. Knight V., McClung H. W., Wilson S. Z. *et al*. Ribavirin small particle aerosol treatment of influenza. *Lancet* 1981; **ii:** 945–9.

59. Hall C. B., McBride J. T., Walsh E. E. *et al*. Aerosolized ribavirin treatment of infants with respiratory syncytial viral infection: a randomized double-blind study. *N Engl J Med* 1983; **308:** 1443–7.

60. Matsumori A., Wang H., Abelmann W. H., Crumpacker C. S. Treatment of viral myocarditis with ribavirin in an animal preparation. *Circulation* 1985; **71:** 834–9.

61. Carswell E. A., Old L. J., Kassel R. L. *et al*. An endotoxin-induced serum factor that causes necrosis of tumors. *Proc Natl Acad Sci (USA)* 1975; **72:** 3666–70.

62. Mestan J., Digel W., Mittnacht S. *et al*. Antiviral effects of recombinant tumor necrosis factor *in vitro*. *Nature* 1987; **323:** 816–19.

63. Reis L. F. L., Le J., Hirano T. *et al*. Antiviral action of tumor necrosis factor in human fibroblasts is not mediated by B cell stimulatory factor 2/IFN-β₂, and is inhibited by specific antibodies to IFN-β. *J Immunol* 1988; **140:** 1566–70.

64. Rook A. H., Masur H., Lane C. *et al*. Interleukin-2 enhances the depressed natural killer and cytomegalovirus-specific cytotoxic activities of lymphocytes from patients with the acquired immune deficiency syndrome. *J Clin Invest* 1983; **72:** 398–403.

65. Siegel J. P., Rook A. H., Djeu J. Y., Quinnan G. V. Jr. Interleukin 2 therapy in infectious disease: rationale and prospects. *Infection* 1985; **13** (suppl 2): 219–22.

66. Gaulton G. N., Bangs J., Maddock S. *et al*. Characterization of a monoclonal rat anti-mouse interleukin 2 (IL-2) receptor antibody and its use in the biochemical characterization of the murine IL-2 receptor. *Clin Immunol Immunopathol* 1985; **36:** 18–29.

67. Kirkman R. L., Barrett L. V., Gaulton G. N. *et al*. The effect of anti-interleukin-2 receptor monoclonal antibody on allograft rejection. *Transplantation* 1985; **40:** 719–22.

68. Kilbourne E. D., Wilson C. B., Perrier D. The induction of gross myocardial lesions by a coxsackie (pleurodynia) virus and cortisone. *J Clin Invest* 1956; **35:** 362–70.

69. Mason J. W., Billingham M. E., Ricci D. R. Treatment of acute inflammatory myocarditis assisted by endomyocardial biopsy. *Am J Cardiol* 1980; **45:** 1037–44.

70. Fenoglio J. J. Jr., Ursell P. C., Kellogg C. F. Diagnosis and classification of myocarditis by endomyocardial biopsy. *N Engl J Med* 1983; **308:** 12–18.

71. Tomioka N., Kishimoto C., Matsumori A., Kawai C. Effects of prednisolone on acute viral myocarditis in mice. *J Am Coll Cardiol* 1986; **7:** 868–72.

72. Monrad E. S., Matsumori A., Murphy J. C. *et al*. Theraphy with cyclosporine in

experimental murine myocarditis with encephalomyocarditis virus. *Circulation* 1986; **73**: 1058–64.

73. Matoba Y., Matsumori A. Cyclosporine accelerates the development of anti-heart antibody in viral myocarditis in mice. *Circulation* 1987; **76** (suppl IV): 264.

74. O'Connell J. B., Reap E. A., Robinson J. A. The effect of cyclosporine on acute murine coxsackie B3 myocarditis. *Circulation* 1986; **73**: 353–9.

75. Kino T., Hatanaka H., Miyata S. *et al*. FK-506, a novel immunosuppressant isolated from a streptomyces: immunosuppressive effect of FK-506 *in vitro*. *J Antibiot* 1987; **40**: 1256–65.

76. Ochiai T., Nakajima K., Nagata M. Studies of the effects of FK506 on renal allografting in the beagle dog. *Transplantation* 1987; **44**: 729–33.

77. Sawada S., Suzuki G., Kawase Y., Takaku F. Novel immunosuppressive agent, FK506: *in vitro* effects on the cloned T cell activation. *J Immunol* 1987; **139**: 1797–803.

78. Captopril multicenter research group: a placebo controlled trial of captopril in refractory chronic congestive heart failure. *J Am Coll Cardiol* 1983; **2**: 755–63.

79. A cooperative multicenter study of captopril in congestive heart failure: hemodynamic effects and long term response. *Am Heart J* 1985; **110**: 439–47.

80. Kenneth J., Duchen K., Hudes E. M., Mcgiff J. C. The antihypertensive effect of captopril in essential hypertension: relationship to prostaglandins and the kallikrein–kinin system. *J Hypertension* 1987; **5**: 121–8.

81. Suzuki H., Matsumori A. Myocardial injury due to viral myocarditis improved by captopril in mice. *Circulation* 1990; **82** (suppl III): 674.

82. Rezkalla S., Kloner R. A., Khatib G., Khatib R. Beneficial effects of captopril in acute coxsackievirus B_3 murine myocarditis. *Circulation* 1990; **81**: 1039–47.

83. Nucci G., Warner T., Vane J. R. Effect of captopril on the bradykinin-induced release of prostacyclin from guinea-pig lungs and bovine aortic endothelial cells. *Br J Pharmacol* 1988; **95**: 783–8.

84. Westlin W., Mullane K. Dose captopril attenuate reperfusion induced myocardial dysfunction by scavenging free radicals? *Circulation* 1988; **77** (suppl 1): 30–9.

85. Petrone W. F., English D. K., Wong K., McCord J. M. Free radicals and inflammation: superoxide-dependent activation of a neutrophil chemotactic factor in plasma. *Proc Natl Acad Sci (USA)* 1980; **77**: 1159–63.

86. Waagstein F., Hjalmarson A., Varnauskas E., Wallentin I. Effect of chronic beta-adrenergic receptor blockade in congestive cardiomyopathy. *Br Heart J* 1975; **37**: 1022–36.

87. Swedberg K., Hjalmarson A., Waagstein F., Wallentin I. Prolongation of survival in congestive cardiomyopathy by beta-receptor blockade. *Lancet* 1979; **i**: 1374–9.

88. Waagstein F., Caidahi K., Wallentin I. *et al*. Long-term β-blockade in dilated cardiomyopathy: effects of short- and long-term metoprolol treatment followed by withdrawal and readministration of metoprolol. *Circulation* 1989; **80**: 551–63.

89. Gilbert E. M., Anderson J. L., Deitchman D. *et al*. Long-term β-blocker vasodilation therapy improves cardiac function in idiopathic dilated cardiomyopathy: a double-blind, randomized study of bucindolol versus placebo. *Am J Med* 1990; **88**: 223–9.

90. Rezkalla S., Kloner R. A., Khatib G. *et al*. Effect of metoprolol in acute coxsackievirus B3 murine myocarditis. *J Am Coll Cardiol* 1988; **12**: 412–14.

91. Tominaga M., Matsumori A., Okada I. *et al*. β-blocker treatment of dilated cardiomyopathy: beneficial effect of carteolol in mice. *Circulation* 1991; **86**: 2021–8.

6

Pathogenesis of disease: humans

B. Maisch, M. Herzum and U. Schönian

Introduction

> We have examined the course and sequelae of inflammatory processes and abcesses of the heart. But what is the fruit of our investigations? The inflammation of the heart is difficult to diagnose and if we have diagnosed it, can we then treat it better?
>
> (J. B. Senac, 1772; private physician of the ordinary to Louis XV[1])

Two hundred and twenty years after J. B. Senac[1] our knowledge about viral infections of the heart has expanded immensely. In the 18th century inflammation was a common cause of disease. Cardiotropic viruses and bacteria, however, were not yet known as causes of disease. In 1899, more than 100 years later, P. von Schroetter[2] postulated that 'the most important role in aetiology of heart failure is played by inflammatory processes of myocardium'. At that time the incidence of coronary heart disease was underestimated and most disease processes were attributed to inflammation. Such diseases which are now defined as viral myocarditis, pericarditis or myopericarditis were described as early as 1854,[3] long before it was possible to isolate viruses, conduct serological studies or employ molecular biological techniques. Descriptions of myocardial involvement in mumps,[4] influenza, cytomegalovirus and Epstein–Barr virus followed a century later (Table 6.1). Pleuropericarditis occurring as a complication of Bornholm disease or pleurodynia[5] was described long before its viral origin was identified (Table 6.1).

Gore and Saphir[56] classified a large cohort of what was probably fairly heterogenous forms of myocarditis patients in 1947 and reviewed their findings some 20 years later.[66]

In the second half of the 20th century the essential role of viruses in inducing and in some cases in perpetuating heart disease, with its facets of myocardial, pericardial and endocardial involvement as well as the involvement of the vascular endothelium and the conduction system, have been described.

In an attempt to characterize the central haemodynamics of chronic heart disease as well as its aetiology, the World Health Organization/International Society and Federation of Cardiology (WHO/ISFC) task force defined cardiomyopathy in 1980[67] as heart muscle disease of unknown cause and classified cardiomyopathies as being hypertrophic, dilated or restrictive.

Table 6.1 Viral heart disease in humans.

Classification	Virus	Selected references
RNA virus		
Picornavirus	Coxsackie A	6–8
(Enterovirus)	Coxsackie B	0–20, 148, 190–192
	Echovirus	21–22
	Poliovirus	23–28
Orthomyxovirus	Influenza A + B	29–33
Paramyxovirus	Mumps	34
	Measles	35
Arbovirus*	Chikunguna	36, 37
	Dengue	
	Yellow fever	37, 38
Rubivirus	Rubella	39
Rhabdovirus	Rabies	40, 41
Arenavirus	Lymphocytic choriomeningitis	42
DNA virus		
Herpesvirus	Cytomegalovirus	43–47
	Epstein-Barr-Virus	48
	Varicella-zoster	49–52
	Herpes simplex	53
Adenovirus	Adenovirus	36, 54, 55
Poxvirus	Vaccinia	58–60
Hepadnavirus	Hepatitis B	61, 62
Retrovirus	HIV-1	63–65

Updated from Woodruff 1980.[137] See also Chapter 1, Table 1.1.
*The term arbovirus is no longer in use in taxonomy and includes viruses in a number of different families, particularly togaviruses.

More recently, a better understanding of viral heart disease including cardiomyopathy has been achieved. This resulted from development and implementation of techniques in molecular biology, experimental and clinical immunology, virology and biochemistry:

1. Although it is well established that humoral antibody responses directed against certain viruses may be present in patients with acute myocarditis and dilated cardiomyopathy (DCM),[68–70] such molecular biological techniques as dot blot[17] and *in situ* hybridization[18,71] have recently shown that enterovirus RNA can be detected in the myocardium of patients with myocarditis and DCM. Furthermore, employing dot blot hybridization, cytomegalovirus DNA has been detected in the myocytes as well as in the endothelial and interstitial cells of the heart, even after the overt inflammatory process has subsided.[45–47]
2. Both cellular and humoral autoreactivity have been clearly demonstrated in myocarditis[72–105] and dilated heart muscle disease.[85–87,89–115] In addition mediators and soluble factors of inflammation, and *de novo* expression of major histocompatibility antigens have been identified.[116–119] Thus, although immunocardiology is beginning to answer some questions relating to the pathogenesis of myocarditis and perimyocarditis, it remains to be determined whether:
   (a) Histologically validated myocarditis according to the Dallas criteria (see Chapter 3),[120] or essentially similar definitions[86,90,93,121–127] are

identical with or are just a minor part of the newly evolving entity of immune-mediated heart disease?[91,128] How should the latter be defined?

(b) The virus is the only trigger of myocardial lesions induced at a later time by immune cells and antibodies as has been suggested by studies of myocarditis employing animal models[77–79,81,84,128–130,131–141] or whether the virus is killing the myocytes and interstitial cells alone or whether both mechanisms are involved? What might their relative contributions be in the different forms of acute and chronic myocarditis?

This chapter describes current knowledge on viral heart disease in humans in relation to the interplay with the autoimmune system. Different clinical entities will be briefly defined before their pathogenesis in relation to cardiotrophic viruses and autoreactive heart muscle disease is discussed.

Definition of the myocarditis–perimyocarditis syndrome

The interaction of the virus in the heart involves all tissue compartments to a varying extent. In addition to host factors and other such factors as the tissue tropism of the virus, its virulence and its immunoreactivity interact to produce a variable clinical picture. Recently developed diagnostic tests may shed further light on the role of viral infections of the heart although it must be appreciated that access to such investigations may not always be available. Although different tissue compartments of the heart are likely to be involved in virus infections, most patients are usually classified as having a myocarditis, pericarditis or 'cardiomyopathy'. Because of this, it is important to establish a clear definition of the different forms of cardiac disease for clinical and scientific purposes.

Histologically validated myocarditis is defined as active, healing or healed myocarditis[138] according to Aretz *et al.*[120,138] (Table 6.2). It has been suggested recently that acute forms of myocarditis should be subclassified clinically and histologically into fulminant forms which cause either death as a result of acute and severe complications (cardiogenic shock) or result in a virtually complete recovery. Alternatively, chronic forms with incomplete recovery and a poor long-term prognosis may occur.[139,140] Japanese authors have suggested criteria to separate acute from chronic forms.

Chronic myocarditis remains a controversial diagnosis histologically although the clinical features of chronicity are well established.[123] Recent studies on the secondary immunopathogenesis in protracted forms of perimyocarditis and in enteroviral heart disease with viral persistence suggests that an effort to reintroduce this term in a clinical context may be worthwhile.[194] Further subclassification into chronic and chronic persistent forms[110,121,139] has been suggested but this has yet to be generally accepted.

Perimyocarditis is defined as 'pericardial effusion and cardiomegaly or a segmented wall motion abnormality'. Demonstration of pericardial effusion (in the absence of neoplastic, postradiation or postinjury syndromes or uraemia) confirms the presence of an inflammatory, epicardial or pericardial process, cardiac dilation or wall motion abnormality.[90–92] As already pointed

Table 6.2   Criteria for myocarditis and perimyocarditis, dilated cardiomyopathy and postmyocarditic heart muscle disease.

Myocarditis and perimyocarditis
Essential criteria:
1.   Inflammation of the myocardium determined by biopsy/necropsy with infiltrate, focal necrosis, interstitial oedema) with or without fibrosis. According to Daly et al.[138] and Aretz et al.[120] one can distinguish different forms of *myocarditis*:
     Active myocarditis (prominent infiltrate close to myofibres, necrosis ± fibrosis
     Healing myocarditis (scarce (interstitial) infiltrate, fibrosis, no or very little necrosis)
     Healed myocarditis (2nd biopsy: focal fibrosis, no infiltrate; but in 1st biopsy: active inflammation)
     or
2.   Pericardial rubs or pericardial effusion with segmental wall motion abnormality and dysrhythmia after exclusion of coronary artery disease by coronary angiography (= *perimyocarditis*)

Additional criteria
     Positive RNA or DNA probe for cardiotropic viruses
     A more than threefold alteration of titre in complement-fixation or neutralization tests against cardiotropic viruses

Dilated cardiomyopathy
Essential criteria
     Cardiomegaly in laevocardiography (left ventricular end-diastolic volume index >100 ml/m^2 and reduced ejection fraction ($<55\%$)
     Exclusion of coronary artery disease, valvular heart disease, hypertension and other forms of secondary heart muscle diseases, e.g. diabetes mellitus, neuroendocrine disorder, alcohol consumption

Addition criteria
     Indicative histomorphology with hypertrophy and branching of myocytes, diffuse or focal fibrosis

Postmyocarditic heart muscle disease
     Biopsy-proven cellular infiltrate in 1st biopsy and missing infiltrate in 2nd biopsy
     or
     Perimyocarditis proven by clinical criteria (above) at 1st examination; no infiltrate in 2nd biopsy but cardiomegaly with reduced ejection fraction at the 2nd examination

out by Woodruff,[137] viral pericarditis is nearly always associated with underlying epicardial and myocardial lesions which lead to the use of such terms as myopericarditis[9] or more precisely perimyocarditis.[90] Since myocarditis is not always associated regularly with pericardial effusion, both clinical entities, although not identical, overlap. For such patients a biopsy which may provide evidence of active inflammation although not obligatory may be helpful.

Pericarditis is defined as an increase in pericardial fluid in the absence of noninflammatory causes (Table 6.3). Acute forms are distinguished from chronic, chronic-recurring and constrictive forms of pericarditis. In some patients a pericardial rub may be the only clinical manifestation of pericarditis. However, echocardiography provides the most sensitive and reliable diagnostic investigation since it frequently demonstrates the presence of an effusion which may be manifest by a separation of the epicardial and pericardial layers (Table 6.3).[16,142a–b]

Inflammatory heart muscle disease includes myocarditis and pericarditis as well as rejection episodes following cardiac transplantation. The terms chronic and acute (as in Fig. 6.1) which are used in this chapter relate to a

Table 6.3 (Part 1)   Aetiology, pathophysiology and pathogenesis of the acute pericarditis syndrome and present therapeutical options (see also Table 1.1, 3.1 and 3.2).

Aetiological classification	Incidence*	Therapeutic options*
1. **Idiopathic pericarditis**	26*	Physical restraint; aspirin 3 g/d or corticoids in case of recurrence (initial dose: 100 mg/d) PC or PD for diagnostic reasons and in tamponade
2. **Infectious pericarditis**		PC or PD for diagnostic reasons and
2.1 *Viruses*	10*	in tamponade; physical restraint, immunoglobulins; specific therapy is mostly experimental
2.1.2 Coxsackie A and B		(interferon)
2.1.3 Echovirus (e.g. type 4)		
2.1.4 Cytomegalovirus		(Hyperimmune sera and/or
2.1.5 Epstein–Barr (post-transfusion syndrome)		gancyclovir)
2.1.6 Mumps		
2.1.7 Herpes simplex		
2.1.8 Varicella-zoster		
2.1.9 Hepatitis B		(Hyperimmune sera, interferon)
2.2 *Bacteria*	8*	
2.2.1 Tuberculosis	4*	PC; tuberculostatic therapy (isoniazid 300 mg/d and rifampicin 600 mg/d for 9 months) ethnambutol 25 mg/kg/d for 2 months; prednisone 1 mg/kg/d for 2 months, tapered off
2.2.2 Pneumococcus		Sensitive to antibiotics
2.2.3 Staphylococcus		Sensitive to antibiotics
2.2.4 Streptococcus		Sensitive to antibiotics
2.2.5 Gram-negative rods and Haemophilus		Sensitive to antibiotics
2.2.6 Gonococcus		Sensitive to antibiotics
2.2.7 *Legionella pneumophia*		Sensitive to antibiotics
2.2.8 Rickettsiosis		Tetracycline for 3–6 months
2.2.9 Borreliosis		Long-term antibiotics for 3–6 months
2.3 *Fungo-bacterial*	Rare	
2.3.1 Actinomyces		Selected antimycotic treatment
2.3.2 Nocardia		Selected antimycotic treatment
2.4 *Fungal*	Rare	
2.4.1 Candida		Selected antimycotic treatment
2.4.2 Histoplasmosis		Selected antimycotic treatment
2.4.3 Blastomycosis		Selected antimycotic treatment
2.4.5 Coccidioidomycosis		Selected antimycotic treatment
2.5 *Parasitic*	Rare	
2.5.1 Amoebiasis		Metronidazol 3 × 0.5–0.75 mg/d (2 weeks) or dehydroemetin 1 mg/kg 2 × /d (max. dose 1 g)
2.5.2 Echinococcosis		No puncture but surgery, if possible, to eliminate the cysts, otherwise poor prognosis
2.5.3 Toxoplasma gondii		Pyrimetamin and sulphadiazin or spiromycin with limited success, wide pericardiectomy
2.6 *Other inflammatory disorders*	Rare	
2.6.1 Sarcoidosis		See 1.0 or 3.1

Table 6.3 (Part 1) – *contd.*

2.6.2	Amyoloidosis,	
2.6.3	Inflammatory bowel disease	See 1.0
2.6.4	Whipple's disease	See 1.0, PC or PD in case of tamponade
2.6.5	Temporal arteritis	See 1.0 or 3.1
2.6.7	Behçet's syndrome	See 1.0 or 3.1

*See Table 6.3, Part 2.
PC = pericardiocentesis. PD = pericardiectomy.

Table 6.3 (Part 2) Aetiology, pathophysiology and pathogenesis of the acute pericarditis syndrome and present therapeutical options.

Aetiological classification	Incidence*	Therapeutical options*
3. **Immunologically mediated**	30*	
3.1 *Postinfectious, secondary autoimmune* (often relapsing)	14*	Physical restraint; prednisone: initial dose 1.25 mg/kg/d for 4 weeks, 2–3 months 0.3 mg/kg/d, then tapered off, azathioprin: initial dose 2 mg/kg/d for 4 weeks, 2–3 months 0.85 mg/kg/d. In case of recurrence: Colchicin initial dose 3 mg for 2 days, then 2 mg for 2 days, 1 mg for 3–12 months
3.2 *Postcardiac injury syndromes* (delayed hypersensitivity reactions)	16*	
Postcardiotomy syndrome (p10th d) – (DD: early booster 3rd–5th day)	30†	Postoperatively; restraint of physical activity, small effusions: antiphlogistics (aspirin 1–3 g/d for 8–12 weeks); larger effusions: prednisone as in 3.1, azathioprin is rarely needed
3.3 *Postinfarction (Dressler's) syndrome* (DD: pericarditis epistenocardica	5†	Of infarctions; therapy see 3.2 after 1–2 days of infarct only antiphlogistics
3.4 *In systemic connective tissue disease and autoimmune disorders*	7*	
3.4.1 Acute rheumatic fever		Aspirin 6–8 g/d or 1–2 mg/kg/d prednisone
3.4.2 Systemic lupus erythematosus	35†	See 3.1 or cyclophosphamide
3.4.3 Rheumatoid arthritis	30†	See 3.1
3.4.4 Still's disease	7†	See 2.1
3.4.5 Spondylitis ankylosans	1†	See 3.1
3.4.6 Reiter's syndrome	2†	See 3.1
3.4.7 Systemic sclerosis	56†	See 3.1
3.4.8 Mixed connective tissue disease		See 3.1
3.4.9 Wegner's granulomatosis		Cyclophosphamide 2 mg/kg/d and 60 mg prednisone or see 3.1
3.4.10 Churg–Strauss syndrome/vasculitis		See 3.4.9
Panarteriitis nodosa		See 3.4.9
4. **Trauma**	1*	
Haemopericardium		Following trauma, surgery, pacemaker insertion; PC or PD

Table 6.3 (Part 2) – *contd.*   Aetiology, pathophysiology and pathogenesis of the acute pericarditis syndrome and present therapeutical options.

Aetiological classification	Incidence*	Therapeutical options*
Pneumopericardium		Following trauma, surgery, pacemaker insertion; PC or PD (With secondary immunopathogenesis) possible
Postradiation		
5. **Uremia** Untreated renal failure During ineffective hemodialysis	12*	
6. **Neoplastic**	17*	PC for diagnostic purposes, intrapericardial Cisplatinum
7. **Myxoedema**	0.5*	Thyroid hormones
8. **Chylopericardium**	Rare	Surgery to ligate thoracic duct
9. **Hydropericardium**	30*	Diuretics and classic heart failure therapy (4 D's) with ACE inhibitors

Modified from Maisch.[103]
PC = pericardiocentesis. PD = pericardiectomy.
*Incidence of pericarditis in proportion to the total number of pericarditis patients on the Marburg Registry of pericardial diseases 1980–1992.
†Incidence of pericarditis in the course of the systemic disorders (from Maisch[103]).

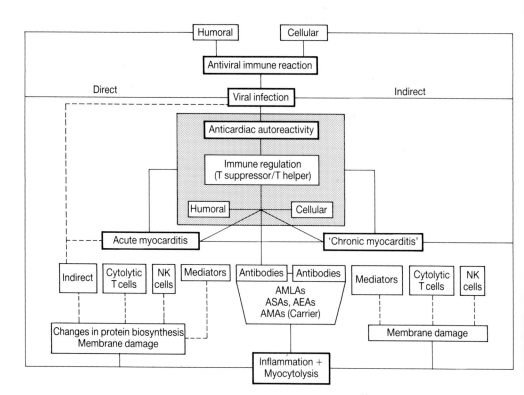

Fig. 6.1   Present status of anti-viral and anti-cardiac autoreactivity in myocarditis and viral heart disease. Reproduced with permission from Maisch.[143]

clinical rather than a histological diagnosis and cover both myocarditis and pericarditis.

Dilated heart muscle disease is either idiopathic (DCM) (Table 6.2), or secondary to other causes, which may be viral myocarditis,[144] a viral perimyocarditis or an autoreactive process (Table 6.2). The diagnostic criteria for perimyocarditis or dilated heart muscle disease are summarized in Table 6.2.

Viral heart disease may be defined if structural abnormalities in inflammatory or dilated heart disease are associated with the presence of virus, viral RNA or DNA in the myocardium. The association of electrical, haemodynamic or structural abnormalities in the heart in the context of an apparent viral illness only provides circumstantial evidence of viral heart disease.

Immune-mediated heart disease or secondary immunopathogenesis refers to patients with either inflammatory heart disease or dilated heart muscle disease with signs of autoimmunity.[128,145] Several forms of this disorder were recently described employing immunological and immunohistopathologic techniques as well as by *in vitro* assays of humoral and cellular autoreactivity (Table 6.4).

Histological diagnosis in viral or autoimmune heart disease in humans

Although the Dallas criteria for myocarditis[120,138] are now widely accepted, problems relating to this classification, as well as other histopathologic definitions, are centred around three issues:[146,147]

1. *Interobserver variability*: Even using the same histopathologic criteria, Shanes *et al.*[147] demonstrated considerable variation in the interpretation of the Dallas criteria by different pathologists.
2. A clinical definition of myocarditis varies widely and may not equate in different centres. For example, Lie[148] when comparing the incidence of myocarditis as a cause of heart failure, observed figures ranging from 2.5 to 67% and concluded that, as different centres produced markedly variable figures, the predictability of a correct diagnosis of myocarditis was extremely low.

Improved diagnostic approaches in viral heart disease in humans

The diagnosis of viral heart disease cannot be established from clinical features alone with sufficient validity. Assessing serum antibody titres in suspected cases is of limited diagnostic value except, perhaps, when certain viruses are prevalent in the community. However, high titres to coxsackie B viruses have been reported in patients with DCM[70] and molecular genetic techniques are now becoming of increasing value in defining the role of enteroviruses[17,71] and cytomegaloviruses,[46,47] and in conducting studies to establish their role in the pathogenesis of acute and chronic heart disease. Employing *in situ* hybridization, Kandolf and Hofschneider[18] demonstrated the presence of enterovirus RNA in endomyocardial biopsies in 19 of 81 patients with suspected myocarditis and 8 of 27 with DCM. Employing a dot

Table 6.4 Immunologic classification of dilated heart muscle diseases.

	Endomyocardial biopsy			Peripheral blood					
	Lymphocytic infiltrate	IgG,M,A,C3 binding	Class II expr. on M[1]	Cardio-LC[2]	NK-cell act[3]	AMLAs[4] or anti-ANT ab	AFAs[5]	matrix ab	ab/AEA[6]
Myocarditis	++	++	+	+	Reduced		++		+
Perimyocarditis	++	++	+	+	Reduced	++		+	
Pericarditis	−	+	+/−	−*	=	+		−	
Postmyoc. HMD†	−	++	−	+	Reduced	++/+		+	
DCM‡	−	+/−	−	+/−	Reduced/=	+	+		+

= unchanged.
− negative.
+ positive finding in more than 50% of patients.
++ positive finding in more than 80% of patients.
1 myocytes.
2 lymphocytotoxicity to isolated rat heart cells by peripheral blood lymphocytes (non-MHC controlled lymphocytotoxicity).
3 Natural killer cell activity to K562 erythroblast cell line (Perlmann & Perlmann 1971)
4 antimyolemmal antibodies.
5 antifibrillary antibodies mostly from the antimyosin type.
6 antiendothelial antibodies.
*No cardiocytotoxicity of peripheral blood lymphocytes but strong lymphocytotoxicity from lymphocytes of the pericardial fluid (unpublished).
†Heart muscle disease.
‡Dilated cardiomyopathy.

blot technique, Archard *et al.*[149] detected enterovirus RNA in a much higher proportion but this technique is less specific since, unlike *in situ* hybridization, it does not demonstrate the presence of viral RNA in relation to the tissue architecture. Nevertheless, the accumulated data from these observations suggests that enteroviruses persist in the myocardium and this may well be of importance in the pathogenesis of DCM.

Whether the virus induces an autoreactive cellular and humoral response or is itself responsible for myocardial necrosis remains unresolved.[102,150] Preliminary data, including results from experimental work in myocarditis, show that even using mice experimentally this issue is controversial. Other cardiopathic agents have been defined in the last few years including cytomegalovirus (CMV), influenza A and B, human T cell lymphotropic virus (HTLV) and a bacterial agent B. burgelorferi which causes Lyme disease and responds to treatment with antibiotics. This organism may be associated with up to 20% of patients with myocarditis.[151]

Immune response and structural alterations

Virus induction of myocardial inflammation has been demonstrated in many patients with myocarditis and dilated cardiomyopathy. However, viral persistence does not prove that myocardial inflammation and destruction or the induction of reparative processes are mediated or caused by the virus which may merely have just left only its 'fingerprints'. Some of the reparative features, e.g. hypertrophy, may be controlled by proto-oncogenes, such as *c-myc* and *c-fos* or by collagen genes, which have been expressed *de novo* in different forms of heart disease first having been described in rejection episodes following cardiac transplantation.[152] For the induction of fibrosis in inflammatory heart disease mediators such as the platelet-derived growth factor (A and B) are likely to be an early competence signal, which is followed by a progression signal, e.g. the insulin-derived growth factor. Activated macrophages produce fibronectin, fibroblast growth factor and interleukin-1, which stimulate collagen synthesis. Although the role of cytokines is beginning to emerge in inflammation it is still mostly speculative in myocarditis. Samsonov *et al.*[153] and Klappacher *et al.*[154,155] recently demonstrated that in dilated cardiomyopathy, as in any other form of congestive failure, the neopterin concentration is increased. Neopterin is released by monocytes under control of activated T lymphocytes via interferon-γ thus reflecting T cell activation. Tumour necrosis factor-alpha (TNFα) has also been found to be increased in advanced stages of heart failure regardless of the cause. In addition, β2-microglobulin levels are also increased in dilated cardiomyopathy, due both to impairment of renal function occurring in advanced heart failure as well as to T cell activation. Preliminary studies on the role of mediators in postviral dilated heart muscle disease and in rejection episodes following heart transplantation demonstrate similar findings.

Antigens of the virus in viral heart disease

Before *in situ* hybridization or dot blot techniques were available the diagnosis of viral infection was dependent primarily on detecting humoral anti-viral responses by complement-fixation tests or microneutralization tests to cardiotropic viruses. The circulating anti-viral antibodies, however, did not permit direct diagnosis of viral heart disease, but only confirmation of a viral infection in an individual with cardiac symptoms.

Antigenic mimicry induced via sensitized T cells and autoantibodies, which may cause cardiac damage independent of any viral infection of the myocardium, is now being increasingly recognized in the pathogenesis of myocardial disease.[156]

Immune mechanisms in viral heart disease in humans

Lymphocyte subpopulations and peripheral blood cells

In our own series[87,90,157] peripheral blood leucocyte counts did not show any significant differences between patients with viral or idiopathic myocarditis, perimyocarditis, pericardial effusion, dilated cardiomyopathy or postmyocarditic heart disease and noncardiac controls. Lymphocytosis was observed in a quarter of the patients who only had an acute inflammation, but the distribution of T lymphocyte subpopulations in patients with myocarditis was not significantly different from a control population. However, a significant increase of OKlal-positive B cells and activated T lymphocytes in perimyocarditis and a marginal decrease in T suppressor cells in post-myocarditic heart muscle disease was demonstrated (Table 6.4). In contrast, in primary dilated cardiomyopathy circulating OKMI-positive monocytes were increased.[90]

Lymphocytes from endomyocardial biopsies

Lymphocytes can be outgrown from the biopsies of patients with suspected myocarditis or dilated cardiomyopathy[158] and can be cultured and expanded in the presence of human recombinant interleukin-2 (IL-2). CD4+ cell populations prevailed in two-thirds of patients when compared to CD8+ cells or a mixed population Schultheiß, (personal communication).[158] They may exert natural killer cell activity and produce lymphokines like IL-2.

T suppressor cell activity

The reports of changes of T suppressor cell activity in myocarditis and dilated cardiomyopathy vary considerably. In contrast to other reports[110,159] our patients with myocarditis (assessed according to Breshnihan and Jasin[160]) *in vivo* spontaneous and Con A generated T suppressor cell activity (assessed according to Hallgren and Yunis[161]) did not differ from sex- and age-matched controls without heart disease.[91] In post-myocarditic dilated heart disease, however, in such selected indicator systems as the autologous irradiated mixed lymphocyte reaction and allogenic mitogen stimulation a significant reduction in T suppressor cell activity was seen. There is, however, a broad variance in T suppressor cell activity, both in controls and in patients with acute inflammatory heart disease. Different indicator systems for the assessment of T suppressor cell activity may not possess the same sensitivity in expressing changes in some of the T suppressor cell subpopulations. Thus antigen-specific T suppressor cell activity cannot be excluded although global changes were not observed.

Cellular effector mechanisms in humans

Natural killer cell activity
Natural killer (NK) cell activity in patients with perimyocarditis was markedly decreased in the acute state in all three lymphocyte/target cell ratios examined. In post-myocarditic dilated muscle heart disease, NK cell activity is virtually normal (Table 6.5); in primary dilated cardiomyopathy however, a significant decrease in NK cell activity is observed.[90,106]

Target cell specific non-major histocompatibility complex restricted lymphocytotoxicity
In contrast, in myocarditis target cell specific non-major histocompatibility complex (MHC) restricted lysis against living adult allogenic rat myocytes is sustained or slightly enhanced (Table 6.5). This also occurs in patients with post-myocarditic dilated heart disease and primary dilated cardiomyopathy, a

Table 6.5 Immunohistological findings in endomyocardial biopsy. Würzburg multicentre study (% positive titres $\geq$ +1).

Clinical diagnosis	N	Trivalent	IgG	IgM	IgA	C3	C3 or IgM
Myocarditis (active/acute)	20	100*†	90*†	55*†	70*†	70*†	85*†
Perimyocarditis (active/acute)	20	100*†	100*†	95*†	90*†	90*†	100*†
Status post-myocarditis (no cardiomegaly)	22	100*†	95*†	32*	32*	36*	45*
Status post perimyocarditis (no cardiomegaly)	15	73*	60*	13	7	33*	40*
Post-myocarditic HMD‡ (cardiomegaly)	28	79*	75*	18	36*	61*†	75*
Dilated cardiomyopathy (idiopathic)	50	60*	56*	48*†	8	12	48*
Dilated HMD‡ with increased alcohol intake	20	60*	60*	15	25*	35*	40*
Noncardiac controls	17	12	12	0	0	0	0
Coronary artery disease	100	43*	41*	11	20*	3	14

*$P < 0.05$ by χ^2 analysis when compared to noncardiac controls.
†$P < 0.05$ by χ^2 analysis when compared to coronary artery disease.
‡HMD, heart muscle disease.
Reproduced with permission from Maisch.[93]

third of patients having increased target cell-specific cytotoxicity. Analysis of antibody-dependent cellular cytotoxicity (ADCC) showed little variation from normal.[99]

Myocardial antigens in autoreactive and postviral heart disease

Autoantigens of the myocyte
Various cardiac antigens have been identified as targets for humoral and cellular autoreactivity. They include components identified by light microscopy on cryostat sections (Fig. 6.2) or antigens characterized biochemically or defined by monoclonal antibodies:

1. Antibodies to the cardiac membrane and its constituents

Circulating antimembrane antibodies
Of particular interest are circulating and biopsy-bound antibodies to the membrane of the cardiomyocyte, the sarcolemma and myolemma, to which cytolytic complement-fixing antibodies (AMLAs; Fig. 6.3a) have been demonstrated in coxsackie B virus, mumps and influenza myocarditis.[86,89,90,99,101,157,162] Recent evidence suggests that antigenic mimicry may play an important role: Epitopes on the sarcolemmal surface[105] and to the adenine nucleotide translocator (ANT)-carrier,[163] which in turn shares antigenic properties with the membrane-bound calcium channel, were found to cross-react with coxsackie B viruses. In absorption experiments it was shown that in viral myocarditis the sarcolemmal fluorescence was greatly diminished,

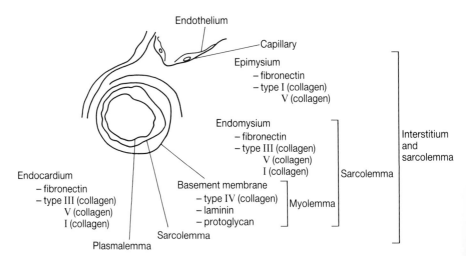

Fig. 6.2 Autoantigens of the heart: Comparison of the classic histological and immunological nomenclature. The myolemma, which can be identified clearly with isolated human heart cells, consists of the plasmalemma, the myolemma and basement membrane and is made up of laminin, proteoglycans, membrane-bound receptors and membrane-specific epitopes. The sarcolemma as identified by immunofluorescence techniques includes the endomysium with fibronectin, type I, II and V collagen. The interstitium comprises the epimysium with its biochemically defined components.

and the cytolytic serum activity could be absorbed by the respective viruses, for example, for coxsackie B and influenza viruses.[90,92,98,99,164]

In addition there was a correlation between the presence of anti-myolemmal antibody titres (AMLAs) and cytolytic serum activity, clearly demonstrating the presence of complement-fixing cytolytic anti-membrane antibodies. In recent work it was shown that the antibodies were cross-reactive with enteroviral core proteins by Western blot analysis.[105]

Antibodies directed against fibronectin, laminin, desmin and vinculin, which are proteins of the extracellular matrix, also stain the 'myolemma' or sarcolemma in isolated heart cells. Monoclonal antibodies to actin, α-actinin and myosin stain both fibrils and sometimes even parts of the membrane (Table 6.5). The incidence of circulating AMLAs and anti-sarcolemmal antibodies in inflammatory and dilated heart muscle disease compared to controls is shown in Table 6.6.

Antibodies to the β-adrenoceptor (BAR) which have been postulated to possess β-blocking activity have recently been shown to be present in patients with dilated cardiomyopathy.[165,166] In contrast β-receptor antibodies that increased the beating frequency of isolated foetal heart cells have been demonstrated.[167] Thus the pathogenic role of BARs *in vivo*, although intriguing, is speculative.

Bound anti-membrane antibodies in endomyocardial biopsy specimens
Anti-membrane antibodies can be found in the peripheral blood and also bound to the sarcolemma (Fig. 6.3b) and the interstitial tissue[93,99,100,168] in the endomyocardial biopsies of patients. In a multicentre study[93] IgG fixation was detected regularly. IgM, IgA and C3 or C1q fixation, however, are of particular diagnostic value indicating secondary immunopathogenesis in the course of an inflammatory or postinflammatory process (Table 6.7).

2. Antibodies to intracellular antigens
Antibodies to **mitochondrial proteins** include the *M7 protein*,[82,83] and its relevant constituent sarcosin dehydrogenase (P. A. Berg, personal communication), and the *anti-nucleotide translocator*,[169–174] which have been found in patients with myocarditis and dilated cardiomyopathy (Table 6.6a–d). The ANT antibodies have also been shown to interfere with the energy metabolism of the myocardial cell in experimental animals *in vitro*. Kühl *et al.*[159,175] have suggested that the anti-nucleotide translocator antibody may cross-react with the calcium channel. Schwimmbeck *et al.*,[174] using synthetic peptides, gave evidence of cross-reactivity between peptides form the adenine nucleotide translocator of the inner mitochondrial membrane and peptides from coxsackie B3 virus. Their findings support the hypothesis that molecular mimicry may be of importance to the pathogenicity of virally induced heart disease.

Antibodies to fibrils (Table 6.6a–d), particularly antibodies to myosin and actin, have been described in human[176] and murine myocarditis.[73] The pathogenetic relevance of anti-myosin antibodies in viral heart disease, however, is still a matter of debate. Cross-reactivity to coxsackievirus proteins, although less likely has not been entirely excluded; cross-reactivity to mitochondrial proteins, although postulated, has also not yet been conclusively demonstrated. Since fibrils lie intracellularly, antibodies directed against them are more likely to be a secondary phenomenon unless sequence homologies to sarcolemmal proteins can be demonstrated.

Table 6.6a Circulating antibodies to the sarcolemma, the extracellular matrix and intermediate filaments (% positive) in healthy controls.

References	n	AMLA (homol)	ASA (homol)	ALA	A-Fibron bands	Z-bands	A-Actin	A-Myosin	A-Tubulin	AIDA	A-Desmin	A-Vimentin	ANT	A-M7	AEA	A-BAR	A-Collagen I	III	IV	V
Maisch et al.[99,100]	200	31	35	nd	nd	5	5	5	0	0	0	0	nd	nd	17	nd	nd	nd	nd	nd
Maisch et al.[105,145]	45	16	18	20	nd	nd	nd	nd	nd	nd	0	nd	nd	nd	nd	nd	nd	nd	nd	nd
Obermayer et al.[177]	25	20	20	nd	nd	0	nd	0	0	nd	4	0	nd	nd	nd	nd	nd	nd	nd	nd
de Scheerder et al.[???]	40	10	5	nd	nd	nd	5	3	nd	nd	nd	nd	nd	0	12	nd	5	5	5	5
Klein et al.[82]	nd	nd	nd	nd	nd	nd	nd	nd	nd	nd	nd	nd	nd	0	nd	nd	nd	nd	nd	nd
Schultheiß et al.[69,73]	nd	nd	nd	nd	nd	nd	nd	nd	nd	nd	nd	nd	nd	nd	nd	nd	nd	nd	nd	nd

Table 6.6b Circulating antibodies to the sarcolemma, the extracellular matrix and intermediate filaments (% positive) in myocarditis and perimyocarditis.

References	n	AMLA (homol)	ASA (homol)	ALA	A-Fibron bands	Z-bands	A-Actin	A-Myosin	A-Tubulin	AIDA	A-Desmin	A-Vimentin	ANT	A-M7	AEA	A-BAR	A-Collagen I	III	IV	V
de Scheerder[94]	12	100	12	nd	nd	nd	58	67	nd	nd	nd	nd	nd	nd	91	nd	35	40	35	35
Klein[82,83]	nd	nd	nd	nd	nd	nd	nd	nd	nd	nd	nd	nd	nd	13	nd	nd	nd	nd	nd	nd
Maisch[99,105,145,164]																				
Viral myocarditis (adults)	44	79–90	75–90	nd	nd	15	7	10–50	0	0	nd	nd	nd	nd	80	nd	nd	nd	nd	nd
Idiopathic myocarditis	144	59	45	nd	nd	nd	0	23	9	0	nd	nd	nd	nd	40	nd	nd	nd	nd	nd
Maisch et al.[90,99] in children	132	100	100	nd	nd	0	0	0	0	0	nd	nd	nd	nd	91	nd	nd	nd	nd	nd
Maisch et al.[164]	nd	nd	nd	30–35	nd	nd	nd	nd	nd	nd	nd	0	nd	nd	nd	nd	nd	nd	nd	nd
Obermayer et al.[177]	25	64	72	nd	nd	16	0	4	0	nd	0	0	nd	nd	72	nd	nd	nd	nd	nd
Schultheiß[69–73]	29	nd	nd	60	nd	20	nd	nd	nd	nd	nd	nd	nd	nd	nd	nd	30	40	35	35

Table 6.6c Circulating antibodies to the sarcolemma, the extracellular matrix and intermediate filaments (% positive) in pericarditis

References	n	AMLA (homol)	ASA (homol)	ALA (homol)	A-Fibron bands	Z-bands	A-Actin	A-Myosin	AIDA	A-Desmin	A-Tubulin	A-Vimentin	ANT	A-M7	AEA	A-BAR	A-Collagen I	III	IV	V
de Scheerder et al.[92]	20	60	60	nd	nd	nd	10	10	nd	nd	nd	nd	nd	nd	70	nd	nd	nd	nd	nd
Maisch et al.[94] Tuberculous pericarditis	10	100	100	nd	nd	0	8	67	0	nd	nd	nd	nd	nd	42	nd	nd	nd	nd	nd
Maisch et al.[94] uremic pericarditis	41	30–83	50–100	nd	nd	0	0	0	0	nd	nd	nd	nd	nd	20–50	nd	nd	nd	nd	nd
Obermayer et al.[177] idiopathic pericarditis	10	80	50	nd	nd	0	nd	nd	nd	0	0	0	0	0	nd	nd	nd	nd	nd	nd

Table 6.6d Circulating antibodies to the sarcolemma, the extracellular matrix and intermediate filaments (% positive) in diluted cardiomyopathy.

References	n	AMLA (homol)	ASA (homol)	ALA (homol)	A-Fibron bands	Z-bands	A-Actin	A-Myosin	AIDA	A-Desmin	A-Tubulin	A-Vimentin	ANT	A-M7	AEA	A-BAR	A-Collagen I	III	IV	V
Klein et al.[82,83]	nd	nd	nd	nd	nd	nd	nd	nd	nd	nd	nd	nd	nd	30	nd	nd	nd	nd	nd	nd
Maisch et al.[94,97]	79	9	10	nd	nd	nd	4	20	2	nd	nd	nd	nd	nd	13	nd	nd	nd	nd	nd
Maisch et al.[100]	30	33	42	nd	nd	nd	10	33	2	nd	nd	nd	nd	nd	45	nd	nd	nd	nd	nd
Schultheiß et al.[69–73]	51	nd	nd	72	nd	nd	nd	nd	nd	nd	nd	nd	nd	nd	nd	nd	12	24	6	24
Obermayer et al.[177]	36	42	31	nd	nd	8	0	8	nd	nd	0	0	nd	nd	31	nd	nd	nd	nd	nd

AMLA Anti-myolemmal antibody; *ASA* anti-sarcolemmal antibody; *ALA* anti-laminin antibody; *A-* anti-; *Fibron* fibronectin; *AIDA* anti-intercalated disc antibody; *ANT* anti-nucleotide translocator; *AEA* anti-endothelial antibody; *Bar* beta-receptor.
Tables 6.6(a–d) are adapted from Maisch[94]

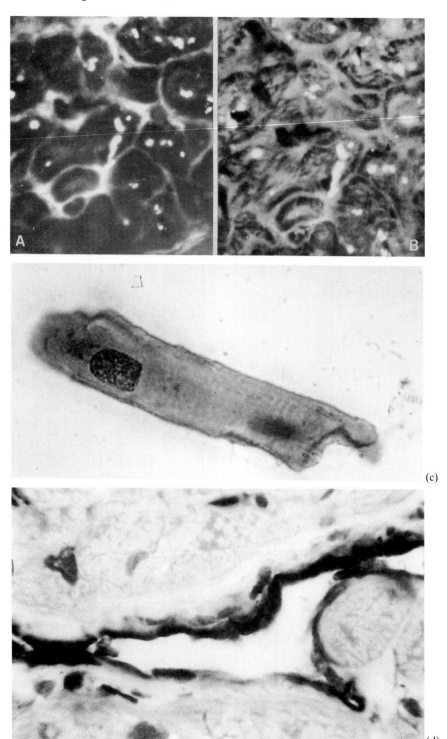

Table 6.7   The Dallas criteria of myocarditis (see also Chapter 3).

1. Active myocarditis: cellular infiltrate in close contact to myofibres, myocytolysis with or without an interstitial oedema
2. Ongoing myocarditis: as in point 1 in a subsequent biopsy
3. Resolving (healing) myocarditis: sparse infiltrate mostly in the interstitial space none or very little myocytolysis in a subsequent biopsy
4. Resolved myocarditis: focal (or diffuse) interstitial fibrosis, which may be rich in cells (mostly fibroblasts) in a subsequent biopsy
5. Borderline myocarditis: sparse infiltrate no myocytolysis: second biopsy recommended

3. Antibodies to the extracellular matrix and to endothelial cells

Further nonorgan-specific but defined antigens include desmin (in myocytes), vimentin, which is present and shows as a marker for fibroblasts and histiocytes, collagen (particularly type III), fibronectin, myosin and actin (reviewed by Maisch 1989).[94]

Table 6.6a–d summarizes the present knowledge on circulating autoantibodies to cardiac epitopes in healthy control patients, and in patients with myocarditis, perimyocarditis, pericarditis and dilated heart muscle disease.

Ubiquitous antigens, which are found in many cells of the body, such as the micro- and intermediate filaments, the macrofilaments or the extracellular matrix constituents, may evoke nonorgan-specific immune responses in contrast to species-specific or even individual-unique epitopes, such as the major histocompatibility complex constituents. The tissue-specific epitopes may be of greater importance in immune disease restricted to the myocardium, whereas in systemic disease, in which the myocardium may also be involved, these or nonspecific proteins (e.g. parts of the cytoskeleton, the extracellular matrix and the microfilaments) may also be involved. Antibodies to the extracellular matrix components have been observed frequently in endomyocardial biopsies[90,94,159,168] but less frequently circulating in the serum of patients with myocarditis.[177]

Renewed interest has also been expressed in relation to the vascular endothelium. *De novo* expression of class I and II antigens of the major histocompatibility complex (Fig. 6.3c) were found in myocarditis.[118,178] In addition anti-endothelial antibodies have been demonstrated in myocarditis. These antibodies which may be cytolytic for living cultured human endothelial cells II (Fig. 6.3d), were demonstrated in endomyocardial biopsy specimens of patients with biopsy-proven myocarditis.

Fig. 6.3   (a) Demonstration of bound anti-myolemmal antibodies (IgG, C3-fixation, IgA) in the endomyocardial biopsy specimen of a 42-year-old male patient with postviral (previous coxsackievirus myocarditis) dilated heart muscle disease. The immunoglobulin binds to the sarcolemma and interstitial space × 800. Anti-human IgG, Medac; dilution 1:1:1000; TRICT-labelled Fab₂-fragments. (b) The identity of bound and circulating (FITC-labelled) anti-sarcolemmal antibodies can be demonstrated in the same patient with a double sandwich technique. × 800. Anti-human IgG, Medac; dilution 1:1000; Fab₂-fragments; serum dilutions 1:320. (c) Demonstration of anti-myolemmal antibodies of the same patient with an isolated intact human atrial cardiocyte × 1200. Anti-human IgG, Medac; dilution 1:1000; Fab₂-fragments; serum dilutions 1:320. (d) *De novo* expression of major histocompatibility complex (MHC) class II antigens at the vascular endothelium in a 29-year-old woman with severe heart failure due to lymphocytic myocarditis. Cytomegalovirus DNA could be demonstrated by *in situ* hybridization.

4. Circulating immune complexes

In viral myocarditis, circulating immune complexes may be present in the majority of patients during the acute phase of the illness.[179] These immune complexes may partly be responsible for some of the systemic features which occur, for example, proteinuria, haematuria or even myalgia, and may be seen in endomyocardial biopsies. By light microscopy, employing indirect immunofluroescence, this deposition cannot be easily distinguished from bound anti-endothelial antibodies.

Autoreactivity of natural antibodies

Figure 6.1 illustrates current views on anti-viral and autoreactive processes in viral heart disease. Autoreactivity, however, is the paradoxical facet of immunoreactivity which is required when a host encounters infection.[180,181] The interactions of viral agents during inflammatory diseases is complex, but the immune response to the invading pathogen is the major host mechanism which determines the severity of the infective disorder, its course, its self-limitation and progression to postinfectious autoimmunity. Coming from Paul Ehrlich's 'horror autotoxicus' and Jerne's[182] 'forbidden clones' it is now believed that autoantibodies, if low in titre or perhaps directed towards external epitopes, although occurring naturally,[183] may be involved in the pathogenesis of myocardial disease.[94]

After a viral infection the extent of the initial immune response in inflammatory myocardial, pericardial and endocardial disease may also be influenced by the genetically determined tropism and virulence of the invading agent as well as the genetic composition of the host.

Antigenic mimicry is an important mechanism by which autoimmune disorders of the heart may result; it may well be that further investigations will reveal additional immunoglobulins belonging to the microheterogeneity of anti-membrane or anti-cardiac antibodies. Their mere presence may be of interest as biological or even prognostic markers, and their possible role may be assessed in relation to their effect on isolated resting or stimulated adult myocytes.[184]

Coxsackievirus-induced myocarditis in humans

The virus (see Chapters 1 and 4)

Many viruses are potentially cardiotropic but enteroviruses, particularly coxsackie B viruses, are most frequently implicated as a cause of myocarditis.[137] coxsackie B viruses are single-stranded RNA viruses of positive sense which are 27–30 nm in diameter and exhibit icosahedral symmetry. The virus attaches to susceptible cells via specific receptors on the cells' surfaces following which it takes over the host's cell machinery in order to synthesize viral RNA and proteins, which eventually results in cell death or a disturbance in its metabolism. Coxsackie B viruses replicate first in the cells of the small gut and the nasopharyngeal mucosa and this may be followed by a viraemia which may result in infection of various organs including the heart and skeletal muscle if the particular virus strain has tropism for the cells in such organs.

This tropism determines, at least in part, the clinical features of infection by coxsackieviruses.

Clinical features

In most cases of human myocarditis and perimyocarditis the patient presents with nonspecific symptoms. Fatigue, precordial discomfort or pain, palpitation, dyspnoea or dyspnoea on exertion or the history of a recent gastro-intestinal infection are prominent features of the disease. In the course of enteroviral myocarditis,[137] acute heart failure with peripheral and pulmonary oedema, dyspnoea at rest and shock is rare, but ominous.

Electrocardiographical changes are frequent, but there is no specific alteration. ST-segments and T-wave abnormalities are observed most often, but A–V block and ventricular arrhythmias are not uncommon.

Echocardiography may disclose left ventricular dilation and pump failure, pericardial effusion and segmental wall motion abnormalities, thereby suggesting heart muscle disease. Texture analysis of the myocardium by echocardiography in order to demonstrate inflammatory process, however, is not yet sufficiently sensitive to substitute for cardiac catheterization. An endomyocardial biopsy is therefore required to establish the diagnosis of myocarditis. Investigations on such specimens are also useful for shedding light on the pathogenesis of inflammatory heart muscle disease, including its aetiology.

Histological studies (see Chapter 3)

The Dallas classification of myocarditis, although still controversial, has proven useful in providing a more generally accepted definition of the histologic features of the disease (Table 6.7).[120]

Aetiological studies

Only on rare occasions is it possible to isolate a coxsackievirus from myocardial tissue.[185,186] Experimental studies in mice have shown that myocardial inflammation is maximal when replicating virus has almost been cleared from cardiac tissue.[187] Serological studies have revealed that a significant proportion of patients have high neutralizing titres to coxsackie B viruses. In relapsing perimyocarditis and DCM, a considerable number of patients were shown to have an enterovirus-specific IgM response in their sera which persisted for up to 10 years after the onset of their initial symptoms.[188] However, a later study failed to confirm these findings.[189] The strongest evidence that coxsackieviruses play a major aetiologic role in human myocarditis has been obtained using hybridization and polymerase chain reaction (PCR) techniques. In patients with the clinical features of myocarditis coxsackie viral RNA was demonstrated in the endomyocardial biopsies of 25 to 52% of cases by *in situ* hybridization and slot blot hybridization, respectively.[18,190] PCR detected coxsackie viral RNA sequences in one out of five patients with biopsy-proven myocarditis or less.[148,191] In endstage idiopathic dilated cardiomyopathy 29% of patients had coxsackie viral-specific RNA sequences in the heart, adding support to the observation that coxsackievirus-induced myocarditis may lead to dilated cardiomyopathy.[192] The significance of persisting coxsackievirus RNA sequences in the heart to the pathogenesis of the disease remains to be clarified. In acute myocarditis, when replicating coxsackievirus can be isolated from the tissue, viral proteins are detectable in the myocardium by specific antisera. In virus culture negative cases, making up for the majority of later stage myocarditis and dilated cardiomyopathy, the presence of viral proteins is much rarer.[193]

Aspects of pathogenesis

A number of factors are likely to be involved in the pathogenesis of coxsackievirus-induced myocarditis. Coxsackieviruses are cytolytic in susceptible cells. *In situ* hybridization studies have shown that in myocarditis the virus infects connective tissue cells as well as the myocytes themselves.[18] It remains to be determined how much the viral infection of the myocyte itself and its sequelae contribute to the clinical features of the disease.

As clinical symptoms of myocarditis are seen mostly after the overt viral disease has subsided, and experimental studies demonstrate humoral and cellular immune reactions towards the myocardium, it has been suggested that the immune system has an important role in inducing coxsackievirus cardiac damage.

As a result of viral infection of the host, humoral immune reactions to the virus and to the cardiocytes develop. Antibodies to the virus are formed to combat infection. However, cross-reactivity of these anti-viral immunoglobulins with cardiac myocytes and sarcolemmal proteins in particular has been demonstrated by immunoabsorption studies with viral proteins and synthetic peptides,[99,163] isolated viral cardiocytes (Fig. 6.4) in a complement-dependent way. This suggests that they have a pathogenic role in inducing the myocyte necrosis seen in histological specimens. Furthermore, anti-idiotypic antibodies to anti-viral antibodies may bind to structures belonging to the virus

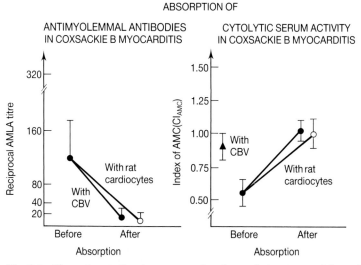

Fig. 6.4 Absorption studies demonstrate that the cytolytic serum activity and anti-myolemmal antibody titre are reduced after absorption of the serum with sarcolemma and enteroviral proteins. Reproduced with permission from Maisch.[99]

receptor on the myocyte cell surface, as has been shown in reovirus infections.[194] Several autoantigens have been described. In experimental coxsackie B3 myocarditis antibodies to cardiac myosin seem to play a major role in mediating late phase myocarditis.[119] In humans anti-myosin antibodies develop in the course of myocarditis; their incidence and pathogenic role in coxsackievirus-induced myocarditis remains to be elucidated. The mitochondrial ADP/ATP translocator is yet another antigenic determinant targetted by humoral immune reactions in human and experimental coxsackievirus myocarditis. A cross-reaction with the calcium channel on the cell surface supports the idea of a pathogenic factor in the pathogenesis of myocarditis.[195]

Knowledge of cellular immune reactions towards the myocardium in coxsackievirus-induced myocarditis stems mainly from experimental models (see Chapter 5) because syngeneic myocardial cells as target cells for cellular immune reactions are barely available in humans. In coxsackie B3 virus-infected mice depletion of T lymphocytes by polyclonal and monoclonal antibodies largely prevent inflammation in the myocardium.[84] Three distinct epitopes expressed on myocardial cells are recognized by cytolytic T lymphocytes (Fig. 6.5). Firstly, CD4+ T cells lyse virally infected cardiocytes trig-

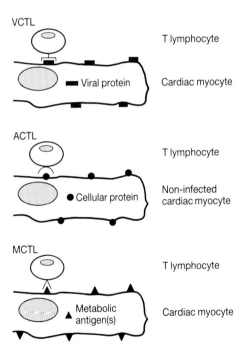

Fig. 6.5 Schematic diagram of the cellular immune response in enteroviral myocarditis as analysed in murine coxsackie B3 virus (CVB3) myocarditis. At least three different receptors for T cells can be postulated. The virus-specific cytolytic T lymphocytes (VCTL) recognize viral proteins on virally infected cardiocytes and lyse them. Restriction by MHC class II antigens is present. The autoimmune cytolytic T cells (ACTL) lyse noninfected cardiac myocytes. It may be that membrane proteins or cardiac myosin is one of the recognized antigens. Restriction by class I MHC antigens is present. The metabolic cytolytic T lymphocytes (MCTL) lyse virally infected cardiac myocytes and react with cellular antigen(s) which are presented after viral or toxic disturbance of the cellular metabolisms.

gered by antigens belonging to coxsackieviruses themselves. A second type of T cell also kills virally infected cells. The recognized antigen appears on the cell surface after infection of the cell with many enteroviruses and actinomycin D, a drug known to inhibit cellular protein synthesis. The findings are suggestive of the formation of an antigen arising from metabolic disturbances by the viral infection of the cell. The third population of cardiocytotoxic T lymphocytes belongs to the CD8+ cytolytic/suppressor cell class which are activated by a yet undefined antigen on normal uninfected cardiac myocyte.[196] Whether a similar pattern exists in human coxsackievirus-induced myocarditis remains to be established.

Therapy of viral and enteroviral myocarditis

Since physical exercise seems to aggravate myocarditis and to promote cardiac dilation,[137] rest and if necessary reduction of cardiac pre- and afterload by vasodilating drugs like angiotensin which convert enzyme inhibitors are promising. As pointed out above, immune reactions to infected and noninfected cardiac tissue are likely to be involved in the pathogenesis of cardiac damage. Therefore, trials with various immunosuppressive drugs have been undertaken, but have yielded ambiguous results so far. A large controlled treatment trial evaluating the usefulness of immunosuppression in myocarditis has just been completed, the results of which will shortly be available.

Influenza virus myocarditis

Influenza is an acute, usually self-limited, febrile illness caused by infection with influenza type A or B virus that occurs in outbreaks of varying severity almost every winter. The attack rates during such outbreaks may be as high as 10–40% over a 5- to 6-week period. The most common clinical manifestations are fever, myalgias and cough, but infection with influenza virus may also produce cardiac disease.

In 1972–1973 during an epidemic with influenza A virus in Sheffield, among 42 patients treated at home, transient ECG changes occurred in 18 cases and permanent changes were found in two cases.[197]

The virus (see also Chapters 1 and 2)

Influenza belongs to the family of orthomyxoviridae, which contains three genera: influenza type A, influenza type B and influenza type C. The morphological characteristics of all influenza virus types and strains are similar (Fig. 1.1). Electron microscopic studies estimate their size to be in the medium range of 80–100 nm in diameter and show them to be enveloped viruses covered with surface projections and spikes. They may exist as spherical or elongated filamentous particles as well.

Eight proteins have been identified in influenza viruses. The surface spikes are glycoproteins which possess either haemagglutinin or neuraminidase activity. The envelope is composed of a lipid bilayer. Within the envelope are eight segmented pieces of nucleocapsid. The nucleocapsid is a double helix formed by a single species of protein, nucleoprotein and by pieces of single-stranded RNA genome. Three other proteins, polymerase proteins, appear to be involved in RNA transcriptase activity. Finally, there is an internal, nonstructural protein of unknown function.

The haemagglutinin is one of the major antigens of the influenza virus. It is the site for attachment of the virus to host cells to initiate infection.

The neuraminidase is another important protein of the influenza virus. The number of infectious units decreases in neuraminidase-defective mutants of the virus and the infectivity titre is reduced accordingly. Viral neuraminidase presumably eliminates receptors on the surface for haemagglutinin that would cause the virus to aggregate and form conglomerates. Thus, neuraminidase appears to protect the virus from its own haemagglutinin.

The inner lipid bilayer portion of the envelope of the influenza virion is derived from the host cell membrane. The matrix or membrane (M) protein is found in close association with the inner surface of the inner lipid layer. The M protein serves as a type-specific antigen.

The nucleocapsid of influenza virus contains the type-specific antigenicity on which the classification of influenza into A, B and C types is based.[198]

Diagnosis of influenza virus myocarditis

The diagnosis of an infection with influenza virus is based on conventional serologic methods such as enzyme immuoassay and complement-fixing tests. Cardiac involvement is probable if after 10 to 30 days of illness cardiac symptoms such as chest pain, dyspnoea, pericardial friction rub and arrhythmia appear. Possible ways of establishing the diagnosis include cultivation of the virus, or the demonstration by *in situ* hybridization of viral RNA in cardiac biopsies.

Pathological findings and pathogenesis

In fatal influenza pneumonia, the tracheobronchial tree shows extensive haemorrhage, hyaline membrane formation and polymorphonuclear cell infiltration.[199,200]

Patients may die suddenly during a mild tracheobronchal infection as a result of haemorraghic pulmonary oedema; haemorrhage and oedema being found in the interstitial myocardial tissue.

The pathological findings include an inflammatory reaction with infiltration of lymphocytes and histiocytes, and interstitial haemorrhage. The myocyte nuclei are enlarged and myocardial fibrils show some fragmentation and loss of striation. Eosinophilc staining is marked and early necrosis can be demonstrated by acid–fuchsin staining.[200]

Immunotyping of the infiltrating cells shows partly a predominance of T helper cells, as well as in part depletion of T cells in the biopsy and in the peripheral blood.

Oseasohn *et al.*[32] reported 27 patients who died of influenza infection. Examination of the heart showed a pale, flabby myocardium and bilateral cardiac dilation. Six patients had subepicardial and subendocardial petechiae and haemorrhagic extravasation. Microscopically, varying degrees of acute inflammation were found in the myocardium of 10 patients, with infiltrates of lymphocytes, monocytes and granular cells. The myocardial fibrils in the vicinity of the exudate were eosinophilic and lost their cross-striations. The infiltrate was found in all portions of the myocardium, including the subepicardial and subendocardial regions. In one case, the inflammatory exudate was accompanied by a haemorrhagic component.

In 1957 Giles *et al.*[22] observed one case of myocarditis among 53 deaths during an influenza epidemic in Britain. Well-marked right-sided and moderate left-sided ventricular hypertrophy and large numbers of neutrophils, eosinophils and plasma cells infiltrating the myocardium and an organizing thrombus which lined the endocardium were observed.

All studies report a predominance of cardiac symptoms in patients with chronic heart disease including valvular heart disease, valve lesions, rheumatic carditis or scars after myocardial infarction.

Immunological mechanisms in influenza myocarditis

In 1982 we described four cases of viral myocarditis associated with a positive complement-fixing test for influenza A and B.[99] In all these patients anti-myolemmal antibodies could be detected by immunofluorescence with titres ranging from 1:20 to 1:80. They could be demonstrated almost immediately after admission to hospital. Nonspecific anti-endothelial antibodies could be detected in three cases. After absorption of the sera with influenza antigens, the anti-myolemmal fluorescence was abolished but not after absorption with other viruses. Antibody-mediated cytolysis of vital heterologous target cells (rat myocytes) had a high score in all cases and disappeared after absorption. Control patients with influenza pneumonitis had no significant titers of anti-myolemmal antibody or cytolysis.[99]

Cytomegalovirus myocarditis

Cytomegalovirus (CMV) has also been implicated as a cause of myocarditis. Acquisition of immunity to this virus is dependent on age and other predisposing factors. In general, the prevalence of antibodies increases progressively with age; a British study showed that 81% of the population aged 35 years or more had CMV antibodies.[201] Infection is usually subclinical although neonatal autopsy studies have shown that 1–2% of patients have evidence of current CMV infection. Although sometimes associated with an infectious mononucleosis-like syndrome in otherwise previously healthy persons, CMV induces severe and sometimes fatal infections in immunocompromised patients, particularly those with leukaemia and lymphoma or during immunosuppression following organ transplantation.

There have been a few sporadic reports implicating CMV as a cause of myocarditis not only in patients in high-risk groups[202] but also occasionally in previously healthy persons.[202,204] In Finland, Klemola *et al.*[205] reported three cases of possible CMV-induced myocarditis in two young adults and an elderly woman; Wilson *et al.*[206] reported a case of a 60-year-old woman who developed CMV-induced myocarditis following a respiratory infection. A further study from Finland[207] reported a CMV myocarditis associated with hepatitis in a 14-year-old boy and Wink and Schmitz[203] isolated CMV from the urine of a 31-year-old man with myocarditis. In 1989 Gowna *et al.*[202] isolated CMV from the explanted heart of a patient who developed DCM following cardiac transplantation.

The virus (see Chapter 1)

Cytomegalovirus belongs to the herpesvirus group. It is a double-stranded DNA virus with an icosahedral capsid consisting of 162 capsomeres; the virus may be surrounded by a lipid-containing envelope. The length of the DNA is 240 kb. Other members of the herpesvirus group are *Herpes simplex* (types 1 and 2), varicella-zoster, Epstein–Barr (EB) and human herpes type 6 viruses. All members of this group may remain latent in the host after initial infection but may reactivate. In the infected cell CMV produces nuclear and paranuclear cytoplasmatic inclusions.

Cytomegalovirus can persist in a host in a latent form despite the presence of an anti-viral the immune response. Virus can be reactivated from cells of infected tissue by cocultivation with susceptible cells without being able to detect the virus directly in disrupted tissue. During certain immune reaction-related events, such as pregnancy, organ transplantation or immune suppressive therapy, reactivation may occur which can be detected by rising titres of CMV antibodies or by virus isolation.[210]

Assessment of a cytomegalovirus infection in humans

In suspected CMV myocarditis, virus isolation from myocardial tissue is of value diagnostically. The virus can be cultured in human diploid fibroblasts. The specific cytopathic effect may not be visible for an interval ranging from 2–3 days to 2–3 weeks, this being dependent on the concentration of virus in the clinical specimen.

A diagnosis may be made serologically by demonstrating a four fold or greater rise in serum antibody titre but patients may present with cardiac features at a point at which antibody levels are not at their maximum. The presence of CMV-specific IgM antibodies provides evidence of a current or recent antigenic stimulus but inconclusive evidence that myocardial involvement is related to CMV infection itself. The demonstration of CMV pre-early, early or late antigens by immunofluorescence in a endomyocardial biopsy is, of course, of more value since this provides direct evidence of CMV involvement of the myocardium.

Employing *in situ* hybridization on endomyocardial biopsies from 20 patients with active myocarditis, 15 in the post myocarditis state and 22 with acute perimyocarditis, CMV DNA was demonstrated in 10% of the patients with active myocarditis and in 7% of those who were in the post myocarditis state. Cytomegalovirus DNA was localized in the nuclei of the endothelium, the interstitial cells and the myocytes (Fig. 6.6).[247] PCR may provide a suitable and perhaps more sensitive alternative for detecting small quantities of viral nucleic acid in myocardial tissue.

Histopathologic changes in cytomegalovirus myocarditis

The cardiovascular manifestations in adults are generally limited to transient electrocardiographic changes; most patients are asymptomatic. Although fatalities are unusual, when they do occur histological examination of the heart may reveal focal lymphocytic infiltration and fibrosis, but without the presence of inclusion bodies.[207]

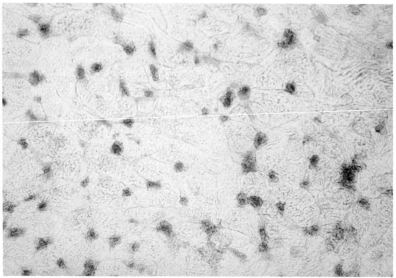

Fig. 6.6   Assessement of cytomegalovirus DNA in an endomyocardial biopsy of a patient with acute myocarditis by *in situ* hybridization

Possible mechanical pathogenesis in cytomegalovirus myocarditis

It is possible that CMV induces cell hyperplasia directly as a result of stimulation by growth factors and cytokines. Virally induced changes in myocardial cells may result in fibrosis. However, indirect mechanisms may be involved, CMV inducing cell damage as a result of adhesion of virus particles to cell surfaces which, in turn, may result in local activation of the immune system, leading to cell damage and necrosis of adjacent cells. Cross-reacting antibodies between CMV and human myocardial tissue may also induce cell damage (molecular mimicry).

Sequence homology between human CMV genes and the gene coding for MHC class molecules in vertebrates has been described. Major histocompatibility complex class 1 molecules bind covalently to β2-microglobulin. Cytomegalovirus may, therefore, bind to the same structure.[210] This finding is in keeping with the detection of CMV bound to β2-microglobulin in the urine of infected patients.[211] The binding of β2-microglobulin to MHC class I antigens and to CMV may result in CMV uptake by the cell. This might result in a loss of specificity of the immune response directed firstly towards the virus which, in turn, may lead to subacute or chronic damage of myocardial tissue.

The expression of antigens or neoantigens in the endothelium or on the myocyte may lead to a secondary immune pathogenesis.

Immunology of cytomegalovirus myocarditis

Fifteen patients with acute CMV infections were studied in order to investigate the role of humoral and cellular immunological effector mechanisms.[99]

Complement-fixation tests were carried out during the acute and postacute phases of the disease which covered a period of several weeks. In contrast to patients with coxsackie B, influenza A and mumps myocarditis, anti-myolemmal (AMLAs), anti-sarcolemmal (ASAs) or anti-endothelial (AEAs) antibodies were rarely detected. The most striking observation, however, was the presence of anti-interfibrillary antibodies, which were present in 13 of 15 patients (Fig. 6.7).

Cytomegalovirus and coronary artery disease
(see Chapter 8)

According to Grattan *et al.*[212] graft sclerosis occurs in more than 10% of patients after heart transplantation if they have previous evidence of infection with CMV compared to only 2% of graft sclerosis without CMV infection.

Among possible direct mechanisms may be included an endothelial cell or media cell hyperplasia, or virus-induced endothelial cell damage leading to insufficient repair and the formation of plaques at the place of repair.

Indirect mechanisms may include the attachment of virus particles at the cell surface which may activate the immune system locally and lead to damage or alteration of the cell surface. Alternatively cross-reacting antibodies may develop which could result in cell damage.

The actual role of CMV must be considered not only from the standpoint of acute infection but also with regard to the effects of long-term alteration of myocardial tissues, including the myocyte, endothelium and interstitial cells. It is also possible that latent virus may be activated and cause cell damage by direct mechanisms or by immunological means.

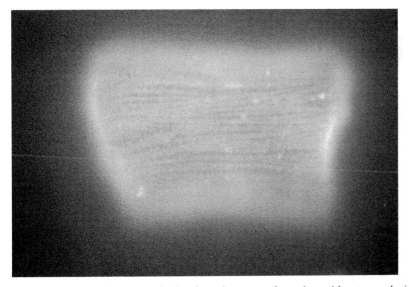

Fig. 6.7 Anti-interfibrillary antibodies from the serum of a patient with cytomegalovirus myocarditis bound on an isolated rat cardiocyte. Fluorescein staining. × 2500.

References

1. Senac J. B. Traité de la structure du coeur, de son action at de ses maladies, 1772. Quoted by Petra Schramm, Editio rarissima 1986.
2. Schroetter P. von. *Die Insuffizienz des Herzmuskels*. Verh Congr Inn Med L, 1899: 17–23.
3. Christian H. A. Nearly ten decades of interest in idiopathic pericarditis. *Am Heart J* 19??; **42**: 645–51.
4. Bengtsson E., Örndahl G. Complications of mumps with special reference to the incidence of myocarditis. *Acta Med Scand* 1954; **149**: 381–8.
5. Sylvest E. *Epidemic Myalgia: Bornholm Disease*. London, Oxford, 1934.
6. Bell E. J., Grist N. R. Coxsackievirus infections in patients with acute cardiac disease and chest pain. *Scott Med J* 1968; **13**: 47–51.
7. Grist N. R., Bell E. J. Coxsackieviruses and the heart. *Am Heart J* 1969; **77**: 295–300.
8. Grist N. R., Bell E. J. A six year study of coxsackievirus B infections in heart disease. *J Hyg* 1974; **73**: 165–74.
9. Smith W. G. Coxsackie B myopericarditis in adults. *Am Heart J* 1970; **80**: 34–46.
10. Javett S. N., Heymann S., Mundel B. *et al*. Myocarditis in new born infant: A study of an outbreak associated with coxsackie group B virus infection in a maternity home in Johannesburg. *J Pediatr* 1956; **48**: 1–22.
11. Kibrick S., Benirschke K. Acute aseptic myocarditis and meningoencephalitis in the newborn child infected with coxsackievirus group B, type 3. *N Engl J Med* 1956; **255**: 883–9.
12. Fletcher E., Brennan C. F. Cardiac complications of coxsackievirus infection. *Lancet* 1957; **i**: 913–15.
13. Fletcher G. F., Coleman M. T., Feorius P. M. *et al*. Viral antibodies in patients with primary myocardial disease. *Am J Cardiol* 1968; **21**: 6–14.
14. Sainani G. S., Krompotic E., Slodki S. J. Adult heart disease due to the coxsackievirus B infection. *Medicine* 1968; **47**: 133–47.
15. Hirschmann S. Z., Hammer G. S. Coxsackievirus myopericarditis: A microbiological and clinical review. *Am J Cardiol* 1974; **34**: 224–32.
16. Jennings R. C. Coxsackie group B fatal neonatal myocarditis associated with cardiomegaly. *J Clin Pathol* 1966; **19**: 325–7.
17. Bowles N. E., Richardson P. J., Olsen E. G. J., Archard L. C. Detection of coxsackie B virus-specific RNA sequences in myocardial biopsy samples from patients with myocarditis and dilated cardiomyopathy. *Lancet* 1986; **1**: 1120–3.
18. Kandolf R., Hofschneider P. H. Viral heart disease. *Springer Semi Immunol Pathol* 1989; **11**: 1–13.
19. Maisch B. Historical retrospective and clinical classification. In: Maisch B. ed. *Recent Advances in Pericardial Disease*. Berlin: Springer-Verlag, in press, 1992.
20. Longson M., Cole F. M., Davies C. Isolation of a coxsackievirus group B, type 5, from the heart of a fatal case of myocarditis in an adult. *J Clin Pathol* 1969; **22**: 654–8.
21. Russell S. J. M., Bell E. J. Echoviruses and carditis. *Lancet* 1970; **i**: 784–5.
22. Monif G. R. G., Lee C. W., Hsiung G. D. Isolated myocarditis with recovery of ECHO type 9 virus from the myocardium. *N Engl J Med* 1976; **277**: 1353–5.
23. Ludden T. E., Edward J. E. Carditis in poliomyelitis: An anatomic study of thirty-five cases and review of the literature. *Am J Pathol* 1949; **25**: 357–81.
24. Dolgopol V. B., Cragen M. D. Myocardial changes in poliomyelitis. *Arch Pathol* 1948; **46**: 202–11.
25. Kipkie G. F., McAuley J. S. M. Acute myocarditis occuring in bulbar poliomyelitis. *Can Med Assoc J* 1954; **70**: 315–17.
26. Laake H. Myocarditis in poliomyelitis. *Acta Med Scand* 1951; **140**: 159–69.

27. Giles C., Chuttleworth E. M. *Post mortem* findings in 46 influenza deaths. *Lancet* 1957; **ii:** 1224–5.
28. Weinstein L., Shelokov A. Cardiovascular manifestations in acute poliomyelitis. *N Engl J Med* 1951; **244:** 281–5.
29. Hamburger W. W. The heart in influenza. *Med Clin North Am* 1938; **22:** 111–21.
30. Finland M., Parker F. Jr., Barnes M. W., Joliffe L. S. Acute myocarditis in influenza infections: Two cases of non-bacterial myocarditis with isolation of virus from the lungs. *Am J Med Sci* 1945; **209:** 455–68.
31. Adams C. W. Post viral myopericarditis associated with the influenza virus: Report of eight cases. *Am J Cardiol* 1959; **4:** 56–67.
32. Oceasohn R., Adelson L., Kaji M. Clinicopathologic study of thirty-three fatal cases of Asian influenza. *N Engl J Med* 1959; **260:** 509–18.
33. Coltman Jr. C. A. Influenza myocarditis: Report of a case with observations on serum glutamic oxaloactic transaminase. *J Am Med Assoc* 1962; **180:** 204–8.
34. Rosenberg G. H., Acute myocarditis in mumps (epidemic parotitis). *Arch Intern Med* 1945; **76:** 257–63.
35. Giustra F. X., Nilsson D. C. Myocarditis following measles. *Am J Dis Child* 1950; **79:** 487–90.
36. Gardinger A. J. S., Short D. Four faces of acute myopericarditis. *Br Heart J* 1973; **35:** 433–42.
37. Cannell D. E. Myocardial degenerations in yellow fever. *Am J Pathol* 1928; **4:** 431–43.
38. Bugher J. C. The pathology of yellow fever. In: Stoker G. K. ed. *Yellow Fever.* New York: McGraw-Hill, 1951: 137–63.
39. Ainger L. E., Lawyer N. G., Fitch C. W. Neonatal rubella myocarditis. *Br Heart J* 1966; **28:** 691–7.
40. Ross E, Amentrout S. A. Myocarditis associated with rabies: Report of a case. *N Engl J Med* 1962; **266:** 1087–9.
41. Cheetham H. D., Hart J., Goghill N. F., Fox B. Rabies with myocarditis: Two cases in England. *Lancet* 1970; **i:** 921–2.
42. Thiede W. H. Cardiac involvement in lymphozytic choriomeningitis. *Arch Intern Med* 1962; **109:** 50–4.
43. Ahvenainen E. K. Inclusion disease or generalized salivary gland virus infection: Report of five cases. *Acta Pathol Microbiol Scand* 1952; **93** (suppl): 159–67.
44. Bodey G. P., Wertlake P. T., Douglas G., Levin R. H. Cytomegalic inclusion disease in patients with acute leukemia. *Ann Intern Med* 1965; **62:** 899–906.
45. Maisch B., Crombach C., Schönian U. Cytomegalovirus infection as a cause of viral myocarditis. *Eur Heart J* 19??; (abstract suppl).
46. Maisch B., Wendl J. Cytomegalovirus DNA in endomyocardial biopsies of patients with (peri)myocarditis. *Eur Heart J* 1989; **9** (suppl 1): 1000 (abs).
47. Schönian U., Crombach M., Maisch B. Does CMV infection play a role in myocarditis? New aspects from *in-situ* hybridization. *Eur Heart J* 1991; **12** (suppl D): 65–8.
48. Hoagland R. J. Cardiac involvement in infectious mononucleosis. *Am J Med Sci* 1956; **232:** 252–7.
49. Hackel D. B. Myocarditis in association with varicella. *Am J Pathol* 1953; **29:** 369–79.
50. Sampson C. C. Varicella myocarditis: report of case. *J Natl Med Assoc* 1959; **51:** 138–9.
51. Tatter D., Gerad P. W., Silverman A. H. *et al.* Fatal varicella pancarditis in a child. *Am J Dis Child* 1964; **108:** 88–93.
52. Moore C. M., Henry J., Benzing G., Kaplan S. Varicella myocarditis. *Am J Dis Child* 1969; **118:** 899–902.
53. Lowry P. J., Thompson R. A., Littler W. A. Humoral immunity in cardiomyopathy. *Br Heart J* 1983; **50:** 390–4.

54. Berkovich S., Rodriguez-Torres R., Lin T. S. Virologic studies in children with acute myocarditis. *Am J Dis Child* 1968; **115:** 207–12.
55. Henson D., Muffson M. A. Myocarditis and pneumonitis with type 21 adenovirus infection: Association with fatal myocarditis and pneumonitis. *Am J Dis Child* 1971; **121:** 334–6.
56. Gore I., Saphir O. Myocarditis: A classification of 1402 cases. *Am Heart J* 1947; **34:** 827–30.
57. Anderson T., Foulis M. A., Grist N. R., Landsman J. B. Clinical and laboratory observations in a smallpox outbreak. *Lancet* 1951; **i:** 1248–52.
58. Dalgaard J. B. Fatal myocarditis following smallpox vaccination. *Am Heart J* 1957; **54:** 156–8.
59. Caldera R., Sarrut S., Mallet R., Rossier A. Existe-t-il des complications cardiaques de la vaccine? *Sem Hop Paris* 1961; **37:** 1281–4.
60. Maut K. Mort subité due à une myocardité focale suivant une vaccination contre la variole. *Ann Med Leg* 1963; **43:** 1–3.
61. Abelmann W. H., Kowalski H. J., McNeely W. F. Cardiovascular studies during acute infectious hepatitis. *Gastroenterology* 1954; **27:** 61–6.
62. Saphir O., Amromin G. D., Yokoo H. Myocarditis in viral (epidemic) hepatitis. *Am J Med Sci* 1956; **231:** 168–76.
63. Besterri R. B. Cardiac involvement in the acquired immune deficiency syndrome. *Int J Cardiol* 1989; **22:** 143–6.
64. Grody W. W., Cheng L., Pang, M., Lewis W. Direct infection of the heart by human immunodeficiency virus (HIV). *Circulation* 1989; **80** (suppl II): 2644 (abs).
65. Lewis W. AIDS: Cardiac findings from 115 biopsies. *Prog Cardiovasc Dis* 1989; **32:** 207–15.
66. Gore I., Kline I. K. Pericarditis and myocarditis. In: Gould S. E. ed. *Pathology of the Heart and Blood Vessels.* 3rd edition. Springfield, Ill: Thomas, 1968: 731–59.
67. Ragosta M., Crabtree J., Sturner W. Q., Thompson P. D. Report of the WHO/ISFC Task force on the definition and classification of cardiomyopathies. *Br Heart J* 1980; **44:** 672.
68. Banatvala J. E. Coxsackie B virus infections in cardiac disease. In: Waterson A. P. ed. *Recent Advances in Clinical Virology 3.* Edinburgh: Churchill Livingstone, 1983: 99–115.
69. Banatvala J. E., Bryant J., Schernthaner G. *et al.* Coxsackie B, mumps, rubella and cytomegalovirus-specific IgM responses in patients with juvenile onset insulin-dependent diabetes mellitus in Britain, Austria and Australia. *Lancet* 1985; **i:** 1409–12.
70. Cambridge G., MacArthur C. G. C., Waterson A. P. *et al.* Antibodies to coxsackie B viruses in congestive cardiomyopathy. *Br Heart J* 1979; **16:** 692–6.
71. Kandolf R., Ameis D., Kirschner P. *et al. In situ* detection of enteroviral genomes in myocardial cells; an approach to the diagnosis of viral heart disease. *Proc Natl Acad Sci USA* 1987; **84:** 6272–6.
72. Alvarez F. L., Neu N., Rose N. R. *et al.* Heart-specific autoantibodies induced by coxsackievirus B: Identification of heart autoantigens. *Clin Immunol Immunopathol* 1987; **43:** 12–23.
73. Beisel K. W. Immunogenetic basis of myocarditis: role of fibrillary antigens. *Springer Semin Immunopathol* 1989; **11:** 31–42.
74. Bolte H. D., Schultheiss P., Cyran J., Goss F. Binding of immunoglobulins in the myocardium (biopsy). In: Bolte H.-D. ed. *Myocardial Biopsy.* Berlin: Springer-Verlag, 1980; 85–92.
75. Bülowius H., Maisch B., Klopf D. *et al.* Lymphozytensubpopulationen bei akuter Perimyokarditis, sekundären und primären dilatativen Herzmuskelerkrankungen, *Z Kardiol* 1983; **72** (suppl I): 16.

76. Eckstein R., Mempel W., Bolte H.-D. Reduced suppressor cell activity in congestive cardiomyopathy and in myocarditis. *Circulation* 1982; **65:** 1224–9.
77. Gauntt C. J., Goeny E. K., Lutton C. M., Pernandes G. Role of natural killer cells in experimental murine myocarditis. *Springer Semin Immunopathol* 1989; **11:** 51–9.
78. Huber S. A., Lodge P. A. Coxsackie B 3 myocarditis: Identification of different pathogenic mechanisms in DBA/2 and Balb/c mice. *Am J Pathol* 1984; **122:** 284–91.
79. Huber S. A., Lodge P. A. Coxsackievirus B3 myocarditis in BALB/c mice: evidence for autoimmunity to myocyte antigens. *Am J Pathol* 1984; **116:** 21–9.
80. Huber S. A., Job L. P., Woodruff J. F. Lysis of infected myofibres by coxsackievirus B₃ immune T-lymphocytes. *Am J Pathol* 1980; **98:** 681–94.
81. Huber S. A., Simpson K., Weller A., Herzum M. Immunopathogenic mechanisms in experimental myocarditis: evidence for autoimmunity to the virus receptor and antigenic mimicry between the virus and the myocardium. In: Schultheiß H. P. ed. *New Concepts in Viral Heart Disease*. Berlin: Springer-Verlag, 1988: 179–87.
82. Klein R., Maisch B., Kochsiek K., Berg P. A. Demonstration of organ specific antibodies against heart mitochondria (anti-M7) in sera from patients with some forms of heart disease. *Clin Exp Immunol* 1984; **58:** 283–92.
83. Klein R., Spiel L., Kleemann U. *et al.* Relevance of antimitochondrial antibodies (anti-M7) in cardiac disease. *Eur Heart J* 1987; **8** (Suppl J): 223–6.
84. Lodge P. A., Herzum M., Olszewski J., Huber S. A. Coxsackie B-3 myocarditis: acute and chronic forms of the disease causes by different immunopathogenic mechanisms. *Am J Pathol* 1987; **128:** 455–63.
85. Maisch B. Cytolytic serum activity in patients with carditis. In: Bolte H. D. ed. *Viral Heart Disease*. Berlin: Springer-Verlag, 1984: 121–30.
86. Maisch B. Diagnostic relevance of humoral and cell-mediated immune reactions in patients with acute myocarditis and congestive cardiomyopathy. In: Chazov E. L., Smirnov V. N., Organov R. G. ed. *Cardiology*. London: Plenum Press, 1984: 1327–38.
87. Maisch B. Humorale immunologische Effektormechanismen bei Perimyokarditis. *Internist* 1984; **25:** 155–64.
88. Maisch B. Rickettsial perimyocarditis – a follow up study. *Heart Vessels* 1985; **2:** 55–9.
89. Maisch B. Surface antigens of adult heart cells and their use in diagnosis. *Basic Res Cardiol* 1986; **80** (suppl 1): 47–52.
90. Maisch B. Immunologic regulator and effector functions in perimyocarditis, postmyocarditic heart muscle disease and dilated cardiomyopathy. *Basic Res Cardiol* 1986; **81** (suppl 1): 217–42.
91. Maisch B. Immunological mechanisms in human cardiac injury. In: Spry J. E. ed. *Immunology and Molecular Biology of Cardiovascular Disease*. In: Shillingfort J. P. ed. *Current status of clinical cardiology*. London: MTP Press, 1987: 225–52.
92. Maisch B. The sarcolemma as antigen in the secondary immunopathogenesis of myopericarditis. *Eur Heart J* 1987; **8** (suppl J): 155–65.
93. Maisch B. The use of myocardial biopsy in heart failure. *Eur Heart J*; **9** (suppl H): 59–71.
94. Maisch B. Autoreactivity to the cardiac myocyte, connective tissue and the extracellular matrix in heart disease and postcardiac injury. *Springer Semin Immunopathol* 1989; **11:** 369–96.
95. Maisch B., Berg P. A., Schuff-Werner P., Kochsiek K. Clinical significance of immunpathological findings in patients with postpericardiotomy syndrome. I. Relevance of antibody pattern. *Clin Exp Immunol* 1979; **38:** 189–97.
96. Maisch B., Berg P. A., Schuff-Werner P., Kochsiek K. Clinical significance of

immunopathological findings in patients with postpericardiotomy syndrome. II. The significance of serum inhibition and rosette inhibitory factors. *Clin Exp Immunol* 1979; **38:** 198–203.

97. Maisch B., Berg P. A., Kochsiek K. Immunological parameters in patients with congestive cardiomyopathy. *Basic Res Cardiol* 1980; **75:** 221–2.
98. Maisch B., Trostel-Soeder R., Berg A., Kochsiek K. Assessment of antibody mediated cytolysis of adult cardiocytes isolated by centrifugation in a continuous gradient of Percoll™ in patients with acute myocarditis. *J Immunol Methods* 1981; **44:** 159–69.
99. Maisch B., Trostel-Soeder R., Stechermesser E. *et al.* Diagnostic relevance of humoral and cell-mediated immune reactions in patients with acute viral myocarditis. *Clin Exp Immunol* 1982; **48:** 533–45.
100. Maisch B., Deeg P., Liebau G., Kochsiek K. Diagnostic relevance of humoral and cytotoxic immune reactions in patients with primary and secondary heart muscle disease. *Am J Cardiol* 1983; **52:** 1072–8.
101. Maisch B., Büschel G., Izumi T. *et al.* Four years of experience in endomyocardial biopsy. An immunohistologic approach. *Heart Vessels* 1985; (suppl I): 59–67.
102. Maisch B., Hauck H., Königer U. *et al.* Suppressor cell activity in (peri)myocarditis and infective endocarditis. *Eur Heart J* 1987; **8** (suppl J): 147–53.
103. Maisch B., Weyerer O., Hufnagel G. *et al.* The vascular endothelium as target of humoral autoreactivity in myocarditis and rejection. *Z Kardiol* 1989; **78:** 95–9.
104. Maisch B., Outzen H., Roth D. *et al.* Prognostic determinants in conventionally treated myocarditis and perimyocarditis – Focus on antimyolemmal antibodies. *Eur Heart J* 1989; **12** (suppl D): 76–80.
105. Maisch B., Bauer E., Cirsi M., Thometzek P. Cytolytic cross-reactive antibodies directed against the cardiac membrane of adult human myocytes in coxsackie B myocarditis – analysis by Western blot, immunofluorescence test and antibody-mediated cytolysis of cardiocytes. In press.
106. Anderson J. L., Carlquist J. F., Hammond E. H. Deficient natural killer cell activity in patients with idiopathic dilated cardiomyopathy. *Lancet* 1982; **ii:** 1124–7.
107. Cambridge G., Campbell-Blay G., Wilmhurst P. *et al.* Deficient 'natural' cytotoxity in patients with congestive cardiomyopathy. *Br Heart J* 1983; **49:** 623 (abs).
108. Das S. K., Callen J. P., Doson V. N., Cassidy J. T. Immunoglobulin binding in cardiomyopathic hearts. *Circulation* 1971; **44:** 612–21.
109. Das S. K., Petty R. E., Meengs W. A., Tubergen D. G. Studies of cell-mediated immunity in cardiomyopathy. In: Sekiguchi M., Olsen E. G. J. eds. *Cardiomyopathy*. Tokyo: University of Tokyo Press, 1980: 375–7.
110. Fowless K. E., Bieber C. P., Stinson E. B. Defective *in vitro* suppressor cell function in idiopathic congestive cardiomyopathy. *Circulation* 1978; **59:** 483–191.
111. Francesini R., Petillo A., Corazza M. *et al.* Lymphocyte response in dilated cardiomyopathy. *IRCS Med Sci* 1983; **II:** 1019–21.
112. Jacobs B., Matsuda Y., Deodhar S. Cell-mediated cytotoxicity to cardiac cells of lymphocytes from patients with primary myocardial disease. *Am J Clin Pathol* 1979; **72:** 1–4.
113. Lowry P. J., Edwards C. W., Nagle R. E. Herpes-like virus particles in myocardium of patient progressing to congestive cardiomyopathy. *Br Heart J* 1982; **48:** 501–4.
114. Lowry P. J., Thompson R. A., Littler W. A. Humoral and cellular mechanisms in congestive cardiomyopathy. *Br Heart J* 1984; **51:** 109 (abs).
115. Yamakawa K., Fukuta S., Yoshinaga T. *et al.* Study of immunological mechanism in dilated cardiomyopathy. *Jpn Circ J* 1987; **51:** 665–75.

116. Hengstenberg C., Rose M., Olsen E. *et al.* Immunological parameters in patients with different heart diseases. *Eur Heart J* 1989; **10** (suppl): 27 (abs).

117. Herskowitz A., Wolgram L. J., Rose N. R., Beisel K. W. Coxsackievirus B3 murine myocarditis: a pathologic spectrum of myocarditis in genetically defined inbred strains. *J Am Cell Cardiol* 1987; **9**: 1311–29.

118. Hufnagel G., Maisch B. MHC antigen expression in endomyocardial biopsies in patients with myocarditis and dilated cardiomyopathy. *Eur Heart J* 1989; **10** (suppl): 28 (abs).

119. Rose N. R., Wolfgram L. J., Herskowitz A., Beisel K. W. Postinfectious autoimmunity: two distinct phases of coxsackievirus B 3-induces myocarditis. *Ann NY Acad Sci* 1986; **475**: 146–56.

120. Aretz H. T., Billingham M. E., Edward W. D. Myocarditis, a histological definition and classification. *Am J Cardiovasc Pathol* 1987; **1**: 3–13.

121. Baughman K. L. Personal communication, Airlie Conference, 1991.

122. Billingham M. E., Mason J. W. Endomyocardial biopsy changes in myocarditis treated with immunosuppressives: In: Bolte H.-D. ed. *Viral Heart Disease*. Berlin: Springer-Verlag, 1984: 200–10.

123. Doerr W. Morphologie der Myokarditis. *Verh Dtsch Ges Inn Med* 1971; **77**: 301–35.

124. Kline I. K., Saphir O. Chronic pernicious myocarditis. *Am Heart J* 1960; **59**: 681–4.

125. Mason J. W., Billingham M. E., Ricci D. R. Treatment of acute inflammatory myocarditis assisted by endomyocardial biopsy. *Am J Cardiol* 1980; **45**: 1037–44.

126. Mills A. S., Hastillo A., Hess M. L. Lymphocytic infection of the myocardium in idiopathic dilated cardiomyopathy: Underestimation of myocarditis with endomyocardial biopsy. *Circulation* 1984; **70** (suppl II): 401 (abs).

127. Mues B., Brisse B., Zwaldo G. *et al.* Myocarditis diagnosis: use of monoclonal antibodies to macrophages in immunocytology. *7th International Congress of Immunology*, Berlin, 1989, *Book of Abstracts* 11–11.

128. Buie C., Lodge P. A., Herzum M., Huber S. A. Genetics of coxsackievirus B3 and encephalomyocarditis virus-induced myocarditis in mice. *Eur Heart J* 1987; **8** (suppl J): 389–401.

129. Godeney E. K., Gauntt C. J. Murine natural killer cells limit coxsackievirus B3 replication. *J Immunol* 1987; **139**: 913–18.

130. Herzum M., Huber S. A., Maisch B. Coxsackie B3 myocarditis: genetic aspects of different immunopathogenic mechanisms in Balb/c and DBA/2 mices. Antigenic specificity of heart-reactive antibodies in DBA/2 mices. In: Schultheiß H. P. ed. *New Concepts in Viral Heart Disease*. Berlin: Springer-Verlag, 1988: 188–94.

131. Neu N., Beisel K., Traystman M. *et al.* Autoantibodies specific for the cardiac myosin isoform are found in mice susceptible to coxsackie virus B3-induced myocarditis. *J Immunol* 1987; **138**: 2488.

132. Rose M. L., Coles M. I., Griffin R. J. *et al.* Expression of class I and class II major histocompatibility antigens in normal and transplanted human heart. *Transplantation* 1986; **41**: 776–82.

133. Wolfgram L. J., Beisel K. W., Rose N. R. Heart-specific autoantibodies following murine coxsackievirus B3 myocarditis. *J Exp Med* 1985; **161**: 1112–21.

134. Wolfgram L. J., Beisel K. W., Herskowitz A., Rose N. R. Variations in the susceptibility to coxsackievirus B3-induced myocarditis among different strains of mice. *J Immunol* 1986; **136**: 1846–152.

135. Wong Y., Woodruff J. J., Woodruff J. F. Generation of cytolytic T-lymphocytes during coxsackievirus B3 infection. I. Model and viral specificity. *J Immunol* 1977; **118**: 1159–64.

136. Wong Y., Woodruff J. J., Woodruff J. F. Generation of cytolytic T-lymphocytes during coxsackievirus B3 infections. II. Characterization of effector cells, a dem-

onstration of cytotoxicity against viral infected myofibers. *J Immunol* 1977; **118:** 1165–9.

137. Woodruff J. F. Viral myocarditis. A review article. *Am J Pathol* 1980; **101:** 425–84.

138. Daly K., Richardson P. J., Olsen E. F. J. *et al.* Acute myocarditis – Role of histological and virological examination in the diagnosis and assessment of immunosuppressive treatment. *Br Heart J* 1984; **51:** 30–5.

139. Fenoglio J. J. Jr., Ursell P. C., Kellogg C. F. *et al.* Diagnosis and classification of myocarditis by endomyocardial biopsy. *N Engl J Med* 1983; **308:** 12–18.

140. Kawai S., Okada R. A histopathological study of dilated cardiomyopathy: With special reference to clinical and pathological comparisons of the degeneration-predominant type and fibrosis-predominant type. *Jpn Circulation J* 1987; **51:** 654–60.

141. McManus B. M., Galinit C. J., Cassung R. S. Immunopathologic basis of myo-cardial injury. *Cardiovasc Clin* 1988; **18:** 163–84.

142. Feigenbaum H. Echocardiographic diagnosis of pericardial effusion. *Am J Cardiol* 1970; **26:** 475–9.

143. Horowitz M. S., Schultz C. S., Stinson E. B. *et al.* Sensitivity and specificity of echocardiographic diagnosis of pericardial effusion. *Circulation* 1974; **50:** 239–46.

143. Maisch B. Retrospective and perspectives in the immunology of cardiac diseases. *Springer Sem Immunopathol* 1989; **11:** 375.

144. Deck W. G., Palacios I. F., Fallon J. T. *et al.* Active myocarditis in the spectrum of acute dilated cardiomyopathies. *Engl J Med* 1985; **342:** 885–97.

145. Maisch B., Schwab D., Bauer E. *et al.* Antimyolemmal antibodies in myocarditis in children. *Eur Heart J* 1987; **8** (suppl J): 167–73.

146. Leatherbury L., Chandra R. S., Shapiro S. R., Perry L. W. Value of endomyo-cardial biopsy in infants, children and adolescents with dilated or hypertrophic cardiomyopathy and myocarditis. *J Am Coll Cardiol* 1988; **12:** 1547–54.

147. Shanes Gahli J., Billingham M. E., Ferrans V. J. *et al.* Interobserver variability in the pathologic interpretation of endomyocardial biopsy results. *Circulation* 1987; **75:** 401–5.

148. Ou J., Sole M. J., Butany J. W., *et al.* The detection of enterovirus RNA in myocardial biopsies from patients with myocarditis and cardiomyopathy using gene by polymerase chain reaction. *Circulation* 1990; **82:** 8–16.

149. Archard L. C., Bowles N. E., Cunningham L. *et al.* Molecular probes for detec-tion of persisting enterovirus infection of human heart and their prognostic value. *Eur Heart J* 1989; **12** (suppl D): 56–60.

150. Burch G. E., Giles T. G. The role of viruses in the production of heart disease. *Am J Cardiol* 1972; **29:** 231–40.

151. Klein J., Stanek G., Bittner R. *et al.* Lyme borreliosis as a cause of myocarditis and heart muscle disease. *Eur Heart J* 1991; **12** (suppl D): 73–5.

152. Kysal A., Haverich A., Heublein B. *et al.* C myc-oncogene expression in myo-cytes in heart allografts. *7th International Congress of Immunology*, Berlin, 1989. *Book of Abstracts*, 814.

153. Samsonov M., Nassonov E., Kostin S. *et al.* Serum neopterin-possible immuno-logical marker of myocardial inflammation in patients with dilated heart muscle disease. *Eur Heart J* 1991; **12** (suppl D): 147–50.

154. Klappacher G., Pacher R., Woluszczuk W., Glogar D. Increased release of neopterin and tumor necrosis factor alpha into the serum of patients with primary dilated cardiomyopathy. *Eur Heart J* 1991; **12** (suppl): 315(A 1616) (abs).

155. Klappacher G., Pacher R., Woluszczuk W., Glogar D. Elevated circulating levels of β2-microglobulin in primary dilated cardiomyopathy. *Eur Heart J* 1991; **12** (suppl): 316(A 1620) (abs).

156. Maisch B. The heart in rheumatic disease. In: Baenkler H.-W. ed. *Rheumatic Disease and Sport. Rheumatology*. Volume 16. Basel: Karger, 1992: 81–117.

157. Maisch B., Maisch S. T., Kochsiek K. Immune reactions in tuberculous and chronic constrictive pericarditis. *Am J Cardiol* 1982; **50**: 1007–13.
158. Kurnick J. T., Leary C., Palacios I. F., Fallon J. T. Culture and characterization of lymphocytic infiltrates from endomyocardial biopsies of patients with idiopathic myocarditis. *Eur Heart J* 1987; **8** (suppl J): 135–9.
159. Kühl U., Ulrich G., Melzner B. *et al.* Characterization of autoantibodies against the Ca^{2+}-channel inducing cytotoxicity by enhancement of calcium permeability. *7th International Congress of Immunology*, Berlin, 1989: 116, 117 (abs).
160. Bresnihan B., Jasin M. E. Suppressor function of peripheral blood mononuclear cells in normal individuals and in patients with systemic lupus erythematosus. *J Clin Invest* 1977; **59**: 106–16.
161. Hallgren H. M., Yunis E. J. Suppressor lymphocytes in young and aged humans. *J Immunol* 1977; **118**: 2004–8
162. Kirsner A. B., Hess E. V., Fowler N. O. Immunologic findings in idiopathic cardiomyopathy. *Am Heart J* 1973; **86**: 625–30.
163. Schwimmbeck P. L., Schultheiß H. P., Strauer B. E. Identification of a main autoimmunogenic epitope of the adenine nucleotide translocator which cross-reacts with coxsackie B3 virus: use in the diagnosis of myocarditis and dilatative cardiomyopathy. *Circulation* 1989; **80** (suppl II): 2642 (abs).
164. Maisch B., Wedeking U., Kochsiek K. Quantitative assessment of antilaminin antibodies in myocarditis and perimyocarditis. *Eur Heart J* 1987; **8** (suppl J): 233–5.
165. Limas C. J., Goldenberg I. F. Autoantibodies against cardiac beta-adrenoceptors in human dilated cardiomyopathy. *Circulation* 1987; **76** (suppl 4): 262–9.
166. Limas C. J., Goldenberg I. F., Limas C. Autoantibodies against beta-adrenoceptors in human idiopathic dilated cardiomyopathy. *Circ Res* 1989; **64**: 97–103.
167. Wallukat G., Boewer V. Stimulation of chronotropic Beta-adrenoceptors of cultures of neonatal rat heart myocytes by the serum of gammaglobulin fraction of patients with dilated cardiomyopathy and myocarditis. *Internationales Symposium: Herzinsuffizienz, Pathogenese und Differentialtherapie*, Berlin, 1988. Universitätsverlag, Berlin A 24 (abs).
168. Hammond E. H., Menlove R. L., Anderson J. L. Immunofluorescence microscopy in the diagnosis and follow-up of patients suspected of having inflammatory heart disease. In: Schultheiß H. P. ed. *New Concepts in Viral Heart Disease. Virology, Immunology and Clinical Management.* Berlin: Springer-Verlag, 1988: 303–11.
169. Schultheiß H. P. The mitochrondrium as antigen in inflammatory heart disease. *Eur Heart J* 1987; **8** (suppl J): 203–10.
170. Schultheiß H. P. The significance of autoantibodies against the ADP/ATP carrier for the pathogenesis of myocarditis and dilated cardiomyopathy: clinical and experimental data. *Springer Sem Immunopathol* 1989; **11**: 15–30.
171. Schultheiß H. P., Bolte H. D. Immunological analysis of autoantibodies against the adenine nucleotide translocator in dilated cardiomyopathy. *J Mol Cell Cardiol* 1985; **17**: 603–17.
172. Schultheiß H. P., Kühl U. Charakterisierung verschiedener Autoantikörper gegen myokardiale Matrixproteine by Myokarditis und dilativer Kardiomyopathie. *Klin Wochenschr* 1987; **65** (suppl IX): 263.
173. Schulze K., Becker B. F., Strauer B., Schultheiß H. P. Antibodies to ADP/ATP carrier – an autoantigen in myocarditis and dilated cardiomyopathy – impair cardiac function. *Circulation* 1990; **81**: 959–69.
174. Schwimmbeck P. L., Schultheiß H. P., Strauer B. E. Identification of a main autoimmunogenic epitope of the adenine nucleotide translocator which cross-reacts with coxsackie B3 virus: use in the diagnosis of myocarditis and dilatative cardiomyopathy. *Circulation* 1989; **80** (suppl II): 2642 (abs).

175. Kühl U., Ulrich G., Schultheiß H.-P. Cross-reactivity of antibodies to the ADP/ ATP translocator of the inner mitochondrial membrane with the cell surface of cardiac myocytes. *Eur Heart J* 1987; **8** (suppl J): 219–22.
176. Wittner B., Maisch B., Kochsiek K. Quantification of antimyosin antibodies in experimental myocarditis by a new solid-phase fluorometric assay. *J Immunol Methods* 1983; **64**: 239–47.
177. Obermayer U., Scheidler J., Maisch B. Antibodies against micro- and intermediate filaments in carditis and dilated cardiomyopathy – are they a diagnostic marker? *Eur Heart J* 1987; **8** (suppl J): 181–6.
178. Hershkowitz A., Neumann D. A., Rose N. R. *et al.* Histocompatibility (MHC) antigens in human myocarditis: new markers of immune-mediated disease. *Circulation* 1989; **80** (suppl II): 2686 (abs).
179. Herzum M., Maisch B., Kochsiek K. Circulating immune complexes in perimyocarditis and infective endocarditis. *Eur Heart J* 1987; **8** (suppl J): 323–6.
180. Boyden S. V. Natural antibodies and the immune response. *Adv Immunol* 1963; **5**: 1–7.
181. Seligman M. The origin and nature of autoantibodies. Introduction. *Ann Inst Pasteur/Immunol* 1986; **137**: 149–50.
182. Jerne N. K. The natural selection theory of antibody formation. *Proc Natl Acad Sci (USA)* 1955; **41**: 849–57.
183. Avrameas S. Natural autoreactive B cells and autoantibodies: the know thyself of the immune system. *Ann Inst Pasteur/Immunol* 1986; **137**: 150–3.
184. Drude L., Wiemers F., Maisch B. Impaired myocyte function *in vitro* incubated with sera from patients with myocarditis. *Eur Heart J* 1991; **12** (suppl D): 36–8.
185. Sutinen S., Kalliomaeki J. L., Pohjonen R., Vastamaeki R. Fatal generalized coxsackie B3 virus infection in an adolescent with successful isolation of the virus from the pericardial fluid. *Ann Clin Res* 1971; **3**: 241.
186. Sutton G., Harding H., Trueheart R., Clark H. Coxsackie B4 myocarditis in an adult: successful isolation of virus from ventricular myocardium. *Aerosp Med* 1971; **38**: 66–9.
187. Huber S. A., Job L. P. Cellular immune mechanisms in coxsackievirus group B, type 3 induced myocarditis in Balb/c mice. In: Spitzer J. J. ed. *Myocardial Injury*. New York: Plenum Publishing Corporation, 1983: 419–508.
188. Muir P., Nicholson F., Tilzey A. J., *et al.* Chronic relapsing pericarditis and dilated cardiomyopathy: serological evidence of persistent enterovirus infection. *Lancet* 1989; **i**: 804–7.
189. Regitz V., Strasser R., Chmielewski G., *et al.* Myocarditis in patients with dilated cardiomyopathy – correlation with clinical, hemodynamic, and biochemical findings. In: Schultheiß H. P. ed. *New Concepts in Viral Heart Disease*. Berlin: Springer-Verlag, 1988: 51–60.
190. Archard L., Bowles N., Olsen E., Richardson P. Detection of persistent coxsackie B virus DNA in dilated cardiomyopathy and myocarditis. *Eur Heart J* 1987; **8** (suppl J): 437–40.
191. Weiss L. M., Movahed L. A., Billingham M. E., Cleary M. L. Detection of coxsackievirus B3 RNA in myocardial tissues by the polymerase chain reaction *Am J Pathol* 1991; **138**: 497–503.
192. Bowles N. E., Rose M. L., Taylor P. *et al.* End-stage dilated cardiomyopathy: persistence of enterovirus RNA in myocardium at cardiac transplantation and lack of immune response. *Circulation* 1989; **80**: 1128–36.
193. Foulis A. K., Farquharson M. A., Cameron S. O. *et al.* A search for the presence of the enteroviral capsid protein VP 1 in pancreases of patients with type 1 (insulin-dependent) diabetes and pancreases and hearts of infants who died of coxsackieviral myocarditis. *Diabetologia* 1990; **33**: 290–8.
194. Noseworthy J. H., Fields B. N., Dichter M. A. *et al.* Cell receptor for the

mammalian reovirus: I. Syngeneic monoclonal anti-idiotypic antibody identifies a cell surface receptor for reovirus. *J Immunol* 1983; **131**: 2533–8.

195. Ulrich G., Kühl U., Melzner B. *et al.* Antibodies against the ADP/ATP carrier crossreact with the Ca-channel – functional and biochemical data. In: Schultheiß H. P. ed. *New Concepts in Viral Heart Disease.* Berlin: Springer-Verlag, 1988: 225–35.
196. Huber S. A., Heintz N., Tracy R. Coxsackievirus B-3-induced myocarditis virus and actinomycin D treatment of myocytes induces novel antigens recognized by cytolytic T lymphocytes. *J Immunol* 1988; **141**: 3214–19.
197. Verel D., Warrack A. J. N., Potter C. W. *et al.* Observations on the A2 England influenza epidemic. *Am Heart J* 1976; **92**: 290–6.
198. Douglas R. G., Betts R. F. Influenza virus. In: Mandell G. L., Douglas R. G., Bennett J. E. eds. *Infectious Diseases.* Second edition. New York: John Wiley, 1985: 846–66.
199. Adams C. W. *et al.* Post viral myopericarditis associated with influenza virus. *Am J Cardiol* 1959; **4**: 56–67.
200. Coltman C. A. Jr. Influenza myocarditis. *J Am Med Assoc* 1962; **180**: 204–8.
201. Stern H., Elek S. D. The incidence of infection with cytomegalovirus in a normal population. *J. Hyg (Camb)* 1965; **63**: 79–87.
202. Gowna T. A. Capehart J. E., Pilcher J. W., Alivizatos P. A. Cytomegalovirus myocarditis as a cause of cardiac dysfunction in a heart transplant recipient. *Transplantation* 1989; **47**: 197–8.
203. Wink K., Schmitz H. Cytomegalovirus myocarditis. *Am Heart J* 1980; **100**: 667–72H.
204. Waris E., Raesaenen O., Kreus K. E., Kreus R. Fatal cytomegalovirus disease in a previously healthy adult. *Scand J Infect Dis* 1972; **4**: 61–7.
205. Klemola E., Kaeaeraeinen L. Cytomegalovirus as a possible cause of a disease resembling infectious mononucleosis. *Br Med J* 1965; **2**: 1099–101.
206. Wilson R. S. E., Morris T. H., Rees J. R. Cytomegalovirus myocarditis. *Br Heart J* 1972; **34**: 865–8.
207. Tiula E., Leinikki P. Fatal cytomegalovirus infection in a previously healthy boy with myocarditis and consumption coagulopathy as presenting signs. *Scand J Med Infect Dis* 1972; **4**: 57–60.
208. Mocarski E. S., Abenes G. B., Manning W. C. *et al.* Molecular genetic analysis of cytomegalovirus gene regulation in growth, persistence and latency in: McDougall J. K. ed. *Cytomegaloviruses.* Berlin: Springer-Verlag, 1990: 47–74.
209. Gao Z. S., Schroeder J. S., Alderman A. L. Clinical laboratory correlates of accelerated coronary artery disease in cardiac transplant patients. *Circulation* 1987; **76**: V56–V61.
210. Smiley M. L., Wlodaver C. G., Grossmann R. A. The role of pretransplant immunity in protection of cytomegalovirus disease following renal transplantation. *Transplantation* 1985; **40**: 157–61.
211. Grattan M. T., Moreno-Cabral C. E., Starnes V. A. *et al.* Cytomegalovirus infection is associated with cardiac allograft, rejection and atherosclerosis. *J Am Med Assoc* 1989; **261**: 3561–6.

7

The role of human immunodeficiency virus in heart disease

A. J. Jacob and N. A. Boon

Introduction

Infection with the human immunodeficiency viruses (HIVs) is widespread and the World Health Organization (WHO) estimates that about 10 million people have been infected.[1] Some 501 000 people worldwide, particularly in the USA (277 000) and Africa (151 000) had been reported to the WHO as suffering from the acquired immune deficiency syndrome (AIDS) by mid-1992.[2] In Western Europe, the highest *per capita* rates of AIDS are found in Switzerland, France and Italy (6–7 cases of AIDS per 100 000 people). By mid 1991, in excess of 15 700 people had been infected with HIV in the UK[3] and of those 6 798 AIDS patients reported by the end of November 1992, 4216 had died.[4] The WHO has estimated that by the year 2000, between 30 and 40 million people will have been infected by HIV with Africa and Southeast Asia particularly affected.[2]

There are four recognized modes of transmission of HIV: penetrative sexual intercourse, injection drug use with contaminated needles and syringes, administration of infected blood and blood products, and transfer of the virus from mother to child (vertical transmission). There is no convincing evidence that casual contact can facilitate the spread of HIVs.[5]

In the western world, homosexuals constitute the largest group of patients who are HIV positive, followed by injection drug users.[2] However, there is evidence that the rate of new HIV infection attributable to heterosexual contact and vertical transmission is rising steeply. These represent major routes of viral transmission in Africa, an area where HIV infection is now widespread and affecting the most productive members of society. This shift towards the heterosexual transmission of HIV is also occurring in Britain and the USA,[6] and, although the baseline is low, people with AIDS acquired by this route now constitute the group with the highest growth rate in the UK.[4] It remains to be seen if public education and modification of risk behaviour will abort the threatened epidemic of HIV infection in western countries.

The origins of HIV are unclear but its similarity to an immunodeficiency virus found in primates has led to speculation that it represents a variant of the Simian immunodeficiency virus which has crossed the species boundary. Sexual practices of certain African tribes, which include the inoculation of monkey blood around the genital area, may have facilitated this transfer from animal to humans.[7]

Opportunistic infection is the principal cause of death for patients with HIV,[2] but the advent of new antimicrobial agents has reduced the mortality from this cause. In a recent report from London, Peters *et al*.[8] studied retrospectively the causes of death in HIV patients over an 8-year period. They found that a progressively smaller proportion of patients were dying of opportunistic infection, and that this was parallelled by a rise in the mortality attributable to malignancy. Clinically significant end-organ damage occurs predominantly in late-stage HIV disease. As fewer people succumb to opportunistic infection, it is likely that as well as malignancy, the prevalence of organ failure including AIDS dementia and heart muscle disease will also increase.

In this chapter, the multiple effects of HIV on the heart with particular emphasis on heart muscle disease which is undoubtedly the most significant cardiac manifestation of HIV in non-African countries will be described.

The immunopathology of human immunodeficiency virus infection

The human immunodeficiency virus is an RNA virus which expresses several defined surface antigens. Two types of HIV are recognised, HIV-1 and HIV-2. HIV-2 is prevalent in West Africa, but has now been imported into Europe, the US and India. HIV-1 and -2 have markedly differing surface antigens but share antigenic components associated with the internal component of the virus (viral core). The structure and classification of HIVs is described in Chapter 1. In view of the comparative rarity of HIV-2 in developed countries, most of the studies on the pathogenesis of infection relate to HIV-1 and, in any case, it is unlikely that there are major differences in the pathogenesis and clinical picture between HIV-1 and HIV-2. One of the surface antigens (the GP 120 protein) binds specifically with cells expressing CD4 receptors, which include T-helper lymphocytes, macrophages and dendritic cells. These cells are then invaded by the virus which proceeds to make two DNA copies of its RNA genome which then associate to form double-stranded DNA. Viral RNA is subsequently degraded and the double-stranded DNA is incorporated into the genome of the host cell. At this stage, HIV enters a latent phase which may last for several years. The factors which promote reactivation of the virus are not known, but may include stimulation of the host cell by secondary organisms. Reactivation results in intracellular replication of HIV, expression of viral antigens at the host cell surface, cytolysis and widespread dissemination of the virus.[9,10] Advancing HIV infection results in a gradual decline in the number of CD4+ lymphocytes with concomitant deterioration in the ability of the patient to mount an effective immune response to other organisms. Progressive immunodeficiency is characterized by recurrent infections, particularly with opportunistic organisms, malignancy and end-organ failure. The term 'AIDS' encompasses these clinical manifestations of HIV disease.

The combination of reduced immune surveillance caused by HIV-induced destruction of T helper lymphocytes and malignant transformation of B lymphocytes by other organisms, particularly the Epstein–Barr virus, may be responsible for the appearance of Kaposi's sarcomata and high-grade B cell lymphomata, the tumours most commonly associated with HIV infection.

These malignancies are relatively rare in non-infected patients but have been found in over half the cases in some AIDS *post mortem* series.[11]

While HIV is primarily an infection of the immune system, it is now apparent that many organs can be damaged directly or indirectly by the virus. Disparate effects on a number of organs including the central nervous system,[12] gastrointestinal tract[13] and cardiovascular system[14] have been described. CD4 cell surface receptors are not essential for HIV ingress as exemplified by the finding of viral genomic material within rectal, epidermal, brain capillary endothelial and colonic cancer cells.[9,15] It is possible that other receptors, hitherto unidentified, or ingestion of antigen–antibody complexes may facilitate the entry of the virus into cells.[9] Once such entry has occurred, however, either immediate cell destruction or incorporation into the host genome and latency ensues.

During the latent period, when the virus lies dormant within blood cells, HIV can be transported around the body in an immunologically protected form. Ingress of the virus into the central nervous system is thought to be mediated in this manner with infected monocytes protecting it from the immune system and carrying it across the blood–brain barrier.[16] These mechanisms offer the means whereby HIV can be propagated throughout the body and enter the component cells of organ systems including the heart.

Cardiac disease is emerging as a significant cause of morbidity, and possibly mortality, in HIV infection. All parts of the heart can be affected. Vascular phenomena such as inflammation, thrombosis and spasm have also been described.[17] The likely effects of HIV upon the cardiovascular system vary depending upon geographical location, risk group and stage of disease. Accurate assessment of the prevalence and nature of HIV heart disease is hampered by two factors. Firstly, cardiac disease may be asymptomatic.[18–20] Secondly, it may present with features which are ascribed incorrectly to other organ systems[21] or opportunistic infection.[18,22,23] This is particularly true of breathlessness which may be attributed mistakenly to respiratory infection. Lipshultz *et al.*[18] studied 31 children using echocardiography and found that the symptoms and signs of heart muscle disease were obscured by hepatosplenomegaly, interstitial lung disease and renal impairment. Moreover, some of the children with greatest myocardial dysfunction failed to show obvious clinical evidence of cardiac involvement. The authors recommended that routine, serial, noninvasive assessment be performed because significant, often occult, cardiac abnormalities were common. The prevalence of cardiac disease will be underestimated in places where high numbers of HIV patients and inadequate diagnostic facilities coexist, regrettably the case in many developing countries. *Post mortem* examinations are not always performed, squandering opportunities to gain valuable information about HIV heart disease. Even when autopsies are done, there is a tendency to ascribe the cause of death to opportunistic infection or malignancy, often in the face of significant heart disease. In the *post mortem* series reported by Cammorasano and Lewis, [11]Stewart *et al.*[21] and Lewis,[24] a total of 77 patients out of 164 (47%) had autopsy evidence of heart disease, yet just four of these patients were said to have died from a direct cardiac cause. These diverse factors result in the morbidity and mortality of HIV heart disease being underestimated, which may not only militate against its prompt recognition and treatment, but also allow potentially deleterious therapies to be administered such as blood transfusions, large intravenous fluid loads containing cotrimoxazole and chemotherapeutic agents for Kaposi's sarcoma derived from anthracyclines.[25]

Myocarditis

Myocarditis is defined histologically as 'a process characterized by an inflammatory infiltrate of the myocardium with necrosis and/or degeneration of adjacent myocytes not typical of the ischaemic damage associated with coronary artery disease.'[26] Its true prevalence in HIV infection is unclear but it has been found in up to 52% of patients in *post mortem* series.[27]

Myocarditis in HIV infection may be caused by the virus itself, either directly or indirectly via autoimmune processes, or by one of many opportunistic organisms.

Cases of myocarditis detected at *post mortem* where there is no evidence of secondary infection may represent situations where HIV is the principal cause of myocyte damage.[27,28] The pathogenetic mechanisms responsible for myocarditis due solely to HIV have not been established although a number of theories have been proposed. Human immunodeficiency virus may enter cardiac myocytes and cause damage either directly or indirectly. For example, by analogy with T helper lymphocytes, HIV-induced destruction may take place by initiation of an intrinsic cellular process leading to apoptosis.[29] The evidence for such viral entry is based upon culture and *in situ* hybridization techniques.[30-33] However, these methods are potentially unreliable because of the possibility of contamination of cardiac muscle preparations by blood cells containing HIV. Furthermore, contradictory results have been obtained from workers who have failed to demonstrate HIV in myocardial biopsies[34] and from *in vitro* experiments using skeletal muscle cell lines[35] which have shown that HIV is unable to gain entry into myocytes. The apparent inconsistency of results and the paucity of published material detailing the direct effects of HIV on the myocardium mean that the role of *primary* HIV infection in the pathogenesis of myocarditis is still a matter of speculation.

Human immunodeficiency virus-induced myocyte damage might also occur indirectly through autoimmune mechanisms. Herskowitz *et al.*[36] found high levels of circulating cardiac autoantibodies in HIV patients with myocarditis and heart muscle disease. This was accompanied by induction of class I major histocompatibility complex antigens within the myocardium suggesting that it was involved in the inflammatory process. It is possible that HIV enters myocytes and either modifies existing surface antigens or exposes previously hidden epitopes provoking the immune system to generate anti-heart antibodies. Another possible mechanism of autoimmune myocyte damage is by 'innocent bystander' destruction, a hypothesis proposed by Ho *et al.*[16] to explain central nervous system destruction in HIV infection. Here, blood cells carrying HIV enter the tissue and release proteolytic enzymes and lymphokines which firstly cause cell destruction and secondly promote the ingress of inflammatory cells which argument the destructive process. Lymphokines such as tumour necrosis factor are found in abnormally high concentrations in the blood of patients with HIV infection[37] and have been shown to cause skeletal myocyte death *in vitro*.[35]

Many opportunistic agents have been implicated in the development of myocarditis including *Toxoplasma gondii*,[38-41] cytomegalovirus,[39]*Crypto-*

coccus neoformans,[11,42]*Histoplasma capsulatum*[39] and *Aspergillus fumigatus*.[43] New infectious cofactors continue to be identified. In particular, several mycoplasma species have been implicated in the pathogenesis of HIV damage to the kidney, liver and spleen.[44] These diverse organisms might cause myocyte damage through the same mechanisms as HIV or by acting synergistically with the virus.[34,45]

Toxoplasma gondii myocarditis has been treated successfully with antibiotics.[46] Similarly, immunosuppressive therapy, although seemingly paradoxical in HIV infection, has also been used with good effect both for HIV-associated skeletal myopathy[47] and myocarditis without any identifiable cause other than the virus itself.[48] It is impossible to be certain, however, if the improvement in cardiac function was a genuine response to treatment or merely part of the natural history of a potentially self-limiting condition. Nevertheless, the fact that some cases of myocarditis are potentially treatable implies that when the condition is suspected, endomyocardial biopsy should be considered for diagnostic and therapeutic purposes.

The diagnosis of myocarditis requires a high index of suspicion based upon symptoms and/or compatible physical findings such as fever, signs of heart failure or a precordial rub. Nonspecific electrocardiographic (ECG) changes may occur such as a sinus tachycardia, conduction defects and repolarization abnormalities,[28] and there may be radiological evidence of cardiac enlargement or pulmonary oedema. Echocardiography offers a practical, noninvasive means of assessing cardiac size and function while also determining the extent of any associated pericardial effusion. The echocardiographic features of myocarditis are nonspecific and often identical to those associated with heart muscle disease. Indeed, differentiation between the two conditions can only be made histologically. Some groups have demonstrated dyskinesia of the left ventricle with[28,48] or without[28,49] dilation, or generalized four chamber enlargement.[46] Wall thickness may also be reduced and lie at the lower end of the normal range. [28]Lipshultz *et al.*[18] studied 31 HIV-positive children echocardiographically and showed that hyperdynamic left ventricular performance was associated with myocarditis. If ventricular dysfunction is demonstrated, consideration should be given to performing a right ventricular endomyocardial biopsy with the aim of submitting a minimum of five biopsies for light and electron microscopy and viral culture. Concomitant serology should also be done in order to try and establish the presence of secondary infection. Unfortunately, serological techniques are of limited value in the context of HIV disease due to widespread immunological dysfunction[10] which may prevent the development of the usual pattern of immune responses both to primary and recrudescent opportunistic infection.

It is likely that a variable proportion of patients with myocarditis suffer irreversible damage of large numbers of myocytes resulting in heart muscle disease and progressive cardiac failure. The relationship between myocarditis and heart muscle disease is discussed further in the following section.

Heart muscle disease

In 1986 Cohen *et al.*[50] described three HIV-positive patients who presented with the symptoms and signs of heart failure. Two of the three patients underwent *post mortem* examinations which showed global dilation of the cardiac chambers without evidence of coronary artery disease or myocarditis. Since then, a number of *in vivo* studies[18,19,21–23,25,50–54] and retrospective *post mortem* analyses[24,27,55] have confirmed the existence of 'HIV heart muscle disease'. This term is preferable to 'HIV cardiomyopathy' since, by definition, cardiomyopathy occurs in the absence of a known causative agent.[56] Estimates of the prevalence of HIV heart muscle disease vary widely with one group[23] reporting that 41% of their patients had left ventricular dysfunction while another[24] showed that only 2% had cardiac dilation at *post mortem*. The consensus of published reports is that it occurs in all major risk groups including homosexuals,[19,22,24,25,53] injection drug users,[23,51,57] and children,[18,21,54,55] particularly[25,52,58] but not exclusively[19] in late stage disease.

The evidence that heart muscle disease represents a specific phenomenon associated with HIV infection as opposed to a nonspecific manifestation of chronic disease in a dying patient is based on two observations. Firstly, cardiac dysfunction has been documented in apparently healthy, well-nourished patients.[52] Secondly, in 1989 Himelman *et al.*[25] studied 70 ambulant and hospitalized HIV patients and compared them to 20 inpatients with acute leukaemia. The hospitalized patients with HIV had more advanced disease than their ambulant counterparts and were of similar nutritional status to those with leukaemia, as evidenced by percentage of predicted ideal body weight and serum albumin. Eight patients with heart muscle disease were identified on the basis of echocardiograms showing four chamber enlargement and diffuse left ventricular hypokinesia. All eight were HIV positive and hospitalized, and remarkably, four of them had the diagnosis of heart muscle disease made only at the time of their ultrasound study. None of the leukaemic patients, despite their parlous condition, had evidence of myocardial dysfunction. Within six months, four of the eight patients had died, indicating that the presence of cardiac dysfunction in late stage HIV infection was a particularly poor prognostic factor.

Human immunodeficiency virus heart muscle disease can cause dilation and dysfunction of one or both ventricles (Fig. 7.1). Some cases of isolated right ventricular dysfunction may, however, arise from pressure or volume overload. Disease of the right ventricle will therefore be discussed separately.

Left and biventricular heart muscle disease

This is the most clinically significant form of HIV heart muscle disease. Symptoms such as fatigue, breathlessness and palpitation, or physical signs consistent with heart failure, including resting tachycardia, elevated jugular venous pressure, gallop rhythm, basal crackles and peripheral oedema, merit formal assessment of the cardiovascular system including echocardiography. In one of the larger echocardiographic studies so far, Corallo *et al.*[23] evaluated 102 patients with late stage HIV disease, the majority of whom were injection drug users. Forty-two patients had a globular left ventricle with diffuse reduction of wall motion. These features were particularly marked in patients with terminal HIV disease and were usually accompanied by a mild to moderate pericardial effusion. Our echocardiographic findings in 173 patients (119 injection drug users, 38 homosexuals, 10 haemophiliacs and six heterosexuals) at various stages of HIV infection have identified 29 patients with heart muscle disease (14 with left ventricular enlargement and global dysfunction, six with

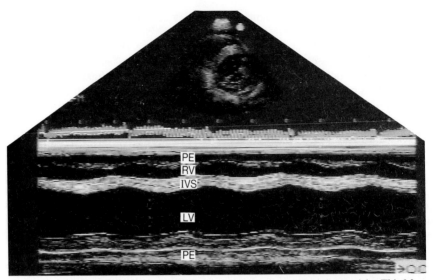

Fig. 7.1 Heart muscle disease with dilation and dysfunction of the left ventricle. This M-mode ultrasound image was taken at the level of the mitral valve papillary muscles in the short axis view. LV = left ventricle. RV = right ventricle. IVS = interventricular septum. PE = pericardial effusion.

isolated left ventricular dilation and nine with isolated dilation of the right ventricle). In common with other similar studies, heart muscle disease was significantly associated with late stage HIV infection. In another study, in a group of eight children, Stewart *et al.*[21] demonstrated reduced left ventricular fractional shortening in all patients accompanied by concentric left ventricular hypertrophy in three and ventricular dilation in five. One child had biventricular dilation and hypofunction and three had associated pericardial effusions. A more recent study[19] of 70 patients, mainly homosexuals, identified eight patients with left ventricular dysfunction (ejection fraction <45% and/ or fractional shortening <28%), three of whom reverted to normal on subsequent examination. Persistent left ventricular dysfunction carried a poor prognosis. Isolated left ventricular dilation has been reported by some workers,[52,57,59] and this may progress to severe biventricular failure.[59] However, this finding has yet to be confirmed by other groups and it is hoped that the prospective study being undertaken in Edinburgh will address this issue since several patients with isolated left ventricular dilation have been identified in the first round of echocardiographic assessments.[57]

Treatment is undertaken with conventional agents including diuretics, digoxin, inotropes and vasodilators.[21,54] Some workers have used serial echocardiography to demonstrate improvements in cardiac function. Regrettably, however, even where there is improvement in the symptoms and signs of heart failure, this is often short lived, with patients dying of either progressive heart failure[25,50] or impairment of other organ systems.[21,25] Persistent echocardiographic evidence of left ventricular dysfunction[19] and clinically overt heart failure[58] are poor prognostic indicators.

The aetiology of HIV heart muscle disease is unknown, undoubtedly complex and probably multifactorial. The most likely causative factors are preceding myocarditis attributable either to HIV itself or secondary infectious agents, nutritional deficiencies, excessive sympathetic drive and the effects of drugs used in the treatment of HIV disease and its complications.

The hypothesis that heart muscle disease is caused by preceding myocarditis is supported firstly by *post mortem* studies which have demonstrated myocarditis in hearts with structural disease[23,27,50] and secondly by analogy with idiopathic dilated cardiomyopathy. Here there is considerable experimental evidence based upon human, animal and *in vitro* work of the pathogenetic role of myocarditis.[60-63] The recent demonstration that some cases of HIV-related left ventricular dysfunction resolve spontaneously[19] is also consistent with the idea that myocarditis, which is potentially self-limiting, serves as the substrate for the subsequent development of HIV heart muscle disease.

The reported prevalence of myocarditis associated with HIV heart muscle disease varies widely. While some groups have failed to identify myocarditis in any of their heart muscle disease patients,[21,24,53] others have found it in nearly all such patients.[27,50] These contradictory findings probably reflect a combination of sampling errors, failure to use standard diagnostic criteria and the transient nature of the underlying inflammatory processes. Moreover, the established Dallas criteria (see p. 43) for the diagnosis of myocarditis based upon an inflammatory infiltrate and adjacent myocardial necrosis[26] may be inappropriate in the context of HIV infection where the capacity to mount an immune response is impaired.[10]

Human immunodeficiency virus heart muscle disease can be likened to idiopathic dilated cardiomyopathy, a condition that may also have a viral aetiology (see Chapters 4 and 9).[61-63] However, studies of the natural history and pathogenesis of HIV-induced heart muscle disease will be easier to perform because the condition occurs in a well-defined group of patients and the virus and its antigens are characterized. Work in this field may, by analogy, help to increase our understanding of the pathogenesis of idiopathic dilated cardiomyopathy and may also lead to new forms of therapy. Identification of the immunological mediators of heart muscle damage may permit the development of specific therapy such as monoclonal antibodies directed against cardiotoxic effector cells and their release products.[64] Alternatively, by analogy with the murine model of myocarditis and idiopathic dilated cardiomyopathy (see Chapter 5 Parts I and II), it may be possible to reduce the severity of heart muscle disease with judicious use of immunosuppressants.[65]

There is increasing interest in the nutritional deficiencies which occur in HIV infection as a result of reduced intake and malabsorption.[66,67] These include, *inter alia*, B group vitamins, zinc, folate and selenium.[68-71] Some of these deficiencies may be mediated by tumour necrosis factor,[72] a cytokine which has been implicated in cellular damage caused by HIV.[35,72] Deficiencies of zinc and some B group vitamins have been associated with reversible impairment of immune function,[68,69] a factor which may influence the inflammatory mechanisms underlying the development of myocarditis and heart muscle disease. Recently, it has been reported that excessive amounts of the products of oxidative metabolism have been found in the blood of HIV-positive patients.[73] This may reflect a defect in naturally occurring antioxidant systems of which the selenoenzyme glutathione peroxidase is an integral part. Preliminary results from Edinburgh suggest that selenium deficiency is widespread in late stage HIV infection and that it is significantly greater in those with HIV heart muscle disease (Jacob *et al.*, unpublished observations). A form of heart muscle disease known as Keshan cardiomyopathy occurs endemically in a Chinese province and its incidence has been reduced by widespread dietary supplementation with selenium.[74] A relationship between selenium deficiency and the development of HIV heart muscle disease has been suggested[75] but requires formal assessment. Similarly, the role of other anti oxidants such as vitamins C and E in the pathogenesis of HIV heart muscle disease merits investigation.

Heart muscle disease may also occur as a result of excessive sympathetic stimulation in a manner analogous to cardiac damage caused by the high circulating level of catecholamines in phaeochromocytoma.[76] Excessive activation of the sympathetic system may be caused by autonomic imbalance related to HIV damage of neural pathways[77] or by stimulation of beta receptors by the group 120 protein.[78]

Some drugs used in the treatment of HIV disease and opportunistic infections may be cardiotoxic. Zidovudine is a thymidine analogue which, by interfering with HIV RNA-dependent DNA polymerase (reverse transcriptase), inhibits elongation of the viral DNA chain and reduces viral replication.[79] It is now widely used in HIV infection and among its recognized side effects is inhibition of mitochondrial DNA replication[80] which can cause or exacerbate a skeletal myopathy characterized by pain, weakness and wasting.[79,81] This is associated with characteristic histological changes including focal necrosis, 'ragged red' sarcoplasm, mitochondrial abnormalities and numerous cytoplasmic bodies.[79] Similar features have been noted in the cardiac muscle of rats given zidovudine.[82] However, to date there is no evidence that zidovudine causes HIV heart muscle disease in humans. In the Edinburgh series, exposure to zidovudine was similar in patients with HIV heart muscle disease and those with structurally normal hearts. Moreover, some patients with severe heart muscle disease had never received zidovudine.[83]

Disease of the right ventricle

Radionuclide[51] and echocardiographic[19,21,84] studies have shown that right ventricular abnormalities are common in HIV infection and may be transient.[20] After pericardial effusion, right ventricular hypertrophy has been described as the commonest cardiac finding at *post mortem*.[24] Dilation and dysfunction of the right ventricle may occur as part of a global myopathic process, characterized echocardiographically by four chamber dilation and loss of function[21,25,50,53] through mechanisms which have already been discussed. However, some cases are related not to intrinsic disease of the heart muscle but rather to the effects of a pressure or volume load (Fig. 7.2). Recurrent respiratory infections, a problem almost universal in HIV-positive patients, can cause pulmonary hypertension and right ventricular failure.[84] Indeed, cor pulmonale has been reported on at least one occasion as being the index diagnosis of congenital AIDS.[85] Right ventricular abnormalities associated with respiratory infection are potentially reversible with antibiotic therapy.[19] Increased right heart pressure may also arise secondary to emboli impacting in the pulmonary microvasculature following the administration of particulate matter during injection drug use or through necrotizing angiitis.[86]

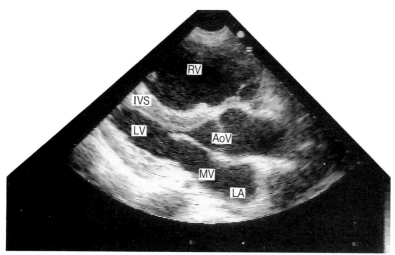

Fig. 7.2 Dilation of the right ventricle. This two-dimensional ultrasound image was taken in the long axis plane. The interventricular septum is shown bulging into the left ventricle during diastole. LV = left ventricle. RV = right ventricle. IVS = interventricular septum. MV = mitral valve. LA = left atrium. AoV = aortic valve.

Finally, Coplan *et al.*[87] have reported four patients who presented with signs of elevated pulmonary artery pressure and appeared to have pulmonary hypertension attributable to HIV *per se.*

In the largest study to date evaluating isolated right ventricular disease in AIDS, Himelman *et al.*[84] described six men presenting predominantly with progressive exertional dyspnoea, all of whom had ECG evidence of right ventricular hypertrophy. Doppler echocardiography demonstrated right atrial and ventricular enlargement, paradoxical septal motion and marked elevation in right ventricular systolic pressure. Cardiac catheterization confirmed that pulmonary artery and right heart pressures were elevated as was the pulmonary vascular resistance. Left ventricular filling pressure and cardiac output were in the low to normal range. These findings occurred in the context of pulmonary infection in five of the six patients. The sixth patient, however, was found to have abnormalities consistent with multiple emboli on selective pulmonary angiography and was treated with oral anticoagulants.

Endocarditis causing damage and dysfunction of the tricuspid valve is also potentially capable of causing right ventricular dilation as a result of excessive volume load. Such a case associated with marantic endocarditis was described by Fink *et al.*[22] However, tricuspid valve incompetence does not always imply preceding endocarditis since it may be the consequence rather than the cause of right ventricular dilation.

Pericarditis and pericardial effusions

The prevalence of pericardial effusion in association with HIV infection varies between 11%[88] and 82%,[89] and has been reported as the commonest cardiac manifestation of HIV disease by one group of workers.[24] While the majority of pericardial effusions in HIV disease are clinically insignificant, some authors using echocardiography have documented large effusions accompanied by collapse of the right atrium and ventricle during late diastole.[90–92] The finding of radiological cardiomegaly is particularly relevant and should prompt early echocardiographic assessment.[22,58]

Pericardial effusions can arise secondary to opportunistic infection, malignant infiltration, myocarditis and heart muscle disease[22,24,25,58] and during intercurrent febrile illness.[19] Effusions not associated with opportunistic infection or malignancy may be accompanied by fluid in other serous cavities and a common metabolic or haemodynamic cause may be responsible.[24] Many such effusions are small, asymptomatic and do not require treatment (Fig. 7.3).[19] Clinically significant pericardial effusions usually occur from secondary infection[88,89,93–95] and malignant infiltration.[96,97] Organisms implicated in the pathogenesis of pericardial effusions in AIDS patients include opportunistic agents,[98] *Staphylococcus aureus*,[99] viruses[90,100,101] and typical and atypical mycobacteria.[88,89,93–95,102] Tamponade due to mycobacterial infection occurs most commonly in Africa[89,93,94] and can be either the index diagnosis of AIDS[103] or occur early in the course of clinically manifest HIV infection.[93] Pericardial disease and effusions may be asymptomatic or present with classical symptoms such as chest pain and breathlessness, and signs including tachycardia, precordial rub, diminished heart sounds, gallop rhythm, pulsus paradoxus and collapse.[90,95,97,103] Nonspecific ECG changes may occur including ST/T wave abnormalities, electrical alternans, prolongation of QTc and abnormal QRS morphology.[92,95,97,101] Another group[99] described a patient with purulent pericarditis which progressed to severe constrictive disease. Here, echocardiography showed considerable thickening of the pericardium and minimal pericardial fluid. Subsequent pericardiectomy resulted in cure. In symptomatic and life-threatening situations, pericardiocentesis and/or pericardial biopsy is indicated. As well as helping to identify any causative

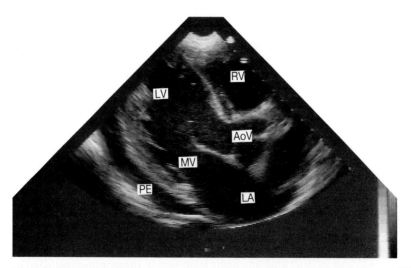

Fig. 7.3 Pericardial effusion in association with biventricular heart muscle disease. This echocardiogram was taken in the long axis plane. LV = left ventricle. RV = right ventricle. PE = pericardial effusion. LA = left atrium. AoV = aortic valve.

organism against which treatment can then be directed,[91] these techniques may also effect a long-term cure.[12]

Pericardial effusions associated with malignant infiltration are likely to increase as the prevalence of lymphoma and Kaposi's sarcoma rises. Treatment is directed at the malignant process together with pericardial drainage if indicated.

Malignant infiltration

Human immunodeficiency virus infection predisposes towards the development of neoplasia, the overall incidence of which has been reported as 39%.[14] Both Kaposi's sarcoma and B cell lymphomata can infiltrate the heart and cause intractable cardiac failure, pericardial effusions and abnormalities of conduction.[14] However, malignant infiltration may also remain clinically silent and be detected only at *post mortem*.[104,105]

Kaposi's sarcoma is an angiosarcoma which, in a recent *post mortem* series, was found in 51% of patients with AIDS. The tumour involved the heart in 19% of these cases.[11] Cardiac infiltration by Kaposi's sarcoma, a tumour found predominantly in homosexuals with HIV infection,[106] usually takes place as part of a metastatic process,[11,96,97,104] but has been reported as a primary phenomenon.[107] The tumour may affect the pericardium, epicardium or myocardium, sometimes with associated coronary artery involvement.[11,24,96,97,104] Concomitant pericardial effusion is common and may cause tamponade.[96,97] Cutaneous Kaposi's sarcoma is often radiosensitive,[97] but at present there is no evidence that such treatment improves survival in patients with cardiac involvement.

Primary cardiac lymphoma is rare in non-HIV patients, accounting for less than 10% of all primary malignant cardiac tumours.[108] It occurs more frequently in those with HIV infection,[105,109,110] but is not as common as cardiac infiltration by Kaposi's sarcoma.[11,14,27,91] Cardiac involvement in disseminated lymphoma is also recognized.[14] The tumour may infiltrate the pericardium, myocardium or endocardium alone or in combination. Intracavitary lymphoma can also occur. Pericardial effusions and intracavitary masses can be visualized readily using echocardiography, facilitating pericardial aspiration or transvenous biopsy to obtain material for histology,[92,105] but the echocardiographic features in cases of myocardial infiltration are nonspecific.[109] Radionuclide scans using ^{67}Ga[110] and magnetic resonance imaging[105] may provide additional diagnostic information. Treatment includes chemotherapy for the underlying malignant process combined with antifailure drugs and pericardial drainage if required.

Endocarditis in human immunodeficiency virus infection

Endocarditis is found in up to 10% of HIV-positive patients at *post mortem*.[24] There are two forms – marantic and infective. The predominant type consists of nonbacterial, thrombotic vegetations (marantic endocarditis) which can affect any or all of the heart valves.[11,24] While this may be a specific complication of HIV, it could be a reflection of the generalized wasting and malignancies which occur in HIV disease.[14] The signs and symptoms of endocarditis may be obscured by ongoing HIV disease in which fevers and anaemia are common. There is no specific therapy for marantic endocarditis.

Infective endocarditis is associated commonly but not exclusively with injection drug use.[14] A range of organisms including bacteria[111] and fungi[43,112,113] can colonize and damage valves, particularly those on the right side of the heart. Echocardiography may show vegetations (Fig. 7.4).[43,111,113] Cox *et al.*[43] described mobile, granular masses within the left ventricular cavity at the level of the insertion of the mitral chordae to the posteropapillary muscle in a patient with *Aspergillus fumigatus* endocarditis who subsequently died with widespread mycotic thromboemboli.

Finally, bacteria may colonize the myocardium itself as exemplified by a case of *Staphylococcus aureus* abscess formation reported by Egan *et al.*[114] Echocardiography showed a lucent area high in the interventricular septum pointing into the right ventricular outflow tract. Open heart surgery was performed and effected a complete cure although the patient died of opportunistic infection 6 months later.

Disorders of rhythm

There are four principal causes of rhythm disturbance in HIV infection – myocarditis and heart muscle disease, abnormalities of the conduction system, derangement of the autonomic nervous system and side effects of drug therapy. Dysrhythmias are undoubtedly responsible for some cases of sudden death occurring in HIV-positive patients.

Myocarditis and heart muscle disease in HIV infection are often complicated by ECG abnormalities and rhythm disturbances including high-grade atrial and ventricular ectopy,[18] ventricular tachycardia[52,115] and sudden death.[48,116]Levy *et al.*[48] studied two patients with myocarditis, one of whom

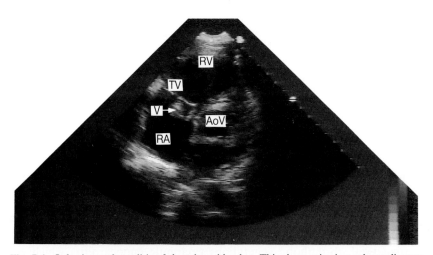

Fig. 7.4 Infective endocarditis of the tricuspid valve. This short axis view echocardiogram was taken at the aortic valve level. AoV = aortic valve. RA = right atrium. RV = right ventricle. TV = tricuspid valve. V = vegetation.

died in the course of an attempted resuscitation from polymorphic ventricular tachycardia, while the other succumbed to a cardiac arrest despite the absence of preceding Holter monitor abnormalities. Similarly, a group of four patients with ventricular tachycardia – one of which proved fatal – were identified by Reilly *et al.*[116] all of whom had myocarditis.

Conduction system abnormalities related to small vessel vasculitis, fibrosis of neural tissue and myocarditis have been described in children. These often, but not invariably, give rise to abnormalities of the ECG and rhythm disturbances.[117,118] The autonomic nervous system can be damaged by HIV[77] and Craddock *et al.*[119] reported a series of five patients who sustained syncopal reactions, one of which progressed to a fatal cardiorespiratory arrest, during percutaneous needle aspiration of the lung. The clinical features of these episodes were suggestive of underlying autonomic neuropathy and, indeed, one of these patients and a further four HIV patients studied had objective evidence of this phenomenon. Dysrhythmias due to excessive sympathetic tone are also recognized.[120]

There have been reports of ventricular arrhythmias associated with adjuvant therapy for opportunistic infection. Pentamadine, used widely for the treatment and prophylaxis of *Pneumocystis carinii* pneumonia, can cause ventricular tachycardia,[121–125] including torsade de pointes, possibly related to its structural similarity with procainamide.[121] This tendency may be enhanced by concomitant electrolyte deficiencies, particularly of magnesium.[121] Patients receiving pentamidine should be monitored for undue prolongation of the QT interval as a guide to potential cardiac toxicity. Recently, ganciclovir, which is used in the treatment of cytomegalovirus infection, has also been shown to provoke ventricular tachydysrhythmias.[126]

References

1. Chin J. Proceedings of the VIIth International Conference on AIDS. Florence, June 1991: Abstract.
2. Carc Calling 1992; **5:** 29.
3. Delamothe T. AIDS update. *Br Med J* 1991; **303:** 208.
4. Communicable Disease Report 1992; **2:** 235.
5. Rogers D. E., Gellin B. G. The bright spot about AIDS: it is very tough to catch. *AIDS* 1990; **4:** 695–6.
6. Berkelman R., Fleming P., Chu S., Hanson D. Women and AIDS: the increasing role of heterosexual transmission in the United States. *Proceedings of the VIIth International Conference on AIDS*. Florence, June 1991: Abstract WC 102.
7. Karpas A. Origin and spread of AIDS. *Nature* 1990; **348:** 578.
8. Peters B. S., Beck E. J., Coleman D. G. *et al.* Changing disease patterns in patients with AIDS in a referral centre in the United Kingdom: the changing face of AIDS. *Br Med J* 1991; **302:** 203–7.
9. Levy J. A. Changing concepts in HIV infection: challenges for the 1990s. *AIDS* 1991; **4:** 1051–8.
10. Robert Y., Samuel B. Immunology of HIV infection. In: Paul W. E. ed. *Fundamental Immunology*. Second edition. New York: Raven Press Ltd, 1989: 1059–79.
11. Cammarosano C., Lewis W. Cardiac lesions in acquired immune deficiency syndrome (AIDS). *J Am Coll Cardiol* 1985; **5:** 703–6.

12. Price R. W., Brew B., Sidtis J. *et al*. The brain in AIDS: Central nervous system HIV-1 infection and AIDS dementia complex. *Science* 1988; **239**: 586–92.
13. Churchill D. R. Gastrointestinal manifestations of AIDS. *Hospital Update* 1991; July: 577–84.
14. Acierno L. J. Cardiac complications in acquired immunodeficiency syndrome (AIDS): A Review. *J Am Coll Cardiol* 1989; **13**: 1144–54.
15. Heyworth M. F., Sullivan K. T., Liu G. H., Kim Y. S. Binding of HIV-1 gp 120 protein to CD4-negative colon cancer cell lines. *Proceedings of the VIIth Conference of AIDS*. Florence, June 1991: Abstract MA 1005.
16. Ho D. D., Pomerantz R. J., Kaplan J. C. Pathogenesis of infection with human immunodeficiency virus. *N Engl J Med* 1987; **317**: 278–86.
17. Joshi V. V., Pawel B., Connor E. *et al*. Arteriopathy in children with acquired immune deficiency syndrome. *Ped Pathol* 1987; **7**: 261–75.
18. Lipshultz S. E., Chanock S., Sanders S. P. *et al*. Cardiovascular manifestations of human immunodeficiency virus infection in infants and children. *Am J Cardiol* 1989; **63**: 1489–97.
19. Blanchard D. G., Hagenhoff C., Chow L. C. *et al*. Reversibility of cardiac abnormalities in human immunodeficiency virus (HIV)-infected individuals: a serial echocardiographic study. *J Am Coll Cardiol* 1991; **17**: 1270–6.
20. Kavanaugh-McHugh A. L., Hutton N., Holt E. *et al*. Echocardiographic abnormalities in pediatric HIV infection: prevalence and serial changes. *Proceedings of the VIIth International Conference on AIDS*. Florence, June 1991: Abstract MB 2402.
21. Stewart J. M., Kaul A., Gromische D. S. *et al*. Symptomatic cardiac dysfunction in children with human immunodeficiency virus infection. *Am Heart J* 1989; **117**: 140–4.
22. Fink L., Reichek N., St John Sutton M. G. Cardiac abnormalities in acquired immune deficiency syndrome. *Am J Cardiol* 1984; **54**: 1161–3.
23. Corallo S., Mutinelli M. R., Moroni M. *et al*. Echocardiography detects myocardial damage in AIDS: prospective study in 102 patients. *Eur Heart J* 1988; **9**: 887–92.
24. Lewis W. AIDS: cardiac findings from 115 autopsies. *Prog Cardiovasc Dis* 1989; **32**: 207–15.
25. Himelman B., Chung W. S., Chernoff D. N. *et al*. Cardiac manifestations of human immunodeficiency virus infection: a two-dimensional echocardiographic study. *J Am Coll Cardiol* 1989; **13**: 1030–6.
26. Aretz T. H., Bllingham M. E., Edwards W. D. *et al*. Myocarditis: a histopathologic definition and classification. *Am J Cardiovasc Pathol* 1987; **1**: 3–14.
27. Anderson D. W., Virmani R., Reilly J. M. *et al*. Prevalent myocarditis at necropsy in the acquired immunodeficiency syndrome. *J Am Coll Cardiol* 1988; **11**: 792–9.
28. Baroldi G., Corallo S., Moroni M. *et al*. Focal lymphocytic myocarditis in acquired immunodeficiency syndrome (AIDS): a correlative morphologic and clinical study in 26 consecutive fatal cases. *J Am Coll Cardiol* 1988; **12**: 463–9.
29. Moore J., Blanc D. F. Immunological incompetence in AIDS. *AIDS* 1991; **5**: 455–6.
30. Grody W. W., Cheng L., Lewis W. Infection of the heart by the human immunodeficiency virus. *Am J Cardiol* 1990; **66**: 203–6.
31. Flomenbaum M., Soeiro R., Udem S. A. *et al*. Proliferative membranopathy and human immunodeficiency virus in AIDS hearts. *J AIDS* 1989; **2**: 129–35.
32. Lipshultz S. E., Fox C. H., Perez-Atayde A. R. *et al*. Identification of human immunodeficiency virus-1 RNA and DNA in the heart of a child with cardiovascular abnormalities and congenital acquired immune deficiency syndrome. *Am J Cardiol* 1990; **66**: 240–50.
33. Calabrese L. H., Proffitt M. R., Yen-Lieberman B. *et al*. Congestive cardiomyo-

pathy and illness related to the acquired immunodeficiency syndrome (AIDS) associated with isolation of retrovirus from myocardium. *Ann Int Med* 1987; **107:** 691–2.

34. Dittrich H., Chow L., Denaro F., Spector S. Human immunodeficiency virus, coxsackievirus, and cardiomypathy (letter). *Ann Int Med* 1988; **108:** 308.

35. Trujillo J. R., Gomez-Lucia E., Lee T. H., Essex M. Retroviral effects on muscle cells. *Proceedings of the VIIth International Conference on AIDS*. Florence, June 1991: Abstract MA 1261.

36. Herskowitz A., Willoughby S., Oliveira M. *et al*. HIV-associated cardiomyopathy: evidence for autoimmunity. *Proceedings of the VIth Conference on AIDS*. San Francisco, June 1990: Abstract FB 510.

37. Lahdevirta J., Maury C. P. J., Teppo A.-M., Repo H. Cachectin/tumor necrosis factor in AIDS. *Am J Med* 1988; **85:** 289–91.

38. Hofman P., Michiels J. F., Mainguene C. *et al*. Cardiac toxoplasmosis in acquired immunodeficiency syndrome (AIDS). A *post mortem* study of 15 cases. *Proceedings of the VIIth International Conference on AIDS*. Florence, June 1991: Abstract MB 2386.

39. Lafont A., Marche C., Wolff M. *et al*. Myocarditis in acquired immunodeficiency syndrome (AIDS): etiology and prognosis. *J Am Coll Cardiol* 1988; **11:** 196A.

40. Vynn Adair O., Randive N., Krasnow N. Isolated toxoplasma myocarditis in acquired immune deficiency syndrome. *Am Heart J* 1989; **118:** 856–7.

41. Roldan E. O., Moskowit L., Hensley G. T. Pathology of the heart in acquired immunodeficiency syndrome. *Arch Pathol Lab Med* 1987; **111:** 943–6.

42. Lewis W., Lipsick J., Cammarosano C. Crytococcal myocarditis in acquired immunodefiency syndrome. *Am J Cardiol* 1985; **55:** 1240.

43. Cox J. N., di Dio F., Pizzolato G. P. *et al*. Aspergillus endocarditis and myocarditis in a patient with the acquired immunodeficiency syndrome (AIDS). *Virch Arch (A) Pathol Anat* 1990; **417:** 255–9.

44. Mycoplasma and AIDS – what connection? (editorial). *Lancet* 1991; **337:** 20–2.

45. Nelson J. A., Ghazal P., Wiley C. A. Role of opportunistic viral infections in AIDS. *AIDS* 1990; **4:** 1–10.

46. Grange F., Kinney E. L., Monsuez J. *et al*. Successful therapy for *Toxoplasma gondii* myocarditis in acquired immunodeficiency syndrome. *Am Heart J* 1990; **120:** 443–4.

47. Simpson D. M., Wolfe D. E. Neuromuscular complications of HIV infection and its treatment. *AIDS* 1991; **5:** 917–26.

48. Levy W. S., Varghese P. J., Anderson D. W. *et al*. Myocarditis diagnosed by endomyocardial biopsy in human immunodeficiency virus infection with cardiac dysfunction. *Am J Cardiol* 1988; **62:** 658–9.

49. Lafont A., Wolff M., Marche C. *et al*. Overwhelming myocarditis due to *Cryptococcus neoformans* in an AIDS patient (letter). *Lancet* 1987; **ii:** 1145–6.

50. Cohen I. S., Anderson D. W., Virmani R. *et al*. Congestive cardiomyopathy in association with the acquired immunodeficiency syndrome. *N Engl J Med* 1986; **315:** 628–30.

51. Raffanti S. R., Chiaramida A. J., Sen P. *et al*. Assessment of cardiac function in patients with the acquired immunodeficiency syndrome. *Chest* 1988; **93:** 592–4.

52. Levy W. S., Simon G. L., Riso J. C., Ross A. M. Prevalence of cardiac abnormalities in human immunodeficiency virus infection. *Am J Cardiol* 1989; **63:** 86–9.

53. Corboy J. R., Fink L., Miller W. T. Congestive cardiomyopathy in association with AIDS. *Radiology* 1987; **165:** 139–41.

54. Steinherz L. J., Brochstein J. A., Robins J. Cardiac involvement in congenital acquired immunodeficiency syndrome. *Am J Dis Child* 1986; **140:** 1241–4.

55. Joshi V. V., Gadol C., Connor E. *et al*. Dilated cardiomyopathy in children with

acquired immunodeficiency syndrome: a pathologic study of five cases. *Human Pathol* 1988; **19:** 69–73.

56. Report of the WHO/ISFC task force on the definition and classification of cardiomyopathies. *Br Heart J* 1980; **44:** 672–3.

57. Jacob A. J., Sutherland G. R., Brettle R. P. *et al.* HIV heart muscle disease – the Edinburgh experience. *Eur Heart J* 1991; **12:** abstract 1215.

58. Monsuez J., Kinney E. L., Vittecoq D. *et al.* Comparison among acquired immune deficiency syndrome patients with and without clinical evidence of cardiac disease. *Am J Cardiol* 1988; **62:** 1311–13.

59. Flavia T., Jacopi F., Maresta A. *et al.* Incidence and natural history of HIV-associated heart disease. *Proceedings of the VIIth International Conference on AIDS.* Florence, June 1991: Abstract MB 2379.

60. Oakley C. M. Cardiomyopathies. *Curr Opin Cardiol* 1990; **5:** 300–2.

61. Richardson P. J., Why H. J. F. Dilated cardiomyopathy. *Curr Opin Cardiol* 1990; **5:** 306–9.

62. Kereiakes D. J., Parmley W. W. Myocarditis and cardiomyopathy. *Am Heart J* 1984; **108:** 1318–26.

63. MacArthur C. G. C., Tarin D., Goodwin J. F., Hallidie-Smith K. A. The relationship of myocarditis to dilated cardiomyopathy. *Eur Heart J* 1984; **5:** 1023–35.

64. Wolff S. M. Monoclonal antibodies and the treatment of Gram-negative bacteremia and shock. *N Engl J Med* 1991; **324:** 486–8.

65. O'Connell J. B., Mason J. W. Immunosuppressive therapy in experimental and clinical myocarditis. *Pathol Immunopathol Res* 1988; **7:** 292–304.

66. Kotler D. P. Malnutrition in HIV infection and *AIDS* 1989; **3** (suppl 1): S175–S180.

67. Nutrition and HIV (editorial). *Lancet* 1991; **338:** 86–7.

68. Beach R. S., Cabrejos C., Mantero-Atienza E. *et al.* Effect of zinc normalization on immunological function in early HIV-1 infection. *Proceedings of the VIIth International Conference on AIDS.* Florence, June 1991: Abstract MC 3128.

69. Baum M. K., Beach R., Mantero-Atienza E. *et al.* Predictors of change in immune function: longitudinal analysis of nutritional and immune status in early HIV-1 infection. *Proceedings of the VIIth International Conference on AIDS.* Florence, June 1991: Abstract MC 3127.

70. Mantero-Atienza E., Solomayor M. C., Shor-Posner G. *et al.* Selenium status and immune function in early HIV-1 infection. *Proceedings of the VIIth International Conference on AIDS.* Florence, June 1991: Abstract MC 3126.

71. Dworkin B. M., Rosenthal W. S., Wormser G. P., Weiss L. Selenium deficiency in the acquired immunodeficiency syndrome. *J Parenteral Enteral Nut* 1986; **10:** 405–7.

72. Beutler B. The presence of cachectin/tumor necrosis factor in human disease states. *Am J Med* 1988; **85:** 287–8.

73. Fuchs J., Jenka S., Ochendorf F. *et al.* Oxidants and antioxidants in HIV infected patients. *Proceedings of the VIIth International Conference on AIDS.* Florence, June 1991: Abstract WB 2166.

74. Keshan Disease Research Group (Chinese Academy of Medical Sciences). Observations on effect of sodium selenite in the prevention of Keshan disease. *Chin Med J* 1979; **92:** 471–6.

75. Zazzo J. F., Chalas J., Lafont A. *et al.* Is nonobstructive cardiomyopathy in AIDS a selenium deficiency-related disease? *J Parenteral Enteral Nut* 1988; **12:** 537–8.

76. Sardesai S. H., Mourant A. J., Sivathandon Y. *et al.* Phaeochromocytoma and catecholamine induced cardiomyopathy presenting as heart failure. *Br Heart J* 1990; **63;** 234–7.

77. Freeman R., Roberts M. S., Friedman L. S., Broadbridge C. Autonomic func-

tion and human immunodeficiency virus infections. *Neurology* 1990; **40:** 575–80.
78. Glulio L., Petrucci T., Patrizio M., Bernardo A. HIV envelope glycoprotein gp120 interacts with astroglial beta-adrenergic receptors. *Proceedings of the VIIth International Conference on AIDS*. Florence, June 1991: Abstract MA 1037.
79. Fischl M. A. State of antiretroviral therapy with zidovudine. *AIDS* 1989; **3** (suppl 1): S137–S143.
80. Arnaudo E., Dalakas M., Shanske S. *et al*. Depletion of muscle mitochondrial DNA in AIDS patients with zidovudine-induced myopathy. *Lancet* 1991; **337:** 508–10.
81. Berger J. R., Sherbert R., Gregorios J. B. Exacerbation of HIV-associated myopathy by zidovudine. *AIDS* 1991; **5:** 229–30.
82. Lamperth L., Dalakas M. AZT-induced myocytotoxicity and cardiac toxicity. *Proceedings of the VIIth International Conference on AIDS*. Florence, June 1991. Abstract WA 63.
83. Jacob A. J., Sutherland G., Brettle R. *et al*. Is zidovudine responsible for HIV heart muscle disease? *Clin Sci* 1991 **81:** 31 (abs).
84. Himelman R. B., Dohrmann M., Goodman P. *et al*. Severe pulmonary hypertension and cor pulmonale in the acquired immunodeficiency syndrome. *Am J Cardiol* 1989; **64:** 1396–9.
85. Hays M. D., Wiles H. B., Gillette P. C. Congenital acquired immunodeficiency syndrome presenting as cor pulmonale in a 10-year-old girl. *Am Heart J* 1991: **121:** 929–31.
86. Citron B. P., Halpern M., McCarron M. *et al*. Necrotizing angiitis associated with drug abuse. *N Engl J Med* 1970; **283:** 1003–11.
87. Coplan N. L., Shimony R. Y., Ioachim H. L. *et al*. Primary pulmonary hypertension associated with human immunodeficiency viral infection. *Am J Med* 1990; **89:** 96–9.
88. Romeu J., Larrousse E., Sirera G. *et al*. Utility of echocardiography in AIDS (letter). *Chest* 1990; **98:** 775.
89. Kagame A., Taelman H., Bogeerts J. *et al*. Pericardial effusion and HIV infection in Kigali, Rwanda. *Proceedings of the VIth International Conference on AIDS*. San Francisco, June 1990: Abstract 2051.
90. Scott P. J., Conway S. P., Da Costa P. Cardiac tamponade complicating cytomegalovirus pericarditis in a patient with AIDS. *J Infect* 1990; **20:** 92–3.
91. Turco M., Seneff M., McGrath B. J., Hsia J. Cardiac tamponade in the acquired immunodeficiency syndrome. *Am Heart J* 1990; **120:** 1467–8.
92. Andress J. D., Polish L. B., Clark D. M., Hossack K. F. Transvenous biopsy diagnosis of cardiac lymphoma in an AIDS patient. *Am Heart J* 1989; **118:** 421–3.
93. Cegielski J. P., Ramaiya K., Lallinger G. J. *et al*. Pericardial disease and human immunodeficiency virus in Dar es Salaam, Tanzania. *Lancet* 1990; **335:** 209–12.
94. Reynolds M., Berger M., Hecht S. *et al*. Large pericardial effusions associated with the acquired immune deficiency syndrome (AIDS). *J Am Coll Cardiol* 1991; **17:** 221A.
95. Woods G. L., Goldsmith J. C. Fatal pericarditis due to *Myocobacterium aviumintracellulare* in acquired immunodeficiency syndrome. *Chest* 1989; **95:** 1355–7.
96. Steigman C. K., Anderson D. W., Macher A. M. *et al*. Fatal cardiac tamponade in acquired immunodeficiency syndrome with epicardial Kaposi's sarcoma. *Am Heart J* 1988; **116:** 1105–7.
97. Stotka J. L., Good C. B., Downer W. R., Kapoor W. N. Pericardial effusion and tamponade due to Kaposi's sarcoma in acquired immunodeficiency syndrome. *Chest* 1989; **95:** 1359–61.
98. Bivet F., Livartowski J., Herve P. *et al*. Pericardial cryptococcal disease in acquired immune deficiency syndrome (letter). *Am J Med* 1987; **82:** 1273.
99. Stechel R. P., Cooper D. J., Greenspan J. *et al*. Staphylococcal pericarditis in a homosexual. *N Y State J Med* 1986; **86:** 592–3.

100. Toma E., Poisson M., Claessens M. *et al*. Herpes simplex, Type 2 pericarditis and bilateral facial palsy in a patient with AIDS. *J Infect Dis* 1989; **160:** 553–4.
101. Freedberg R. S., Gindea A. J., Dieterich D. T., Greene J. B. Herpes simplex pericarditis in AIDS. *N Y State J Med* 1987; **87:** 304–6.
102. D'Cruz I. A., Sengupta E. E., Abrahams C. *et al*. Cardiac involvement, including tuberculous pericardial effusion, complicating acquired immune deficiency syndrome. *Am Heart J* 1986; **112:** 1100–2.
103. Dalli E., Quesada A., Juan G. *et al*. Tuberculous pericarditis as the first manifestation of acquired immunodeficiency syndrome. *Am Heart J* 1987; **114:** 905–6.
104. Silver M. A., Macher A. M., Reichert C. M. *et al*. Cardiac involvement by Kaposi's sarcoma in acquired immune deficiency syndrome (AIDS). *Am J Cardiol* 1984; **53:** 983–5.
105. Goldfarb A., King C. L., Rosenzweig B. P. *et al*. Cardiac lymphoma in the acquired immunodeficiency syndrome. *Am Heart J* 1989; **118:** 1340–4.
106. Krigel R. L., Friedman-Kien A. E. Kaposi's sarcoma in AIDS. In: DeVita V. T., Hellman S, Rosenberg S. A. eds. *AIDS*. Philadelphia: J. B. Lippincott Co., 1985.
107. Autran B. R., Gorin I., Leibowitch M. *et al*. AIDS in a Haitian woman with cardiac Kaposi's sarcoma and Whipple's disease. *Lancet* 1983; **i:** 767–8.
108. McAllister H. A., Fenoglio J. J. Jr. Tumors of the cardiovascular system. In: McAllister H. A., Fenoglio J. J. eds. *Atlas of Tumor Pathology*. Washington DC: Armed Forces Institute of Pathology, 1978: 111–19.
109. Balasubramanyam A., Waxman M., Kazal H. L., Hi Lee M. Malignant lymphoma of the heart in acquired immune deficiency syndrome. *Chest* 1986; **90:** 243–6.
110. Constantino A., West T. E., Gupta M., Loghmanee F. Primary cardiac lymphoma in a patient with acquired immune deficiency syndrome. *Cancer* 1987; **60:** 2801–5.
111. Kinney E. L., Monsuez J.-J., Kitzis M., Vittecoq D. Treatment of AIDS-associated heart disease. *Angiology* 1989; **40:** 970–6.
112. Stool E., Gathe J. Jr, Plot D. *et al*. Fusariosis with endocarditis in a patient with AIDS. *Proceedings of the VIIth International Conference of AIDS*. Florence, June 1991: Abstract MB 2390.
113. Henochowicz S., Mustafa M., Lawrinson W. E. *et al*. Cardiac aspergillosis in acquired immune deficiency syndrome. *Am J Cardiol* 1985; **55:** 1239–40.
114. Egan T. M., Maitland A., Sinave C. *et al*. Myocardial abscess in a patient with AIDS-related complex: pericardial patch repair. *Ann Thor Surg* 1990; **49:** 481–2.
115. Olson L. J., Gertz M. A., Edwards W. D. *et al*. Senile cardiac amyloidosis with functional impairment; diagnosis by myocardial biopsy and immunohistochemistry. *J Am Coll Cardiol* 1987; **9:** 154A.
116. Reilly J. M., Cunnion R. E., Anderson D. W. *et al*. Frequency of myocarditis, left ventricular dysfunction and ventricular tachycardia in the acquired immune deficiency syndrome. *Am J Cardiol* 1988; **62:** 789–93.
117. Bharati S., Lev M. Pathology of the heart in AIDS. *Prog Cardiol* 1989; **2/2:** 261–72.
118. Bharati S., Joshi V. V., Connor E. M. *et al*. Conduction system in children with acquired immunodeficiency syndrome. *Chest* 1989; **96:** 406–13.
119. Craddock C., Pasvol G., Bull R. *et al*. Cardiorespiratory arrest and autonomic neuropathy in AIDS. *Lancet* 1987; **i:** 16–18.
120. Lipshultz S. E., Luginbuhl L., McIntosh K. Dysrhythmias, unexpected arrest and sudden death in pediatric HIV infection. *Proceedings of the VIIth International Conference on AIDS*. Florence, June 1991: Abstract TU B 36.
121. Wharton J. M., Demopulos P. A., Goldschlager N. Torsades de pointes during administration of pentamidine isethionate. *Am J Med* 1987; **83:** 571–6.

122. Pujol M., Carratala J., Mauri J., Viladrich P. F. Ventricular tachycardia due to pentamidine isethionate (letter). *Am J Med* 1988; **84:** 980.
123. Mitchell P., Dodek P., Lawson L. *et al.* Torsades de pointes during intravenous pentamidine isethionate therapy. *Can Med Assoc J* 1989; **140:** 173–4.
124. Loescher T. H., Loeschke K., Niebel J. Severe ventricular arrhythmia during pentamidine treatment of AIDS-associated pneumocystis carinii pneumonia (letter). *Infection* 1987; **45:** 455.
125. Stein K. M., Haronian H., Mensah G. A. *et al.* Ventricular tachycardia and torsades de pointes complicating pentamidine therapy of *Pneumocystis carinii* pneumonia in the acquired immunodeficiency syndrome. *Am J Cardiol* 1990; **66:** 888–9.
126. Cohen A. J., Weiser B., Afzal Q., Fuhrer J. Ventricular tachycardia in two patients with AIDS receiving ganciclovir (DHPG). *AIDS* 1990; **4:** 807–9.

8

The role of cytomegalovirus in human atherosclerosis

J. L. Melnick and E. Adam

Introduction

Atherosclerosis places an enormous burden on society with the high morbidity and mortality and the financial losses associated with the disease. Recent progress has been made in diagnosis, chemotherapy, and surgical intervention, but these procedures are not simple and remain expensive. If atherosclerosis is to become a preventable illness, a better understanding is required of the primary causes and pathogenesis of the disease.

Atherosclerotic lesions usually become apparent in adult patients as a result of complete occlusion of a strategic blood vessel and the resulting complications. Yet, lesions often begin to form in adolescence, or sometimes even in young children. Such lesions may persist, or regress. However, they often progress and cause the serious clinical manifestations associated with ischaemic disease.[1-3] Risk factors, such as high blood pressure, smoking and high serum cholesterol, that enhance the progression of the atherosclerotic lesion, have been identified and their control inhibits the progression of the primary lesion.[4] This chapter will not address these enhancing risk factors but will be concerned with possible mechanisms through which the primary lesion is initiated and maintained.

It was the Fabricants'[5,6] reports on induction of atherosclerosis in chickens by an avian herpesvirus (Marek) that stimulated many of the subsequent investigations on human atherosclerosis reviewed in this chapter.

The structure of the arterial wall has been described in detail.[2,3] There are three layers in the wall – the intima, the media and the adventitia, each separated by thin sheets of elastic fibres. The innermost layer, the intima, is believed to be the one most directly involved in the initiation of atherogenesis. Surrounding the epithelial layer are occasional smooth muscle cells and connective tissue fibres. This major component of the vessel wall is known as the media, consisting chiefly of smooth muscle cells, which may be present in several layers depending upon the size of the vessel. Surrounding the media is the adventitia, made up of fibroblasts and smooth muscle cells embedded in connective tissue.

This chapter will not deal with the disease process, arteriosclerosis, this being a loss of the elasticity of the arterial wall that accompanies aging, but will focus on atherogenesis, the beginning of the process leading to atherosclerosis in which the intima is chiefly affected. The lesion itself, known as the atherosclerotic plaque, consists of lipid deposits, leucocytes, smooth muscle cells and connective tissue, often characterized by calcification, haemorrhage, and necrosis.[3]

Atherogenesis is believed to follow a response to injury[2] but the agent or agents of injury remain elusive. Recent evidence supports the hypothesis that cytomegalovirus may act as such an agent. This hypothesis is compatible with the view that a transforming event causes a single smooth muscle cell to begin dividing and to form a monoclone of proliferating cells, similar to a benign neoplasm.[7] The Benditts[7] suggested that an infectious agent might be a good candidate for initiating monoclonal atherosclerosis, as a nonspecific injury would be expected to cause a nonspecific polyclonal response. The subsequent demonstration that DNA from atherosclerotic plaques, but not from a normal artery, could transform murine 3T3 cells to malignancy is consistent with the monoclonal hypothesis of atherogenesis.[8]

Animal model systems

In 1950, Paterson and Cottral[9] called attention to the development of coronary atherosclerosis in chickens ill with Marek's lymphomatosis. Subsequently the aetiological agent of Marek's disease was discovered to be a herpesvirus, known as Marek's disease virus (MDV). A vaccine was developed for the disease and is currently in widespread use in the poultry industry. Subsequently, Fabricant et al.[5] observed that inoculation of MDV into pathogen-free chickens caused atherosclerosis as well as lymphomatosis.

Upon visual examination, 14% of the chickens infected with the herpesvirus developed atherosclerosis, but upon microscopic examination the rate increased to 65%, but remained zero for the control, noninfected animals. Cholesterol acted as a risk factor by accelerating the disease process. Thus feeding chickens with a cholesterol-rich diet increased the rate of visible and microscopic disease and enhanced the fatty nature of the lesions. In contrast, uninfected chickens failed to develop atherosclerotic plaques regardless of the amount of cholesterol fed to them.

Arterial smooth muscle cells at the periphery of the lesion contained viral antigens as revealed by immunofluorescence. Benditt et al.[10] added to these findings by demonstrating nucleic acid sequences of MDV in arteries of infected chickens.

A vaccine for MDV has been developed; it is a live herpesvirus of turkeys, antigenically related to MDV. It causes neither lymphomatosis nor atherosclerosis in chickens, but vaccinated chickens are completely resistant to MDV-induced atherosclerosis.[11]

A second avian model system for herpesvirus-related atherosclerosis is provided by the Japanese quail. Strains of quail were extensively inbred by Shih et al.[12] and selected for either susceptibility or resistance to atherosclerosis induced by dietary cholesterol. Dot hybridization experiments using a library of viral DNA probes showed that DNA extracted from arteries or from embryos of susceptible quail contained sequences related to MDV, the avian herpesvirus, whereas DNA from tissues of resistant quail did not. It is not known which viral genes are carried by the susceptible quail or whether they are derived from MDV itself or from a related herpesvirus of quail. However, these results implicate herpesviruses (or viral genes) in the aetiology of atherosclerosis in at least two avian species. It would be worthwhile to determine whether atherosclerosis-prone strains of pigeons also carry herpesvirus genes.

Cholesterol accumulation in Marek's disease virus-infected cells

The mechanism of MDV-induced atherogenesis was investigated by infecting smooth muscle cells cultured from normal chicken arteries with the virus.[13] Marek's disease virus-infected cells had significantly more cholesterol and cholesteryl esters than did mock-infected cells. Similar lipid analyses were performed on arterial tissues from MDV-infected chickens,[14] and uninfected control chickens. After 4 months, the MDV-infected birds had a two- to three-fold increase over the control chickens in total aortic lipids, especially cholesterol, cholesteryl esters and phospholipid, suggesting that alterations in cholesterol metabolism were due specifically to the virus infection and occur during early stages of the disease.

Infection by MDV changed the activity of important enzymes involved with lipid metabolism: infection resulted in a rise in cholesterol ester synthetic activity but prevented the normal age-related rise in cholesterol ester hydrolase activity. Together, these activities promote cellular lipid accumulation. It is evident that a herpervirus can initiate atherosclerosis in at least one animal model and that the virus induces basic changes in aortic smooth muscle cell lipid content and changes in enzyme activity involved in cellular lipid metabolism. Furthermore, it was demonstrated that all of these changes could be prevented by vaccination.

The herpesvirus family(see also Chapter 1)

Many characteristics of the human herpesviruses, and of cytomegalovirus in particular, are consistent with a role in atherogenesis.[15,16] All are widely distributed in the population, and childhood infections are common. The herpesvirus family contains several important human pathogens. They possess a large number of genes, some of which have proved to be susceptible to anti-viral chemotherapy. The outstanding property of herpesviruses is their ability to establish lifelong persistent infections in their hosts and to undergo periodic reactivation. It is their frequent reactivation in immunosuppressed patients which is now recognized to lead to serious health complications. The reactivated infection may be clinically quite different from the primary infection.

Herpesviruses of humans include *Herpes simplex* virus types 1 and 2 (HSV-1 and HSV-2), varicella-zoster virus (VZV), cytomegalovirus (CMV), Epstein–Barr virus (EBV) and human herpesvirus 6 (HHV-6).

A useful division of Herpesviridae into subfamilies is based on biologic properties of the agents (Table 8.1). Alphaherpesviruses (HSV, VZV) are fast-growing, cytolytic viruses that tend to establish latent infections in neurons. Betaherpesviruses (CMV) are slow-growing and cytomegalic (involving massive enlargements of infected cells) and become latent in secretory glands and kidneys. Gammaherpesviruses (EBV) infect lymphoid cells. Another herpesvirus, human B-lymphotropic virus, has been recovered re-

Table 8.1 Classification of human herpesviruses. Family: Herpesviridae.*

Subfamily	Biological Properties			Examples	
	Growth cycle	Cytopathology	Latent infections	Official name	Common name
Alphaherpesvirinae	Short	Cytolytic	Neurons	Human herpesvirus 1 Human herpesvirus 2 Human herpesvirus 3	Herpes simplex virus type 1 Herpes simplex virus type 2 Varicella-zoster virus
Betaherpesvirinae	Long	Cytomegalic	Salivary glands, kidneys	Human herpesvirus 5	Cytomegalovirus
Gammaherpesvirinae	Variable	Lymphoproliferative	Lymphoid tissue	Human herpesvirus 4	Epstein–Barr virus

*A recently recognized member, human herpesvirus 6 (HHV-6) is a human B cell lymphotropic virus often recovered from patients with lymphoproliferative illnesses. It possesses a genome that resembles that of cytomegalovirus more than that of the gammaherpes Epstein–Barr virus.

cently from patients with lymphoproliferative disorders. It has been designated human herpesvirus 6 (HHV-6). Surprisingly, its genome resembles that of cytomegalovirus.

There is little antigenic relatedness among the members of the herpesvirus family. Only *Herpes simplex* virus types 1 and 2 share a significant number of common antigens. This is not surprising, since there is approximately 50% homology between these two viral genomes.

Although infection is usually inapparent, a wide range of diseases are associated with the herpesviruses. Primary infection and reactivated disease caused by a given virus may involve different cell types and present different clinical pictures.

Herpes simplex virus type 1 and HSV-2 infect epithelial cells and establish latent infections in neurons. Type 1 virus is classically associated with oropharyngeal lesions and causes recurrent attacks of 'fever blisters'. Type 2 primarily infects the genital mucosa and is mainly responsible for genital herpes. Both viruses may also cause neurological disease; HSV-1 is the leading cause of sporadic encephalitis in the USA.

Varicella-zoster virus causes chickenpox (varicella) on primary infection and establishes latent infection in neurons. Upon reactivation, the virus causes 'shingles' (zoster), usually localized to a single dermatome area innervated by a single spinal nerve.

Epstein–Barr virus replicates in epithelial cells of the oropharynx and parotid gland and establishes latent infections in lymphocytes. It causes infectious mononucleosis and appears to be closely involved in the pathogenesis of two human cancers, one a lymphoma (Burkitt's Lymphoma) and the other a carcinoma (nasopharyngeal carcinoma).

Human herpesvirus 6 also infects lymphocytes. It is acquired typically in early infancy and causes exanthem subitum (roseola infantum). Target cells for latent infections and the consequences of reactivations are not known as yet.

Cytomegalovirus replicates in epithelial cells of the respiratory tract, salivary glands and kidneys, and persists in lymphocytes. It may cause infectious mononucleosis. In newborns, cytomegalic inclusion disease may occur. If acquired *in utero* CMV may cause congenital defects and mental retardation. In the USA the prevalence of antibodies to CMV is about 10–15% in the adolescent population, it may rise to 40 or 50% by the age of 35, and may exceed 60 to 70% in adults over the age of 65 years, an age-related pattern similar to that of atherosclerosis. The site of latency for CMV is unknown, although this virus has been isolated from a variety of tissues throughout the body, including lymphocytes that have prolonged contact with cells lining the blood vessel walls.

Because of the features of the herpesvirus family relating to latency and transformation, and since an avian herpesvirus has been observed to induce atherosclerosis in chickens, studies focussed on possible infection of arterial smooth muscle cells by CMV or other human herpesviruses. It was thought that such infections might stimulate smooth muscle cells to proliferate and thereby contribute to the formation of atherosclerotic plaques in humans. Another model system is being developed by Nachtigal et al.[17] using rabbit aortic smooth muscle cells and the early region of the genome of papovavirus SV40, a virus that is also characterized by being tumourigenic and producing latency.

Transformed clones were obtained which accumulated cholesteryl esters after incubation with low-density lipoprotein.

Viruses associated with human atherosclerosis

In the 1960s, the contemporary knowledge of human herpesviruses, when considered together with the new evidence linking a herpesvirus to induction of atherosclerosis in chickens, led several research groups to investigate the possibility of herpesvirus involvement in human atherosclerosis. These studies are summarized below.

An attempt was made to detect viruses in human atheromatous lesions. From 60 biopsy specimens, a single virus isolate was made, this being a member of the paramyxovirus group.[18] As a part of this study, biopsy specimens were also grown in cell culture, but none spontaneously yielded infectious virus.[19]

About 15 years later, in light of the Fabricants' work, the possibility that virus was present in biopsies of atheromatous lesions was reinvestigated. Again, biopsy arterial fragments were placed in culture, but this time attempts were made to detect a latent virus[20,21] by examining the cellular outgrowth for viral antigens and viral nucleic acid sequences. Immunocytochemical techniques were used to screen the biopsies of arterial tissue for evidence of infection with HSV-1, HSV-2 and CMV. This approach was based on the premise that cells which are abortively or persistently infected with a virus may express one or more proteins coded by the viral genome, even if little or no infectious virus is produced. Atherosclerotic plaque tissues were obtained primarily from patients undergoing endarterectomy to relieve stenosis of the carotid arteries. They therefore represented patients with advanced stages of the disease. A few plaque tissues from abdominal aortas, iliac arteries and femoral arteries were also obtained. In addition, punch biopsies of the ascending aortas were obtained from patients undergoing coronary artery bypass surgery. These 'uninvolved' tissues showed minimal atherosclerotic changes upon histological examination. By direct electron microscopic examination of biopsy specimens from the proximal aorta of patients with atherosclerosis, virions of the herpesvirus family could at times be detected, but only after a painstaking, meticulous search.[22] Observed in smooth muscle cells in uninvolved areas in 10 of 60 patients examined, they had the features of incomplete virions.[23,24] The virions were relatively few in number, but when present they were often present in a cluster. Sections from more than 300 plaque tissues and 60 'uninvolved' aortic punch biopsies were reacted with hyperimmune antisera to HSV-1, HSV-2 and CMV. None of these tissues gave a positive reaction with any of the viral antisera, indicating that complete virions were not being formed, at least not in detectable amounts.

Production of viral proteins is often higher in actively growing cells than in quiescent cells such as those in differentiated tissue. Therefore, explant cultures were established from both the plaque tissues and the 'uninvolved' aortic tissues of the above patients. Cells like those of small muscle were successfully grown from finely minced pieces of 54 arterial samples. These cells were tested during their first or second passage in culture for both CMV and HSV-1 antigens, and in some cases for HSV-2 antigens. Twenty of the 54 arterial outgrowths yielded cells containing CMV-specific proteins, whereas none contained HSV1 or HSV-2 proteins. If CMV is indeed a direct cause of atherosclerosis, it may seem somewhat surprising that a higher percentage of cultures from the 'uninvolved' aorta tissues (52%) contained CMV antigens than did cultures from advanced atherosclerotic plaques (29%). However, in the chickens infected with the avian herpesvirus, as discussed above, viral antigens were found in smooth muscle cells of the media during the early stages of pathogenesis. But in advanced disease, viral antigens were found only in smooth muscle cells at the periphery of atherosclerotic plaques, but not in the lesions themselves. Thus, CMV may be an initiating factor that is no longer active in advanced complex plaques. These plaques contain few viable cells (as indicated by the low rate of success in establishing explant cultures), and it is likely that the cells that did grow were derived from tissue peripheral to the necrotic areas of the plaques.

Seventeen of the cell cultures were also examined for the presence of CMV and HSV nucleic acids by *in situ* hybridization using viral DNA probes.[15] The results were similar to those described above, except that some cultures that were negative for CMV antigens proved positive for CMV nucleic acid sequences, reflecting the greater sensitivity of the *in situ* hybridization reaction.

The *in situ* hybridization technique was used by Benditt *et al.*[10] to detect nucleic acid sequences specific for HSV-2, CMV and EBV in small pieces of ascending aortic tissue removed during coronary bypass surgery. In the initial series of experiments, HSV sequences were detected in 11 of 160 tissue samples. In most cases there was little intimal thickening, and positive cells were scattered in the media. In the second series of experiments, four tissue samples were selected because they contained abnormally thickened intima. Sections cut from these tissues were hybridized with DNA probes for HSV-2, CMV and EBV. Two tissues reacted with the HSV-2 probe; none reacted with any of the other probes. The cells containing HSV nucleic acid sequences were located in discrete foci of increased cellularity within or adjacent to the intima.

The next study to be reported was conducted in Chicago by Yamashiroya *et al.*[25] They demonstrated the presence of HSV and CMV genomic sequences and antigens in the coronary arteries and thoracic aortas of 20 young trauma victims between 15 and 35 years of age. Each had been in good health prior to being killed in an accident. Fresh arterial tissue was removed at autopsy and studied by *in situ* DNA hybridization and by immunoperoxidase methods.

Among the 20 subjects, either HSV or CMV latency was detected in the coronary arteries of eight subjects, and in the thoracic aortas of seven subjects. None of the specimens were positive for EBV. It is noteworthy that the positive HSV/CMV findings were often present in areas of the arterial wall showing early atheromatous changes: focal areas of intimal thickening with smooth muscle proliferation and lymphocytic infiltration. No complete infectious virus could be detected, in keeping with our earlier studies.

In recent investigations carried out in Holland by Hendrix *et al.*[26,27] femoral or abdominal arterial samples were obtained (1) from 44 patients undergoing vascular surgery (mean age, 66 years) and (2) from an autopsy-control group of 34 patients (mean age 69 years), who died from nonatherosclerosis-associated diseases and in whom abdominal aorta specimens were removed 12 hours *post mortem*. Demonstration of sequence homology to CMV nucleic acid in smooth muscle cells in the arterial media was achieved by use of an 'immediate early' 7Kb fragment as well as a 2.9Kb fragment from the late genomic region. Initially, both *in situ* hybridization and homology by dot blotting with extracted DNA were used in Bruggeman's laboratory.[28] Subsequently the more sensitive polymerase chain reaction (PCR) was added in an extended study.[27,28]

The dot blot DNA hybridization detected viral genome in a low percentage (18–29%) of samples, regardless of whether an early or late viral DNA probe was used, and regardless of the source of the tissue specimen. These findings are similar to those obtained in other laboratories.[20,21,25] The *in situ* DNA hybridization technique demonstrated viral nucleic acid in 44% of the atherosclerotic patients and in 58% of the autopsy-control groups, when the early probe was used, but only in 12–15% with the late probes. Only the more sensitive polymerase chain reaction permitted differences to be detected between the two groups of patients by demonstrating CMV DNA in 90% of arterial tissues of the surgical patients compared to 53% of the autopsy-control group. Identical case-control differences were found using both immediate early and late sequence primers, as both sequences were found in all the samples that were positive by the polymerase chain reaction. As in studies by other investigators, no infectious virus was isolated from the arterial specimens.

In the studies that had been conducted in Houston and Chicago, the CMV probe consisted of a mixture of late sequences of DNA of the Towne strain of CMV. In the Dutch study, in addition to a late sequence, an 'immediate early' 7Kb fragment (of AD-169 strain) was selected, because the investigators felt it would be more apt to detect transcripts present not only during reproductive viral cycles but also during latent infection (as is the case with HSV latency in neurons).

With the early probes, the *in situ* DNA hybridization technique resulted in an increase in the percentage of positive specimens relative to the dot blot technique, which Hendrix *et al.*[27] believe is largely due to the formation of RNA–DNA hybrids. A similar phenomenon was not observed when the late probe was used. When both techniques were used, with the early probe or with the late probe, no significant differences were observed between the group with severe atherosclerosis and the control group. However, the highly sensitive PCR detected viral DNA in 90% of the vessel wall samples derived from atherosclerotic patients, using either early or late primer, while in the control group only 53% were positive – a difference suggesting that the virus might play a role in the pathogenesis of atherosclerosis. Since no differences were found with the sensitive PCR, using the early or the late primer, the suggestion was made that the whole CMV genome was present in the arterial wall.

Our laboratory has also begun to employ PCR in searching for CMV nucleic acid in arterial tissue from patients undergoing vascular surgery.[29] The tests utilizing a 'late' CMV gene probe were carried out in 1990 with tissues that had been stored frozen, some from as long ago as 10 years when we began these investigations. Recent samples stored for less than 1 year yielded a positive rate of 77% both by gel electrophoresis and by slot blot analysis. However, in samples stored between 1980 and 1985, only 38 to 44% were positive, while those stored from January 1987 to October 1989 yielded a positive rate of 50 to 55%. Thus, the findings from the Netherlands were confirmed, but it was found that the rate of positive findings decreased markedly when tissue that was used had been subjected to long-term storage in the frozen state.

Seroepidemiological studies

In another approach to the problem, the association of infections by CMV, HSV-1 and HSV-2 with atherosclerosis was studied in a group of patients who underwent surgery for atherosclerotic vessel disease and a control group with high cholesterol levels but with no clinical evidence of disease.[16] The surgical patients were pair-matched by age, sex, race and socioeconomic status with control subjects who were participants in a lipid research programme extending over a period of 5 years. Blood samples for determination of antibody levels were taken both from the atherosclerosis patients before surgery, and from the control subjects at the end of the 5-year study period.

Two pair-matched male case-control groups were followed: group A included 134 pairs of patients who underwent cardiovascular surgery and controls who did not have clinical signs of atherosclerosis disease; group B consisted of 46 pairs in which the surgical cases were matched with controls who, during the 5-year observation period, developed myocardial infarction, suffered events compatible with myocardial infarction, or actually required cardiovascular surgery.

As shown in Table 8.2, the prevalence of antibodies to HSV-1 and HSV-2 was similar among the surgical cases and the control groups, but differences in CMV antibody were noted, particularly in the rates of high levels of CMV antibody in surgical patients compared with their matched controls. In group A, the 134 patients (70% with high antibody levels) differed significantly (P<0.001) from their matched group A controls (43% with high levels), none of whom had experienced a cardiovascular event. However, in group B the 46 surgical patients did not differ in the rate of high levels of CMV antibody (80%) from that of their matched controls (72%) – those who had developed a diagnosed cardiovascular event in the 5-year observation period. Another

Table 8.2 Prevalence of high levels of cytomegalovirus antibodies in male pairs of surgical patients with atherosclerosis and their matched controls, and in female surgical patients matched with male controls.*

	Significance of differences between groups	
Group†	Control group A 58/134‡ (43%)	Control group B 33/46 (72%)‡
Male surgical group A 94/134 (70%)	P <0.001	P >0.9
Male surgical group B 37/46 (80%)	P <0.001	P >0.5
Female surgical group 52/69 (76%)	P <0.001	P >0.8

*From Melnick *et al.*[16]
†In group A matched pairs, the controls did not have any recorded cardiovascular event. In group B matched pairs, the controls developed myocardial infarction during the observation period, or suffered events compatible with myocardial infarction, or actually required cardiovascular surgery.
‡Number with cytomegalovirus antibodies over number tested.

group, in this instance 69 female patients who had cardiovascular surgery, did not differ significantly in prevalence of high levels of CMV antibody (76%) from 69 matched male surgical cases (70%), but they had a significantly greater frequency (P< 0.001) of high antibody levels than the 69 male control patients free of cardiovascular disease (46%). Like the male patients, the female patients with atherosclerosis showed no difference in antibody levels when compared with group B controls (72%), all of whom had developed myocardial infarction or cardiovascular symptoms compatible with coronary insufficiency during the 5 years of observation. These data have been confirmed in Italy by Musiani *et al.*[30] They studied 36 patients with angiographically documented atherosclerosis and 36 matched control patients. They reported significantly higher titres of antibody against CMV (and EBV) antigens and a significant increase in CMV- and EBV-reactivated infections in the atherosclerotic patients compared to controls. Moreover, serological signs of concomitant EBV and CMV infections occurred more frequently in atherosclerotic patients than in controls.

Coronary atherosclerosis in heart transplant patients

Soon after renal transplants became accepted treatment, an association was noted between CMV infection and rejection of the transplanted kidney.[31] It is now recognized that glomerulopathy in the kidney transplant occurs during CMV viraemia.[32] Consequently, CMV infection was investigated to determine whether it played a role in the graft atherosclerosis that frequently occurs after heart transplantation.[33,34] In an extended study, 387 consecutive patients who received heart transplants underwent surveillance for evidence of CMV infection which involved assessing: (1) pre- and post-transplant IgM and IgG anti-CMV titres, (2) virus isolation from throat, urine and/or leucocytes, (3) presence of CMV inclusion bodies in cells from patients or from the virus isolation cultures, and (4) leucopenia, fever and malaise characteristic of CMV disease. All patients received immunosuppressive therapy. Cytomegalovirus infection occurred soon after transplantation, with a peak at 7 weeks. Of 387 heart recipients, 122 (32%) showed evidence of CMV infection. They were compared with the remaining 265 transplant patients who formed the non-CMV group for purposes of comparison. Transplant patients in the CMV group developed atherosclerosis earlier and more often. As shown in Table 8.3, infections were the most common cause of death, but these were followed by cardiac atherosclerosis, which occurred four times more frequently in the CMV group. Figure 8.1 indicates that the actuarial death rate from cardiac atherosclerosis was 30% in the CMV group over a 10-year follow-up period, compared to only 10% in the non-CMV group.

These important observations on cardiac transplant patients have been confirmed by investigators in Pittsburgh,[35] Minneapolis[36] and Berlin.[37]

Even though CMV infection has been associated in heart transplant patients with graft occlusion and ischaemic injury, the precise mechanism has not been established. Pober[38] has indicated that the affected arteries exhibit concentric accumulation of smooth muscle cells and extracellular matrix, but they lack the foam cells and extracellular lipid accumulation of typical athero-

Table 8.3   Cause of death in the post-transplant period among 387 consecutive heart recipients.*

Cause of death	CMV group (122 patients) (%)	Non-CMV group (265 patients) (%)
Infection	19.7	8.6
Graft atherosclerosis	9.9	2.4
Rejection	5.5	5.2
Nonspecific graft failure	1.1	2.3
Lymphoid malignancy	2.2	1.4
Nonlymphoid malignancy	1.1	1.9
Pulmonary embolus	2.2	0
Other	3.3	5.2

*Reproduced with permission from Grattan.[34]
CMV = cytomegalovirus.

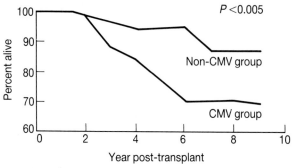

Fig. 8.1   Results from Stanford University Medical Center on cardiac transplant patients. The deaths indicated in this graph were due to graft atherosclerosis. Reproduced with permission from Grattan.[34]

sclerosis. He suggests that graft arteriosclerosis is a more descriptive term for the nature of the lesion – perhaps brought on by the effect of CMV on the drug-suppressed immune system. However, as described in the following section, CMV may directly affect the biology of the arteries.

Cytomegalovirus infection of endothelial cells

The fact that CMV and HSV imprints were detected in arterial tissues that showed minimal atherosclerotic changes suggests that virus infection could be an early event in the atherosclerotic process, particularly since one of the features reported for CMV infection is the accumulation of cholesterol within the host cells. Another important property of CMV is its capacity to infect but not kill endothelial cells.[39–41] Viral glycoproteins appear at the surface of the infected endothelial cells, which then demonstrate a spectacular increase in adherence of polymorphonuclear leucocytes. Thus the inflammatory type of response in the endothelial intima set off by a viral blood-borne infection may be the initiating event in atherogenesis.[40,41] In many respects, the biological properties of CMV are compatible with an atherogenic potential. In contrast, HSV-1 and HSV-2 cause rapid cytolytic infections in human endothelial and smooth muscle cell cultures.

Further support comes from the study by Myerson *et al.*[42] who identified and enumerated cells which appeared normal morphologically but were found to carry a latent CMV infection. In patients with disseminated CMV infection, typical cytomegalic cells were present in lungs and other organs, and virus was isolated from lungs and kidneys. However, by use of biotin-labelled viral DNA probes, occult virus was detected in many other tissues, particularly in scattered foci of endothelial cells of the blood vessels. In spite of this, the cells containing the latent CMV infection appeared normal. There was hardly any local tissue destruction, but hyperplasia was sometimes found.

Does CMV play a role in human atherosclerosis?

The investigations reviewed here provide solid evidence that a member of the herpesvirus family can cause atherosclerosis in chickens. *In vitro* experiments as well as studies of arteries from infected birds suggest that a virus-induced alteration of cellular metabolism, which results in the accumulation of cholesterol and cholesteryl esters, may be the primary mechanism in the development of viral atherosclerosis. In addition, the fact that the same virus induces a malignant lymphoma suggests that it may also have the potential to stimulate the proliferation of arterial smooth muscle cells, a prominent feature of atherogenesis.

The evidence for involvement of one or more members of the herpesvirus family in human atherosclerosis is much more circumstantial.[16,28,43] The findings of viral antigens and nucleic acid sequences in arterial smooth muscle cells suggest that CMV infection of the arterial wall may be a common occurrence in patients with severe atherosclerosis. Although certainly suggestive, these findings by themselves do not demonstrate a viral role in the pathogenesis of atherosclerosis. However, they lead to an attractive working hypothesis of the steps involved (Table 8.4).

Table 8.4 Hypothesis of cytomegalovirus (CMV) initiation and development of atherosclerosis.*

1. Systemic CMV infection
2. Infection of arterial endothelium. Viral glycoproteins appear at the surface of infected cells
3. Polymorphonuclear leucocyte adherence (inflammatory response) leading to damaged endothelium
4. Leakage of CMV from infected endothelial cells and exposure of neighbouring smooth muscle cells within the arterial wall
5. Latent and persistent infections of smooth muscle cells, detected by tracing viral genes or antigens
6. Cell-to-cell spread of CMV within scattered foci along the blood vessels
7. CMV may transform cells and cause smooth muscle cells to proliferate locally, without destroying them, and may induce changes in cellular metabolites, including accumulation of cholesterol
8. At sites of CMV latency, the arterial lesion may be periodically activated, followed by viral infection of the nearby endothelial cells of the intima. This would result in another bout of adherence of polymorphonuclear leucocytes. Virus from the damaged endothelial cells leads to local proliferation of smooth muscle cells. This benign transformation, coupled with risk factors such as hypercholesterolaemia or hypertension, may lead to the formation of atheroma and ultimately to clinically apparent atherosclerosis

*Modified from Melnick *et al*.[16]

Of special importance are the recent findings that heart transplant patients who are immunosuppressed and become infected with CMV are particularly prone to develop atherosclerosis in the transplanted organ.[34–37]

In seroepidemiological studies, high levels of CMV antibodies were found to be associated with clinically manifest atherosclerotic disease, suggesting that a periodically activated latent infection or continuously active infection is present in patients with atherosclerosis.[16] Since CMV DNA, but not infectious virus, is found in arterial cells, the artery itself might be the site of latency.[28,44]

The biological properties of CMV are consistent with pathogenic involvement at several levels of the atherogenic process. Many of these properties are shared by other herpesviruses, and data linking CMV to atherosclerosis by no means exclude the possible involvement of other herpesviruses. Rather, the studies reviewed here should provide a basis for further investigation of the role of viruses in human atherogenesis, and of their ultimate control by means of vaccination or chemotherapy.

References

1. McMillian G. C. Development of arteriosclerosis. *Am J Cardiol* 1973; **31:** 542–6.
2. Ross R. The pathogenesis of atherosclerosis. An update. *N Engl J Med* 1986; **314:** 488–500.
3. Ross R., Glomset J. A. The pathogenesis of atherosclerosis. *N Engl J Med* 1976; **295:** 369–77; 420–5.
4. The National Institutes of Health Consensus Development Conference: Lowering blood cholesterol to prevent heart disease. *J Am Med Assoc* 1985; **253:** 2080–6.
5. Fabricant C. G., Fabricant J., Litrenta M. M., Minick C. R. Virus induced atherosclerosis. *J Exp Med* 1978; **148:** 335–40.
6. Fabricant C. G. Viruses. Causal factors in atherosclerosis. *Microbiol Sci* 1986; **3:** 50–2.
7. Benditt E. P., Benditt J. M. Evidence for a monoclonal origin of human atherosclerotic plaques. *Proc Natl Acad Sci (USA)* 1973; **70:** 1753–6.
8. Penn A., Garte S. J., Warren L. *et al.* Transforming gene in atherosclerotic plaque DNA. *Proc Natl Acad Sci (USA)* 1986; **83:** 7951–5.
9. Paterson J. C., Cottral G. E. Experimental coronary sclerosis. III: Lymphomatosis as a cause of coronary sclerosis in chickens. *Arch Pathol* 1950; **49:** 699.
10. Benditt E. P., Barrett T., McDougall J. K. Viruses in the etiology of atherosclerosis. *Proc Natl Acad Sci (USA)* 1983; **80:** 6386–9.
11. Fabricant C. G., Fabricant J. Marek's disease virus-induced atherosclerosis and evidence for a herpesvirus role in the human vascular disease. In: Calnek B. N., Spencer J. L. eds. *International Symposium on Marek's Disease.* Philadelphia: American Association of Avian Pathologists, 1985: 391–407.
12. Shih J. C. H., Pullman E. P., Kao K. J. Genetic selection, general characterization, and histology of atherosclerosis-susceptible and -resistant Japanese quail. *Atherosclerosis* 1983; **49:** 41–53.
13. Fabricant C. F., Hajjar D. P., Minick C. R., Fabricant J. Herpesvirus infection enhances cholesterol and cholesteryl ester accumulation in cultured arterial smooth muscle cells. *Am J Pathol* 1981; **105:** 176–84.
14. Hajjar D. P., Fabricant C. G., Minick C. R., Fabricant J. Virus-induced atherosclerosis: Herpesvirus infection alters aortic cholesterol metabolism and accumulation. *Am J Pathol* 1986; **122:** 62–70.
15. Petrie B. L., Adam E., Melnick J. L. Association of herpes virus/cytomegalovirus

infections with human atherosclerosis. In: Melnick J. L. ed. *Progress in Medical Virology*. Volume 35. Basel: S. Karger AG, 1988: 21–42.

16. Melnick J. L., Adam E., DeBakey M. E. Possible role of cytomegalovirus in atherogenesis. *J Am Med Assoc* 1990; **263:** 2204–7.

17. Nachtigal M., Legrand A., Nagpal M. L. *et al*. Transformation of rabbit vascular smooth muscle cells by transfection with the early region of SV40 DNA. *Am J Pathol* 1990; **136:** 297–306.

18. Behbehani A. M., Melnick J. L., DeBakey M. E. Continuous cell strains derived from human atheromatous lesions and their viral susceptibility. *Proc Soc Exp Biol Med* 1965; **118:** 759–63.

19. Behbehani A. M., Melnick J. L., DeBakey M. E. A paramyxovirus isolated from human atheromatous lesion. *Exp Molec Pathol* 1965; **4:** 606–19.

20. Melnick J. L., Petrie B. L., Dreesman G. R. *et al*. Cytomegalovirus antigen within human arterial smooth muscle cells. *Lancet* 1983; **ii:** 644–7.

21. Petrie B. L., Melnick J. L., Adam E. *et al*. Nucleic acid sequences of cytomegalovirus in cells cultured from human arterial tissue. *J Infect Dis* 1987; **155:** 158–9.

22. Gyorkey F., Melnick J. L., Guinn G. A. *et al*. Herpesviridae in the endothelial and smooth muscle cells of the proximal aorta in arterioclerotic patients. *Exp Molec Pathol* 1984; **40:** 328–39.

23. Becker P., Melnick J. L., Mayor H. D. A morphologic comparison between the developmental stages of herpes zoster and human cytomegalovirus. *Exp Molec Pathol* 1965; **4:** 11–12.

24. Szilagyi J. F., Cunningham C. Identification and characterization of a novel non-infectious herpes simplex virus-related particle. *J Gen Virol* 1991; **72:** 661–8.

25. Yamashiroya H. M., Ghosh L., Yang R., Robertson A. L. Jr. Herpesviridae in the coronary arteries and aorta of young trauma victims. *Am J Pathol* 1988; **130:** 71–9.

26. Hendrix M. G. R., Dormans P. H. J., Kitslaar P. *et al*. The presence of cytomegalovirus nucleic acids in arterial walls of atherosclerotic and nonatherosclerotic patients. *Am J Pathol* 1989; **134:** 1151–7.

27. Hendrix M. G. R., Salimans M. M. M., van Boven C. P. A., Bruggeman C. A. High prevalence of latently present cytomegalovirus in arterial walls of patients suffering from grade III atherosclerosis. *Am J Pathol* 1990; **136:** 23–8.

28. Bruggeman C. A., van Dam-Mieras M. C. E. The possible role of cytomegalovirus in atherogenesis. In: Melnick J. L. ed. *Progress in Medical Virology*. Volume 38. Basel: S. Karger AG, 1991: 1–26.

29. Melnick J. L., Adam E., DeBakey M. E. Cytomegalovirus and atherosclerosis. *Proc. 10th Paavo Nurmi Symposium Supplement, European Heart Journal*, 1993 (in press).

30. Musiani M., Zerbini M. L., Muscari A. *et al*. Antibody patterns against cytomegalovirus and Epstein–Barr virus in human atherosclerosis. *Microbiologia* 1990; **13:** 35–41.

31. Lopez C., Simmons R. L., Mauer S. M. *et al*. Virus infection may trigger rejection in immunosuppressed renal transplant recipients. *Proc Clin Dialysis Transplant Forum* 1972; **2:** 107.

32. Richardson W. P., Colvin R. B., Cheeseman S. H. *et al*. Glomerulopathy associated with cytomegalovirus viremia in renal allografts. *N Engl J Med* 1981; **305:** 57–63.

33. Grattan M. T., Moreno-Cabral C. E., Starnes V. A. *et al*. Cytomegalovirus infection is associated with cardiac allograft rejection and atherosclerosis. *J Am Med Assoc* 1989; **261:** 3561–6.

34. Grattan M. T. Accelerated graft atherosclerosis following cardiac transplantation: Clinical perspectives. *Clin Cardiol* 1991; 14 (suppl. II): 16–20.

35. Pahl E., Fricker F. J., Armitage J. *et al*. Coronary arteriosclerosis in pediatric

heart transplant survivors: Limitation of long-term survival. *J Ped* 1990; **116:** 177–183.

36. McDonald J. L., Rector R. S., Braunlin E. A. *et al*. Association of coronary artery disease in cardiac transplant recipients with cytomegalovirus infection. *Am J Cardiol* 1989; **64:** 359.

37. Loebe M., Schuler S., Spiegelsberger S. *et al*. Cytomegalievirus-infektion und koronarsklerose nach herztransplantation. *Dtsch Med Wochenschr* 1990; **115:** 1266.

38. Pober J. S. Immunologic basis of cardiovascular disease: An overview. *Clin Cardiol* 1991; 14 (suppl. II): 1–2.

39. Visser M. R., Jacob H. S., Goodman J. L. *et al*. Granulocyte-mediated injury to *Herpes simplex* virus-infected human endothelium. *Lab Invest* 1989; **60:** 296–304.

40. Smiley M. L., Mar E.-C., Huang E.-S. Cytomegalovirus infection and viral-induced transformation of human endothelial cells. *J Med Virol* 1988; **25:** 213–26.

41. Span A. H. M., van Boven C. P. A., Bruggeman C. A. The effect of cytomegalovirus infection on the adherence of polymorphonuclear leucocytes to endothelial cells. *Eur J Clin Invest* 1989; **19:** 542–8.

42. Myerson D., Hackman R. C., Nelson J. A. *et al*. Widespread presence of histologically occult cytomegalovirus. *Human Pathol* 1984; **15:** 430–9.

43. Cunningham M. J., Pasternak R. C. The potential role of viruses in the pathogenesis of atherosclerosis. *Circulation* 1988; **77:** 964–6.

44. Melnick J. L., Adam E., DeBakey M. E. Accelerated graft atherosclerosis following cardiac transplantation: Do viruses play a role? *Clin Cardiol* 1991; **14** (suppl. II): 21–26.

9

The laboratory diagnosis of enterovirus-induced heart disease

P. Muir and R. Kandolf

Introduction

A viral aetiology for acute heart disease may be suspected on clinical grounds, particularly if there is a recent history of an acute viral-type illness. However, a diagnosis of viral heart disease cannot be established solely on such criteria, since a preceding viral illness may be absent or unrecorded, particularly if mild, and may in any case be coincidental and unrelated to cardiac symptoms. In addition, the histological features of endomyocardial biopsy specimens from patients with suspected viral heart disease are usually not virus-specific and are indistinguishable from those seen in inflammatory heart disease of nonviral origin. Furthermore, biopsy specimens may appear normal as myocardial lesions may be focally restricted. A virological diagnosis may therefore be of great value in differentiating heart disease of viral aetiology from that due to other causes. This is particularly true of patients with chronic viral heart disease, which usually cannot be associated with a past history of viral illness.

In some cases cardiac symptoms may develop during the acute phase of virus replication. For example, acute myocarditis with cardiac failure is frequently present in infants with fulminant enterovirus infection. In addition, enteroviruses are capable of producing life-threatening arrhythmias or congestive heart failure of acute onset in adults. The clinical features of acute viral myocarditis or pericarditis typically develop several days or weeks after the initial virus infection, which may have been associated with a febrile illness with lethargy or nonspecific symptoms, or may have been asymptomatic. Some acute forms of enteroviral heart disease may evolve into a chronic form of dilated cardiomyopathy (DCM). Again, the original acute infection may have been asymptomatic. This immediately presents a problem to the virologist, since traditional diagnostic methods aim either to isolate virus from clinical specimens in cell culture, or to demonstrate seroconversion, or at least a rising antibody titre to the infecting virus.

Attempting to isolate virus is usually inappropriate for diagnosing acute viral heart disease, as patients are rarely viraemic or excreting infectious virus in stool or nasopharyngeal secretions beyond the acute phase of virus infection. In any case, for such ubiquitous viruses as enteroviruses, virus excretion may not necessarily indicate systemic infection. Enteroviruses have only very rarely been cultured from cardiac tissue or pericardial fluid.[1] Endomyocardial biopsy specimens may be available from patients with suspected myocarditis, but biopsy specimens are not usually available from patients with acute pericarditis unless there is some complication which warrants invasive diagnostic techniques. Similarly, attempts to demonstrate seroconversion or rising antibody titres are frequently unsuccessful, as anti-viral IgG titres have often already reached their maximal levels by the time patients present with cardiac symptoms.

Demonstrating viral involvement in chronic cardiac disease is even more difficult, as infectious virus cannot be cultured from cardiac tissue, and viral antigens are usually not detected using conventional serotype-specific antisera. Measurement of virus-specific neutralizing antibody titres in these patients has provided some epidemiological evidence of an enteroviral aetiology[2] but neutralizing antibody titres are not useful for diagnosis in individual cases because of the high prevalence of high titre enterovirus-specific neutralizing antibody in the general population. However, the potential biological significance of some traditional diagnostic assays, in particular the virus neutralization test, should not be overlooked, as this may represent an important anti-viral function of antibody *in vivo*.

Because of these diagnostic problems, there is considerable demand for alternative methods for the diagnosis of viral heart disease. Fortunately, during the last decade there have been considerable improvements in serological reagents and methods, as well as major advances in the application of molecular biological techniques to the diagnosis of infectious disease. This has resulted in new serological techniques to demonstrate antibody class-specific responses as well as antigen- or epitope-specific antibody responses. These techniques may provide useful serological determinants of acute or chronic virus infection. In addition, techniques for detecting low amounts of viral antigen or nucleic acid in the absence of detectable infectious virus are available. This chapter describes some of the new techniques which have arisen from recent developments and their application to the diagnosis of the commonest viral cause of heart disease, namely, the enteroviruses. Many of the principles discussed are of general importance to the diagnosis of infectious disease. In addition to reviewing currently available techniques, newer methods which are currently under development and which may become useful for future diagnosis of enteroviral heart disease are also discussed.

This chapter describes: (a) detection of enterovirus-specific IgM responses; (b) detection of enteroviral nucleic acid; and (c) the use of synthetic and recombinant antigens in the diagnosis of enterovirus infection.

Detection of enterovirus-specific IgM

Principles of IgM detection

The diagnostic significance of IgM lies in the relatively short duration of virus-specific IgM responses. IgM responses normally decline several weeks or months after the source of the antigenic stimulus has been eliminated, and are therefore useful as markers of a current or recent antigenic stimulus. In contrast, virus-specific IgG responses persist for many years, often for life.

Anti-viral IgM responses were originally measured by traditional serological methods such as virus neutralization, passive haemagglutination, immunodiffusion or complement-fixation using serum depleted of IgG by absorption with staphylococcal protein A or by sucrose density centrifugation.[3] These assays have practical limitations as they are labour-intensive, time-consuming and usually relatively insensitive.

With newly available μ-chain-specific antisera, which reacted only with IgM, it became possible to develop solid-phase immunoassays for detection of virus-specific IgM in whole serum. These solid-phase assays are of two basic types, as illustrated in Fig. 9.1. In the indirect immunoassay, viral antigen is bound to a solid phase, either directly by passive adsorption (Fig. 9.1a) or via an antigen-specific capture antibody (Fig. 9.1b). Viral antigen is reacted first with patient serum, then with a labelled anti-human IgM detector antibody. The solid phase is washed after each step to remove unbound reactants. Indirect immunofluorescence, enzyme-linked immunosorbent assay (ELISA) and radioimmunoassay (RIA) are based on this principle. However, indirect immunoassays are subject to interference from virus-specific IgG when using whole serum which, being present in excess, competes with IgM for antigen, and gives rise to a false negative result. In addition, the presence of IgM class rheumatoid factor, which binds to the Fc component of antigen-bound IgG, may give rise to false positive results. These problems are not encountered in the IgM capture assay, in which IgM is bound to the solid phase via an anti-human IgM antibody, and IgG is removed by washing before antigen is added. Viral antigen reacts with any bound virus-specific IgM and may itself be labelled with enzyme or radioisotope (Fig. 9.1c), or it may be detected by subsequent reaction with a labelled specific antibody (Fig. 9.1d*i*) or an unlabelled specific antibody followed by an appropriate labelled anti-species antibody (Fig. 9.1d*ii*). Because of the problems encountered with the indirect immunoassay, IgM capture assays are generally more sensitive and specific than indirect IgM assays. The IgM capture principle is currently used in many commercial and inhouse assays for detection of virus-specific IgM.

Enterovirus-specific IgM detection

Current methods for demonstrating enterovirus-specific IgM are based on the IgM capture principle. Typically, solid phase-bound virus-specific IgM is detected by sequential reaction with antigen prepared from one enterovirus serotype, then with serotype-specific mouse antiserum, and finally with horse radish peroxidase-conjugated anti-mouse IgG, according to the principle shown in Fig. 9.1d*ii*.[4,5] Consideration of the technical aspects of this assay, including antigen preparation, determination of cut-off levels and interpretation of results is given elsewhere.[6] A number of other enterovirus-specific IgM capture assays have also been described, using ^{35}S-labelled viral antigen as in Fig. 9.1c,[7] ^{125}I-labelled enterovirus-specific mouse antibody as in Fig. 9.1d*i*[8] or enterovirus-specific rabbit antiserum and enzyme-labelled anti-rabbit IgG, as in Fig. 9.1d*ii*.[9]

Enterovirus serology is complicated by the large number of serotypes; over 70 are known which cause infection in humans, and additional strains are under investigation as possible new prototypes. It is clearly inappropriate to

Indirect IgM immunoassays

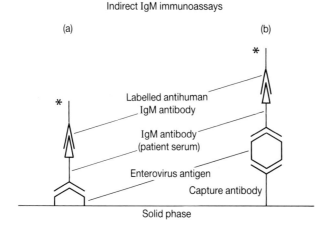

IgM capture immunoassays

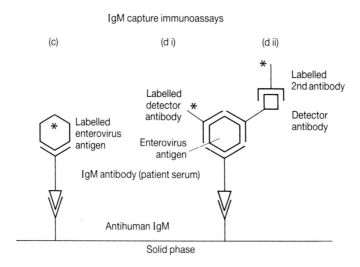

Fig. 9.1   Methods of IgM detection. In the indirect IgM immunoassay, antigen is bound to the solid phase, either (a) directly or (b) via an antigen-specific capture antibody, then reacted sequentially with patient's serum then a labelled anti-human IgM antibody. In the IgM capture assay, IgM antibody is bound to the solid phase via an anti-human IgM antibody, then reacted with labelled antigen (c) or unlabelled antigen which is detected with an antigen-specific detector antibody which (d*i*) may itself be labelled or (d*ii*) may be detected with an appropriate anti-species labelled antibody.

employ this number of serological assays, using antigens prepared from 70 or more serotypes and the same number of serotype-specific antisera. Fortunately, there are antigenic determinants which are common to all or most serotypes.[10,11] These determinants are present on defective or disrupted virus particles[12] as well as viral structural precursors and nonstructural viral proteins.[13,14] The use of viral antigens prepared from naturally infected cell cultures which contain such antigenic components allows detection of an IgM response to an enterovirus infection without using the homologous antigen in many cases.[5,6,12] However, some patients may not mount a detectable IgM response to these shared determinants. In these instances the IgM response is serotype-specific and can only be detected using antigen prepared from the homologous serotype. In practice, therefore, it is common to employ a limited number of antigens prepared from selected serotypes, usually the coxsackie virus B1–5 serotypes (CVB1–CVB5) which are commonly implicated in viral heart disease. This allows the diagnosis of CVB1–CVB5 infections and a proportion of infections caused by other enterovirus serotypes as well. A serotype-specific IgM response to one of the CVB1–CVB5 serotypes will be identified in this assay system as a monotypic reaction with only one of the five antigens used. A heterotypic reaction with multiple serotypes indicates an IgM response to enterovirus-group determinants which may have been induced by a CVB or other enterovirus serotype. This broad specificity is not a problem, as serotypic identification of infecting enterovirus is not necessary for clinical purposes. The increased diagnostic potential of a broadly reactive assay is in fact advantageous.

Pooling of antigens and antisera to facilitate detection of enterovirus-specific IgM using a single assay remains an option but requires further investigation. The relative dilution of serotype-specific determinants resulting from pooling of antigens may reduce the sensitivity of detection of monotypic IgM responses.

Production of synthetic and recombinant enteroviral antigens is described below. Use of such antigens for enterovirus-specific IgM assays, rather than viral antigens derived from naturally infected cells, will allow greater control of antigen composition, and this may prove to be the way forward towards a standard, single assay system for enterovirus-specific IgM detection. It is likely that a single assay system would require a cocktail of synthetic or recombinant antigens representative of the enterovirus serotypes, unless an antigen which consistently induces an immune response in patients with acute infections can be identified, possibly among the highly conserved nonstructural antigens. The potential advantages of a second generation assay are attractive. In addition to being less time-consuming and more easily standardized, such an assay would be safer than current assays which use high titre infectious virus as antigen. An antigen preparation not requiring tissue culture propagation would also be more economical. Finally, a standard, synthetic or recombinant antigen may be more amenable to direct conjugation with enzyme, thus obviating the need for expensive animal antiserum to detect antigen and further simplifying the assay protocol.

Enterovirus-specific IgM responses in patients with acute disease

The rate of detection of enterovirus infection has been greatly improved by the introduction of enterovirus-specific IgM capture ELISA,[5,6] even in patients with acute-phase symptoms such as aseptic meningitis,[9,15] where virus isolation might be expected to be more successful. In patients with acute symptoms, enterovirus-specific IgM can usually be detected within a week of the onset of symptoms, sometimes as early as 1–3 days after onset of disease. Acute myocarditis usually presents days or weeks after the initial virus infection, and in patients presenting with acute cardiac symptoms, enterovirus-specific IgM can be detected at the time of clinical presentation.[16] By detecting enterovirus-specific IgM, 33–50% of cases of acute myopericarditis have been found to be associated with enterovirus infection.[5,16–18] The variation in proportion of patients with enterovirus-specific IgM observed in these studies may reflect the stringency of the diagnostic criteria applied, the relative sensitivity and specificity of the enterovirus-specific IgM assays used, or differences in the relative prevalence of enteroviruses compared with other aetiological agents of myopericarditis in the study populations. Enterovirus-specific IgM responses in patients with self-limiting acute cardiac disease usually become undetectable by IgM capture ELISA within 6 months.[5,18]

Enterovirus-specific IgM responses in patients with chronic cardiac disease

Although IgM responses are normally transient in patients with acute viral infection, a persistent virus infection may be accompanied by a prolonged virus-specific IgM response, reflecting the ongoing antigenic stimulus. IgM responses may therefore also be useful in the diagnosis of chronic viral disease. Two forms of chronic heart disease have been associated with enterovirus infection, namely, DCM and recurrent or chronic relapsing pericarditis (CRP). Serological studies of these patient groups have been limited, however, in one study, 28 of 86 (33%) patients with DCM and 9 of 14 (64%) patients with CRP had enterovirus-specific IgM responses during the chronic phase of disease, compared to 10 of 84 (12%) age-matched controls.[18] Demonstration of IgM persistence may be of great importance in differentiating persistent enterovirus infection from incidental asymptomatic infections in patients with chronic disease, particularly where enteroviruses are prevalent in the population. In two recent surveys, enterovirus-specific IgM was detected in about 20% of healthy adults and 8% of children,[19,20] indicating that asymptomatic infection is common at certain times and in certain age groups. However, follow-up studies showed these responses to be short-lived; almost all became undetectable within 12 months.[20] In contrast, a sequential study of patients with DCM revealed that IgM responses were present up to 19 months before cardiac transplantation and persisted up to 4 years after transplantation. IgM responses in patients with CRP persisted throughout the duration of symptoms – up to 10 years. In some patients, monotypic IgM responses were observed throughout the follow-up period, which strongly suggests that these patients had a persistent enterovirus infection, rather than repeated infections with different enterovirus serotypes.

Comparison of enterovirus-specific IgM responses in patients with acute pericarditis who subsequently suffered from recurrences with IgM responses of patients with self-limiting pericarditis showed that the level of specific IgM was significantly higher in the former group.[18] This may possibly reflect a greater antigenic stimulus or an abnormal response to virus infection in these patients. However, it remains to be determined whether this is a reliable prognostic marker of a subsequent relapsing course.

The persistence of enterovirus-specific IgM responses in patients with DCM is of interest in view of the fact that infectious virus or viral structural antigens are not usually detectable in the end-stage cardiomyopathic heart using conventional methods. It is possible that persistence of the IgM response reflects a productive persistent infection in the heart which is only detected by advanced techniques such as *in situ* hybridization. Virus infection may also persist at extracardiac sites. The persistence of enterovirus-specific IgM responses after cardiac transplantation supports this hypothesis, although this may also be due to enterovirus persistence in residual recipient atrial tissue.

Enterovirus-specific serum IgA responses in patients with acute enterovirus infection, like IgM responses, are usually transient.[21] Enterovirus-specific IgA is less useful than enterovirus-specific IgM as a marker of acute infection, as it is detected less frequently, but may provide information on local immune responses at mucosal sites, which may influence the outcome of infection.[22] IgA is synthesized mainly in gut mucosal tissue, and enterovirus-specific IgA responses may reflect the presence of virus in the gut, which is the initial site of enterovirus replication. Enterovirus-specific IgA responses were found to persist in some patients with chronic cardiac disease, often in the absence of a persistent IgM response,[18,21] suggesting that gut mucosal tissue may be a possible site of viral persistence. Further studies, discussed below, using molecular techniques for the detection of enteroviral RNA in patient tissue will help to clarify this subject.

Detection of enteroviral nucleic acid

Development of an *in situ* hybridization assay for detection of enteroviral RNA

Molecular genetic techniques provide powerful tools with which to define the role of enteroviruses in disease induction and to study the molecular basis of pathogenicity. Cloning of viral complementary DNA (cDNA) obtained by reverse transcription of viral RNA allows enterovirus group-specific cDNA probes to be generated and used to detect viral RNA in clinical specimens by RNA/cDNA hybridization.[23–27] This review focusses on the development and application of enterovirus group-specific *in situ* hybridization,[28–30] which is the method of choice for diagnosing enteroviral heart disease using endomyocardial biopsies.

A major prerequisite for the introduction of *in situ* hybridization for diagnosis of enteroviral heart disease was molecular cloning and characterization of the RNA genome of a cardiotropic CVB3[25] which had been propagated in cultured human heart cells.[31] Full-length, reverse-transcribed CVB3 cDNA generated replication-competent, infectious CVB3 upon transfection of viral cDNA into mammalian cells. Because of the high degree of nucleic acid sequence identity shared among enterovirus serotypes, detection of the most commonly implicated agents of human viral heart disease, including coxsackie A and B viruses and the echoviruses, in a single assay using cloned CVB3 cDNA as a hybridization probe became possible. The broad spectrum of enteroviruses detected by CVB3 cDNA greatly facilitates diagnosis of enteroviral heart disease, since from the clinical point of view, serotypic identification of the implicated enterovirus is of secondary importance. This could in theory be carried out later by hybridization with serotype-specific cDNA probes, although such probes are currently available only for a limited number of serotypes.

Highly specific hybridization conditions have been established for the detection of enteroviruses. When radioactively labelled, cloned CVB3 cDNA corresponding to 95.4% of the viral genome (nucleotides 66 to 7128) was hybridized to electrophoretically resolved CVB3 RNA and to total RNA from human heart cells, specific hybridization occurred only with viral RNA.[25] In addition, no hybridization with restriction endonuclease-digested human cellular DNA was detected under conditions appropriate for detection of single copy genes.

The feasibility of using the *in situ* hybridization technique,[32,33] in which tissue sections are treated to expose and immobilize nucleic acid, then reacted with a specific labelled probe, to detect enteroviral RNA was established using infected cultured cells and then applied to myocardial tissue from CVB3-infected mice.[28] Uninfected Vero cells exhibited essentially no autoradiographic silver grains when hybridized to ^{3}H-labelled or ^{35}S-labelled CVB3 cDNA. In contrast, an intense autoradiographic signal was observed when the same probe was hybridized to Vero cells infected with various enteroviruses (CVB1, CVB3, CVB5, echovirus 11).

Using myocardial tissue sections from CVB3-infected mice, *in situ* hybridization proved to be a powerful tool, not only for establishing an unequivocal diagnosis of myocardial infection, but also for understanding its pathogenesis (Fig. 9.2). Autoradiographic silver grains, which indicate hybridization between viral RNA and the radiolabelled CVB3 cDNA probe, are clearly localized to individual infected myocytes (Fig. 9.2A). These cells are easily identified by interference contrast microscopy in unstained sections because of their characteristic size and morphology. In this model system of enteroviral heart disease, myocardial infection was found to be multifocal and randomly distributed in heart muscle (Fig. 9.2B). Myocardial cross-sections revealed a transmural disseminated infection of the myocardium, as demonstrated in Fig. 9.2C for the left ventricle. Infected myocytes were often found in clusters within areas of severe myocardial lesions and fibrosis (Fig. 9.2D). Furthermore, progression of infection could be observed from areas with myocardial fibrosis to as yet uninfected myocytes (Fig. 9.2E and F), demonstrating cell-to-cell spread of virus. However, viral RNA was also found in isolated myocytes in apparently normal myocardial tissue, primarily in the early stage of infection (Fig. 9.2G). In addition, viral RNA also appeared to be located within small interstitial myocardial cells, possibly fibroblasts (Fig. 9.2B and E). Labelling of myocardial cells did not occur when myocardial tissue sections were probed with radiolabelled plasmid vector control DNA[25] or with the cloned *Eco*R1 J fragment of the genetically unrelated cytomegalovirus.[34] In addition, no labelling of myocardial cells occurred when myocardial sections of uninfected mice were probed with a radiolabelled CVB3 cDNA probe (Fig. 9.2H).

Sensitivity of enteroviral RNA detection was maximized by a number of improvements in methodology including optimized hybridization conditions to prevent nonspecific probe binding, and the use of radiolabelled, cloned cDNA fragments of about 100 nucleotides in length.[28] Quantification of the CVB3 genome copy number in infected cells by RNA blot analysis and comparison with results of *in situ* hybridization using cells from the same culture indicated that as few as 20 viral genome copies are easily detectable within 2 weeks of autoradiographic exposure. Clearly positive hybridization signals with infected mouse myocardial tissue were observed after only 2 days of exposure to the ^{35}S-labelled cDNA probe, indicating a high copy number of replicating viral genomes in myocardial cells (Fig. 9.2G). Furthermore, overexposed myocardial sections showed extremely low background hybridization, confirming the high specificity of *in situ* hybridization for detection of enteroviral RNA. However, a number of precautions should be observed in order to guarantee this high specificity. Homopolymer tails, either poly(A) and poly(T) tails from cloned viral cDNA or poly(G) and poly(C) tails from the cloning vector, hybridize to poly(rA), poly(rC) and poly(rG) transcripts. Care should therefore be taken to ensure that such sequences are excluded from cDNA probes. Appropriate measures should be taken to ensure that cross-hybriziation of the cDNA probe with human myocardial RNA or DNA does not occur. In particular routine use of vector probes as controls is strongly recommended. In addition, the hybridization signal should be clearly localized to myocardial cells, and adjacent sections should remain positive throughout the depths of infected foci, unless only an occasional cell is infected. The ability to perform such specificity controls represents an advantage of *in situ* hybridization over slot blot or spot hybridization methods.

In situ detection of enteroviral RNA in myocardium from patients with myocarditis and dilated cardiomyopathy

In situ hybridization has already proved to be a valuable tool for assessing the presence of enteroviral RNA in endomyocardial biopsy samples obtained from patients with suspected myocarditis or DCM.[29,30] Replicating enterovirus was detected in 23 of 95 patients (24%) with clinically suspected acute myocarditis, including 10 of 33 patients (30%) with DCM of recent onset. Myocardial tissue from 53 control patients, with specific heart diseases not consistent with a primary viral aetiology (e.g. ischaemic, hypertrophic or metabolic cardiomypathies) was negative by *in situ* hybridization in all cases.

Replicating enteroviral RNA was detected not only in the early stages of clinically obvious myocarditis, but also in chronic DCM, indicating that enteroviruses may persist in the human heart. Of 48 patients with chronic DCM, eight patients (17%), including four of 19 (21%) who underwent heart transplantation because of end-stage DCM, were found to have myocardial enterovirus infection. The concept of enterovirus persistence in chronic DCM, evolving from acute or subacute infections, is substantiated by our finding of enterovirus persistence in sequential biopsies from patients with ongoing disease. The negative results obtained in the control group of patients with other specific heart muscle diseases strongly support an aetiological role for enteroviruses in myocarditis and DCM.

The number of infected myocardial cells appears to be related to the severity of clinical symptoms, at least during the acute phase of enterovirus infection. In patients with mild myopericarditis or healing myocarditis, only a few myocardial cells were found to express enteroviral RNA, but numerous infected cells were found in patients with acute heart failure. As expected, the most extensive pattern of myocardial infection was observed in fatal cases of fulminant myocarditis. Figure 9.3 illustrates the pattern of acute

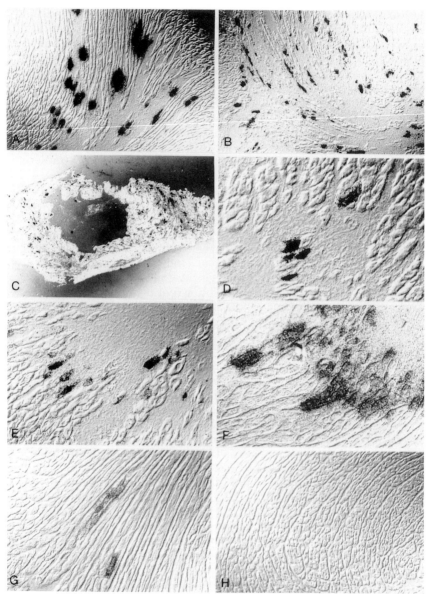

Fig. 9.2 Autoradiographs of (A–G) coxsackievirus B3 (CVB3)-infected or (H) uninfected mouse myocardial tissue hybridized *in situ* with (B–E) ³H-labelled or (A,F,G,H) ³⁵S-labelled cloned CVB3 cDNA. Days after infection of athymic mice were (A) 56, (B–E) 23, (F) 42, and (G) 4. Exposure times were (A,H) 9 days, (B–E) 6 weeks, (F) 4 days and (G) 2 days. Note that since silver grains are positioned at various levels within the photographic emulsion, some grains are not observed and appear out of focus in photography. Interference contrast microscopy of unstained sections: (A,G,H) × 200, (B) × 100, (C) × 25, (D,E) × 400 and (F) × 650. Reproduced with permission from Kandolf *et al.*[28]

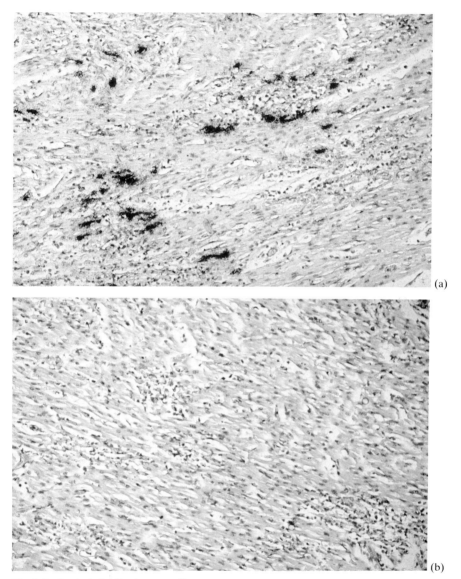

Fig. 9.3 *In situ* hybridization of an ^{35}S-labelled enterovirus group-specific cDNA probe to the paraffin-embedded autopsy heart tissue of an infant who died of acute enterovirus infection. (a) Autoradiographic silver grains can be clearly localized to distinct infected myocytes, thereby providing the possibility for an unequivocal diagnosis of myocardial enterovirus infection. (b) Hybridization to myocardial cells was not observed when myocardial tissues were hybridized with the ^{35}S-labelled plasmid vector control probe, demonstrating the specificity of *in situ* hybridization. Haemotoxylin and eosin × 75.

enterovirus infection in the autopsy heart of an infant who died of fulminant enterovirus-induced myocarditis. The autoradiographic silver grains, which indicate hybridization between viral RNA and radiolabelled cDNA probe, are clearly localized to numerous infected myocardial cells, thereby providing an unequivocal diagnosis of myocardial infection (Fig. 9.3a). Infected myocytes are easily identified because of their characteristic size and morphology. Infected myocytes are also seen adjacent to inflammatory cells, which provide the basis for the histopathological diagnosis of myocarditis. No hybridization was observed when myocardial tissue sections were probed with the radiolabelled plasmid vector control DNA probe (Fig. 9.3b). Another important observation was that replicating enteroviral RNA was found not only in myocytes but also in small interstitial cells, possibly myocardial fibroblasts, which agrees with previous *in vitro* findings in cultured human heart cells and persistently infected human myocardial fibroblasts.[31]

The use of computer-assisted digital image processing allows hybridization signals to be quantified and related to other parameters, such as the extent of myocardial tissue damage and degree of inflammation. In CVB3-induced chronic myocarditis in an immunocompetent murine model a strong spatial and temporal correlation between viral replication and myocardial lesions was observed, indicating that myocardial injury evolves as a consequence of multifocal organ infection.[35] Importantly, no inflammatory lesions were found to evolve independently of virus replication, indicating that persistent infection is essential for development of chronic myocardial disease.

Studies in persistently infected immunocompetent mice indicate that restricted replication of enteroviral RNA may play a role in persistence of virus in myocardium.[35] Using strand-specific RNA probes for *in situ* hybridization of either the viral genomic plus strand RNA or the complementary viral minus strand RNA,[36] it has been shown that, after the acute phase of infection, the amount of viral plus strand RNA present in persistently infected myocardial cells is similar to the amount of minus strand RNA. However, in acutely infected myocardial cells, viral plus strand RNA is synthesized in great excess. Approximately equal amounts of plus and minus strand enteroviral RNA have been found in myocardium from patients with DCM using slot blot hybridization.[37] Restricted replication may explain the common failure to isolate infectious virus from patients after the acute phase of virus replication. However, it remains to be determined whether restriction of viral replication is due to selection of replication-defective mutants, or to viral or cellular control mechanisms, which may be reversible. Reactivation of productive viral replication might explain the clinical phenomenon of recurrence or progression to chronic cardiac disease.

Detection of enteroviral RNA using the polymerase chain reaction

The recently developed PCR[38] offers new possibilities for rapid and sensitive detection of infectious agents. In this assay, a pair of oligonucleotide primers which hybridize specifically to sequences of opposite polarity on the target DNA separated by up to several hundred nucleotides, is used to direct sequential rounds of DNA polymerase-mediated replication of the region flanked by these primers. Each round of DNA replication is followed by thermal denaturation and cooling to allow reannealing of primers to the target DNA prior to the next round of replication using a thermostable DNA polymerase. Theoretically, the specific region of DNA is amplified up to a million-fold or more, thereby greatly enhancing detection. This may be accomplished by gel electrophoresis in which the amplified DNA product is identified by its expected size.

As an additional confirmation of specificity, the PCR product may be visualized by hybridization with a probe specific for the amplified sequence. This may be accomplished by Southern blot hybridization, in which electrophoretically resolved DNA is immobilized by transfer to a solid membrane, then hybridized with a labelled probe,[39] or by oligomer hybridization, in which target DNA is hybridized with the probe prior to electrophoresis.[40] As well as confirming the specificity of PCR, the use of a specific probe to detect PCR product also increases sensitivity. For amplification of RNA sequences, the initial step is reverse transcription of RNA to generate cDNA, which may then be amplified in the normal way.

A number of primer pairs and amplification protocols have been described for group-specific amplification of enteroviral RNA.[41–43] Group-specific detection of enteroviruses by PCR entails amplification of highly conserved regions of the enterovirus genome, typically within the noncoding regions near the 5' and 3' termini of the genome. Highly conserved sequences which may serve as enterovirus group-specific primer sequences can be identified by comparison of nucleotide sequences of different potentially cardiotropic enterovirus serotypes, a number of which have been published.[44–50] Enterovirus group PCR assays cited above successfully detected a broad spectrum of enterovirus serotypes. In addition, serotype-specific identification of enterovirus serotypes of known sequence can be acheived by direct sequencing of PCR products.[51] Because of the high number of potentially cardiotropic serotypes and limited sequence data, serotype-specific PCR is unlikely to be practical for clinical purposes.

In spite of current interest in PCR technology and applications, to date there have been relatively few reports on application of PCR to detect enteroviruses in heart muscle. In one study, enteroviral RNA was detected in endomyocardial biopsy samples from only 5 of 48 patients with myocarditis or DCM.[52] However, the sensitivity of the PCR used was not determined by reconstitution experiments using myocardial RNA to which known amounts of enteroviral RNA had been added. Sensitivity of enterovirus PCR may be limited by the efficiency of reverse transcription. Such considerations must be borne in mind when attempting to detect low amounts of enteroviral RNA, particularly in patients with long-standing chronic heart disease. The approach adopted by Weiss *et al.*[53] of using a CVB3 serotype-specific PCR is not practical for the diagnosis of enteroviral heart disease in humans, as discussed above. Finally, PCR does not allow correlation of morphology with results, as with *in situ* hybridization, but may provide a rapid detection method, provided that sensitivity as well as specificity is satisfactory.

The use of synthetic and recombinant antigens in the diagnosis of enterovirus infection

Production of synthetic and recombinant enterovirus antigens

It is now possible to produce synthetic antigens, either as recombinant polypeptides encoded by a plasmid expression vector into which part of the enterovirus genome has been inserted[13] (see below), or as chemically synthesized oligopeptides[54] using amino acid sequences derived from published nucleotide sequences of enterovirus genomes. Because the antigenic structure of poliovirus is well resolved,[55] it is possible to predict positions of some antigenic determinants of other enterovirus serotypes by nucleic acid and amino acid sequence alignment,[48] secondary structure predictions[56,57] and hydrophobicity prediction.[58] The location and antigenicity of predicted determinants can then be confirmed, either using the 'pepscanning' approach in which overlapping synthetic oligopeptides corresponding to the amino acid sequences of interest are tested by indirect ELISA,[54] or by construction of an antigenic chimera, in which a predicted epitope from one enterovirus serotype is inserted into the corresponding position of another serotype by site-directed mutagenesis, in order to assess its effect on antigenicity and immunogenicity.[59] This second method may be advantageous in comparison to the use of synthetic peptides, as conformational presentation of the predicted epitope, being expressed within a complete polypeptide as part of a complete virion, is more likely to resemble the natural conformation of the epitope. Provided the conformational structure of antigenic determinants is preserved, synthetic and recombinant antigens may be both immunogenic and antigenic.

Such antigens may be of great value as serological reagents. As discussed above, their use may improve and simplify existing serological assays. It may also be possible to identify antibody responses to specific enteroviral polypeptides which distinguish between the acute and chronic phases of enterovirus infection. This would be invaluable for serological diagnosis of acute and chronic enteroviral heart disease.

Antisera raised against recombinant enterovirus antigens

Synthetic and recombinant antigens may also be used to raise antisera for detection of enteroviral antigens. Although there is considerable antigenic homology the use of hyperimmune antisera to detect group-specific antigens has met with limited success, probably due to antigenic heterogeneity within as well as between serotypes. Compared with hyperimmune antisera obtained by immunization of rabbits with purified enteroviral virions,[60] antisera raised against bacterially synthesized CVB3 proteins revealed a much broader spectrum of cross-reactivity within the enteroviruses.[13,14] Several subgenomic fragments from infectious recombinant CVB3 cDNA were inserted into an expression plasmid. Plasmids were constructed which expressed either the structural proteins VP4, VP2 and VP3, or VP1, or the RNA-dependent RNA polymerase of CVB3. Polyclonal antisera raised in rabbits against the purified expression products from these clones reacted with numerous representative enterovirus serotypes. This offers a unique possibility for rapid identification of enteroviral agents of heart disease by antigen detection. In one study, a rabbit antiserum raised against recombinant VP1 was successfully used to demonstrate the presence of enteroviral VP1 antigen in myocardium from 12 of 20 infants who died from suspected CVB-induced myocarditis.[61] The use of these antibodies in combination with *in situ* hybridization in a double-labelling assay[62] may allow simultaneous *in situ* detection of enteroviral RNA and antigens at the single cell level. This would be of great value in determining the level of virus gene product expression in infected myocardial cells at different stages of myocarditis or DCM. Furthermore, these antisera have provided the basis for development of an enterovirus-specific ELISA, which was found to be useful for serological diagnosis.

Comment and outlook

Diagnosis of acute and chronic enteroviral heart disease has been greatly assisted in recent years by the availability of new assays described in this chapter for detection of enterovirus-specific IgM in serum and enteroviral nucleic acid in autopsy, biopsy or explanted cardiac tissue by *in situ* hybridization. As a result, we have a clearer picture of the incidence of enteroviral involvement in acute heart disease, and the association between enteroviruses and chronic cardiac disease, which was largely circumstantial being based on retrospective measurement of IgG titres, has been strengthened. Data from different research groups employing different diagnostic techniques are in general agreement regarding the incidence of enteroviral involvement in human heart disease. The cumulative experience from those employing techniques to detect enteroviral RNA in myocardium indicates that about 25% of patients with myocarditis or DCM had myocardial enterovirus infection.[27,30,52,53,63–68] However, there is still a need to compare different techniques in the same study population in order to determine the interrelationship between results from different diagnostic methods, to compare sensitives, and to determine which method(s) is most appropriate for diagnosis of different forms of enteroviral heart disease. Methods of detecting viral nucleic acid or antigen in cardiac tissue require invasive tissue sampling and may underestimate enteroviral involvement due to sampling error resulting from the focal distribution of lesions and enterovirus infection. These problems are not encountered using serological diagnostic methods, although it is possible, at least in theory, that virus may persist in a low grade or defective manner in the absence of a detectable humoral response. Conversely, the detection of such a response is not conclusive proof of cardiac involvement. It is likely, therefore, that virological and serological detection methods will complement one another.

In addition to establishing a diagnosis, demonstration of an enteroviral aetiology may influence management of patients with heart disease, with particular respect to the use of immunomodulating or antiviral agents discussed in detail elsewhere in this book. Clearly, corticosteroids are contraindicated in the presence of myocardial infection, since increased viral replication[69] and inhibition of the endogenous interferon system may follow their use.[28] Antiviral agents such as interferon may provide protection against myocardial enterovirus infection. The protective role of interferon-β (IFN-β) in CVB3-infected cultured human heart cells has been described.[28,31] In addition, the synergistic interaction between interferon-β and interferon-γ has been assessed in persistently infected cultured human myocardial fibroblasts with a view towards low-dose combination treatment.[70]

It is important to stress that all diagnostic assays described in this chapter are enterovirus group-specific rather than coxsackievirus- or serotype-specific, unless stated otherwise. Designation of an assay as coxsackievirus-specific, when it is capable of detecting infection with other enteroviruses, perpetuates a common belief that coxsackievirus are the most important human heart pathogens and thereby limits the scope of investigation that might demonstrate otherwise. The attention focussed upon coxsackieviruses, particularly CVB, in the past probably reflects the fact that these serotypes were initially isolated from infants with myocarditis, and could be propagated in cell culture more readily than other serotypes. Serotypic identification, although not essential for diagnosis, may provide valuable epidemiological information regarding the spread of enteroviruses and may provide information on the cardiotropic potential of different serotypes and subtypes. Sequencing of enterovirus PCR products derived from cardiac tissue may also allow identification of specific mutations which might be implicated in cardiotropism or enterovirus persistence.

Improvement of existing techniques and development of new techniques, partly in response to increasing appreciation of enteroviral involvement in human heart disease, has contributed to the rapidly changing state of the art in the field of enterovirus diagnosis. It is likely that some techniques discussed here which are currently awaiting or undergoing development and trial will be in widespread use within a few years. In addition, it should be possible to adapt many of the techniques described above for detection of other pathogenic viruses, as discussed elsewhere in this book. The value of these techniques, whether realized or potential, should not be underestimated. As indicated, their usefulness is not restricted to the detection of enteroviruses in patients with heart disease. They may also provide information on extent and distribution of virus infection within organs and tissues, the stage of infection – whether acute or persistent – the replicative state of the virus, and the nature of the patient's immune response to the infection. These factors may have additional implications for patient management and therapy in individual cases, and will undoubtedly influence the design of preventive and therapeutic regimens.

Acknowledgements

Myocardial tissue from autopsy hearts was kindly provided by A. Foulis, Department of Pathology, University of Glasgow. Endomyocardial biopsies were obtained from E. Erdmann and H-P. Schultheiss, Department of Internal Medicine I, University of Munich. This manuscript was written with support from grant 1900929 from The British Heart Foundation, grant Ka 593/2–2 from the Deutsche Forschungsgemeinschaft and grant 321–7291-BCT-0370 'Grundlagen und Anwendungen der Gentechnologie' from the German Ministry for Research and Technology. RK is Professor of Molecular Pathology.

References

1. Grist N. R. Coxsackievirus infections of the heart. In: Waterson A. P. ed. *Recent Advances in Clinical Virology* 1. Edinburgh: Churchill Livingstone, 1977; **141:** 40.
2. Cambridge G., MacArthur C. G. C., Waterson A. P. *et al*. Antibodies to coxsackie B viruses in primary congestive cardiomyopathy. *Br Heart J* 1979; **41:** 692–6.
3. Herrmann K. L. Antibody detection. In: Lennette E. H., Halonen P., Murphy

F. A. eds. *Laboratory Diagnosis of Infectious Diseases. Principles and Practice.* Volume II. *Viral, Rickettsial and Chlamydial Diseases.* New York: Springer-Verlag, 1988: 76–101.

4. El-Hagrassy M. M. O., Coltart D. J., Banatvala J. E. Coxsackie-B-virus-specific IgM responses in patients with cardiac and other diseases. *Lancet* 1980; **ii:** 1160–2.
5. McCartney R. A., Banatvala J. E., Bell E. J. Routine use of μ-antibody-capture ELISA for the serological diagnosis of coxsackie B virus infections. *J Med Virol* 1986; **19:** 205–12.
6. Muir P. Coxsackie B virus. In: Wreghitt T. G., Morgan-Capner P. eds. *ELISA in the Clinical Microbiology Laboratory.* London: Public Health Laboratory Service, 1990: 98–109.
7. Torfason E. G., Frisk G., Diderholm H. Indirect and reverse radioimmunoassay and their apparent specificities in detection of antibodies to enteroviruses in human sera. *J Med Virol* 1984; **13:** 13–1.
8. Morgan-Capner P., McSorley C. Antibody capture radioimmunoassay (MA-CRIA) for coxsackie B4 and B5-specific IgM. *J Hyg* 1983; **90:** 333–49.
9. Day C., Cumming H., Walker J. Enterovirus-specific IgM in the diagnosis of meningitis. *J Infect* 1989; **19:** 219–28.
10. Melnick J. L., Wenner H. A., Philips C. A. Enteroviruses. In: Lennette G. H., Schmidt N. J. eds. *Diagnostic Procedures for Viral, Rickettsial and Chlamydial Infections.* Eighth edition. Washington DC: American Public Health Association, 1979: 341–543.
11. Yolken R. H., Torsch V. M. Enzyme-linked immunosorbent assay for detection and identification of coxsackieviruses A. *Infect Immun* 1981; **31:** 742–50.
12. Muir P., Banatvala J. E. Reactivity of enterovirus-specific IgM with infective and defective coxsackie B virions in patients with monotypic and multitypic IgM responses. *J Virol Methods* 1990; **29:** 209–24.
13. Werner S., Klump W. M., Schönke H. *et al.* Expression of coxsackievirus B3 capsid proteins in *Escherichia coli* and generation of virus-specific antisera. *DNA* 1988; **7:** 307–16.
14. Werner S., Schönke H., Klump W. *et al.* Generation of enterovirus group-specific antisera using bacterially synthesized coxsackievirus B3 proteins. In: Schultheiss H.-P. ed. *New Concepts in Viral Heart Disease.* Berlin: Springer-Verlag, 1988: 125–36.
15. Bell E. J., McCartney R. A., Basquill D., Chaudhuri A. K. R. μ-antibody capture ELISA for the rapid diagnosis of enterovirus infection in patients with aseptic meningitis. *J Virol Med* 1986; **19:** 213–17.
16. Frisk G., Torfason E. G., Diderholm H. Reverse radioimmunoassays of IgM and IgG antibodies to coxsackie B viruses in patients with acute myopericarditis. *J Med Virol* 1984; **14:** 191–200.
17. Banatvala J. E. Coxsackie B virus infections in cardiac disease. In: Waterson A. P. ed. *Recent Advances in Clinical Virology 3.* Edinburgh: Churchill Livingstone, 1983: 99–115.
18. Muir P., Nicholson F., Tilzey A. J. *et al.* Chronic relapsing pericarditis and dilated cardiomyopathy: serological evidence of persistent enterovirus infection. *Lancet* 1989; **i:** 804–7.
19. Miller N. A., Carmichael H. A., Calder B. D. *et al.* Antibody to coxsackie B virus in diagnosing postviral fatigue syndrome. *Br Med J* 1991; **302:** 140–3.
20. Muir P., Nicholson F., Banatvala J. E., Bingley P. J. Coxsackie B virus and postviral fatigue syndrome. *Br Med J* 1991; **302:** 658–9.
21. Muir P., Singh N. B., Banatvala J. E. Enterovirus-specific serum IgA antibody responses in patients with acute infections, chronic cardiac disease and insulin-dependent diabetes mellitus. *J Med Virol* 1990; **32:** 236–42.
22. Dhar R., Ogra P. L. Local immune responses. *Br Med Bull* 1985; **41:** 28–33.

23. Hyypiä T., Stålhandske P., Vainionpää R., Pettersson U. Detection of entero-viruses by spot hybridization. *J Clin Microbiol* 1984; **19:** 436–8.
24. Tracy S. A comparison of genomic homologies among the coxsackievirus B group: use of fragments of the cloned coxsackievirus B3 genome as probes. *J Gen Virol* 1984; **65:** 2167–72.
25. Kandolf R., Hofschneider P. H. Molecular cloning of the genome of a cardiotropic coxsackie B3 virus: full-length reverse-transcribed recombinant cDNA generates infectious virus in mammalian cells. *Proc Natl Acad Sci (USA)* 1985; **82:** 4818–22.
26. Rotbart H. A., Levin M. J., Villareal L. P. *et al.* Factors affecting the detection of enteroviruses in cerebrospinal fluid with coxsackievirus B3 and poliovirus type 1 cDNA probes. *J Clin Microbiol* 1985; **22:** 220–4.
27. Bowles N. E., Richardson P. J., Olsen E. G. J., Archard L. C. Detection of coxsackie-B-virus-specific RNA sequences in myocardial biopsy samples from patients with myocarditis and dilated cardiomyopathy. *Lancet* 1986; **i:** 1120–3.
28. Kandolf R., Ameis D., Kirschner P. *et al. In situ* detection of enteroviral genomes in myocardial cells by nucleic acid hybridization: An approach to the diagnosis of viral heart disease. *Proc Natl Acad Sci (USA)* 1987; **84:** 6272–6.
29. Kandolf R. The impact of recombinant DNA technology on the study of entero-virus heart disease. In: Bendinelli M., Friedman H. eds. *Coxsackieviruses – A General Update.* New York: Plenum Press, 1988: 293–318.
30. Kandolf R., Hofschneider P. H. Enteroviral heart disease. *Springer Sem Immuno-pathol* 1989; **11:** 1–13.
31. Kandolf R., Canu A., Hofschneider P. H. Coxsackie B3 virus can replicate in cultured human foetal heart cells and is inhibited by interferon. *J Mol Cell Cardiol* 1985; **17:** 167–81.
32. Wolf H., zur Hausen H., Becker V. E. B. Viral genomes in epithelial nasopharyn-geal carcinoma cells. *Nature New Biol* 1973; **244:** 245–7.
33. Haase A., Brahic M., Stowring L., Blum H. Detection of viral nucleic acids by *in situ* hybridization. *Meth Virol* 1984; **7:** 189–226.
34. Nelson J. A., Fleckenstein B., Galloway D. A., McDougall J. K. Transformation of NIH 3T3 cells with cloned fragments of human cytomegalovirus strain Ad169. *J Virol* 1982; **43:** 83–91.
35. Klingel K., Hohenadl C., Canu A. *et al.* Ongoing enterovirus-induced myocarditis is associated with persistent heart muscle infection: Quantitative analysis of virus replication, tissue damage, and inflammation. *Proc Natl Acad Sci (USA)* 1992; **89:** 314–18.
36. Hohenadl C., Klingel K., Mertsching J. *et al.* Strand-specific detection of entero-viral RNA in myocardial tissue by *in situ* hybridization. *Mol Cell Probes* 1991; **5:** 11–20.
37. Archard L. C., Bowles N. E., Cunningham L. *et al.* Molecular probes for detec-tion of persistent enterovirus infection of human heart and their prognostic value. *Eur Heart J* 1991; **12** (suppl D) 56–9.
38. Saiki R. K., Gelfand D. H., Stoffel S. *et al.* Primer-directed enzymatic amplifica-tion of DNA with a thermostable DNA polymerase. *Science* 1988; **239:** 487–91.
39. Southern E. M. Detection of specific sequences among DNA fragments separated by gel electrophoresis. *J Mol Biol* 1975; **98:** 503–17.
40. Kellog D. E., Kwok S. Detection of human immunodeficiency virus. In: Innis M. A., Gelfand D. H., Sninsky J. J., White T. J. eds. *PCR Protocols: A Guide to Methods and Applications.* San Diego: Academic Press, 1990: 337–47.
41. Chapman N. M., Tracy S., Gauntt C. J., Fortmueller U. Molecular detection and identification of enteroviruses using enzymatic amplification and nucleic acid hybridization. *J Clin Microbiol* 1990; **28:** 843–50.
42. Olive D. M., Al-Mufti S., Al-Mulla W. *et al.* Detection and differentiation of picornaviruses in clinical samples following genomic amplification. *J Gen Virol* 1990; **71:** 2141–7.

43. Rotbart H. A. Enzymatic RNA amplification of the enteroviruses. *J Clin Microbiol* 1990; **28:** 438–42.
44. Chang K. H., Auvinen P., Hyypiä T., Stanway G. The nucleotide sequence of coxsackievirus A9; implications for receptor binding and enterovirus classification. *J Gen Virol* 1989; **70:** 3268–80.
45. Hughes P. J., North C., Minor P. D., Stanway G. The complete nucleotide sequence of coxsackievirus A21. *J Gen Virol* 1989; **70:** 2943–52.
46. Iizuka N., Kuge S., Nomoto A. Complete nucleotide sequence of the genome of coxsackievirus B1. *Virology* 1987; **156:** 64–73.
47. Jenkins O., Booth J. D., Minor P. D., Almond J. W. The complete nucleotide sequence of coxsackievirus B4 and its comparison to other members of the Picornaviridae. *J Gen Virol* 1987; **68:** 1835–48.
48. Klump W. M., Bergmann I., Müller B. C. *et al.* Complete nucleotide sequence of infectious coxsackievirus B3 cDNA: Two initial 5' uridine residues are regained during plus-strand RNA synthesis. *J Virol* 1990; **64:** 1573–83.
49. Lindberg A. M., Stålhandske P. O. K., Pettersson U. Genome of coxsackievirus B3. *Virology* 1987; **156:** 50–63.
50. Ryan M. D., Jenkins O., Hughes P. J. *et al.* The complete nucleotide sequence of enterovirus type 70: relationships with other members of the Picornaviridae. *J Gen Virol* 1990; **71:** 2291–9.
51. Innis M. A., Myambo K. B., Gelfand D. H., Brow M. A. DNA sequencing with *Thermus aquaticus* DNA polymerase and direct sequencing of polymerase chain reaction-amplified DNA. *Proc Natl Acad Sci (USA)* 1988; **85:** 9436–40.
52. Jin O., Sole M. J., Butany J. W. *et al.* Detection of enterovirus RNA in myocardial biopsies from patients with myocarditis and cardiomyopathy using gene amplification by polymerase chain reaction. *Circulation* 1990; **82:** 8–16.
53. Weiss L. M., Movahed L. A., Billingham M. E., Cleary M. L. Detection of coxsackievirus B3 RNA in myocardial tissues by the polymerase chain reaction. *Am J Pathol* 1991; **138:** 497–503.
54. Smyth M. S., Hoey E. M., Trudgett A. *et al.* Chemically synthesized peptides elicit neutralizing antibody to bovine enterovirus. *J Gen Virol* 1990; **71:** 231–4.
55. Hogle J. M., Chow M., Filman D. J. Three-dimensional structure of poliovirus at 2.9 Å resolution. *Science* 1985; **229:** 1358–65.
56. Chou P. Y., Fasman G. D. Empirical predictions of protein conformation. *Ann Rev Biochem* 1978; **47:** 251–76.
57. Garnier J., Osguthorpe D. J., Robson B. Analysis of the accuracy and implications of simple methods for predicting the secondary structure of globular proteins. *J Mol Biol* 1978; **120:** 97–120.
58. Kyte J., Doolittle R. F. A simple method for displaying the hydropathic character of a protein. *J Mol Biol* 1982; **157:** 105–32.
59. Reimann B.-Y., Zell R., Kandolf R. Mapping of a neutralizing antigenic site of coxsackievirus B4 by construction of an antigenic chimera. *J Virol* 1991; **65:** 3475–80.
60. Mertens T. H., Pika U., Eggers H. J. Cross antigenicity among enteroviruses as revealed by immunoblot technique. *Virology* 1983; **129:** 431–42.
61. Foulis A. K., Farquharson M. A., Cameron S. O. *et al.* A search for the presence of the enteroviral capsid protein VP1 in pancreases of patients with type 1 (insulin-dependent) diabetes and pancreases and hearts of infants who died of coxsackieviral myocarditis. *Diabetologia* 1990; **33:** 290–8.
62. Brahic M., Haase A. T., Cash E. Simultaneous *in situ* detection of viral RNA and antigens. *Proc Natl Acad Sci (USA)* 1984; **81:** 5445–8.
63. Easton A. J., Eglin R. P. The detection of coxsackievirus RNA in cardiac tissue by *in situ* hybridization. *J Gen Virol* 1988; **69:** 285–91.
64. Bowles N. E., Rose M. L., Taylor P. End-stage dilated cardiomyopathy: persist-

ence of enterovirus RNA in myocardium at transplantation and lack of immune response. *Circulation* 1989; **80:** 1128–36.

65. Kandolf R., Canu A., Klingel K. *et al.* Molecular studies on enteroviral heart disease. In: Brinton M. A., Heinz F. X. eds. *New Aspects of Positive Strand RNA Viruses.* Washington DC: American Society of Microbiology, 1990: 340–8.

66. Tracy S. Wiegand V., McManus B. *et al.* Molecular approaches to enteroviral diagnosis in idiopathic cardiomyopathy and myocarditis. *J Am Coll Cardiol* 1990; **15:** 1688–94.

67. Tracy S., Chapman N. M., McManus B. M. *et al.* A molecular and serological evaluation of enteroviral involvement in human myocarditis. *J Mol Cell Cardiol* 1990; **22:** 403–14.

68. Archard L. C., Freeke C., Richardson P. *et al.* Persistence of enterovirus RNA in dilated cardiomyopathy: a progression from myocarditis. In: Schultheiss H.-P. ed. *New Concepts in Viral Heart Disease.* Berlin: Springer-Verlag, 1988: 349–62.

69. Kilbourne E. D., Horsfall F. L. Lethal infection with coxsackievirus of adult mice given cortisone. *Proc Soc Exp Biol Med* 1951; **98:** 503–17.

70. Heim A., Canu A., Kirschner P., *et al.* Synergistic interaction of interferon-β and interferon-γ in coxsackievirus B3-infected carrier cultures of human myocardial fibroblasts. *J. Infect Dis* 1992; **166:** 958–65.

10

Prospects for treatment and prevention of virally induced heart disease

W. Al-Nakib

Viral infections of the heart that are targets for treatment and prevention

The most common cause of primary myocardial disease in adults and children is that due to coxsackie B viruses.[1] Other enterovirus infections, such as those caused by coxsackie A and echoviruses may also result in cardiac abnormalities but to a much lesser extent.[1] Initially the evidence implicating enteroviral involvement in cardiac disease was circumstantial and based on the finding of a relatively high proportion (about 50%) of patients with acute myocarditis having transient enterovirus IgM responses when compared with matched controls.[1,2] However, growing evidence suggests that following an acute or subacute episode of carditis due to an enterovirus infection, the virus persists in the cardiac tissues causing a chronic dilated cardiomyopathy (DCM).[1] Evidence for this came from studies that showed a persistent enterovirus IgM response in these patients thereby suggesting a continuous antigenic stimulus[3,4] and the presence of viral antigens by immunofluorescence in the diseased cardiac tissues.[5] More recently, using recombinant DNA techniques, including *in situ* hybridization and the polymerase chain reaction (PCR), enterovirus RNA was demonstrated in a relatively high proportion of endomyocardial biopsy specimens from patients with myocarditis and DCM but not from other heart diseases.[6,7]

Rubella virus is a major cause of congenital heart disease.[8] Infection during the first 12 weeks of pregnancy often damages the fetal cardiac tissues and results in perinatal mortality or permanent defects such as persistence of patent ductus arteriosis, proximal (valvular) or peripheral pulmonary artery stenosis or a ventricular septal defect.[8]

Another virus that frequently invades the myocardium is mumps virus. Evidence implicating mumps virus in infection of the myocardium has been obtained by documenting the appearance of abnormalities in electrocardiograms,[9] by isolating the virus directly from myocardial tissues or by demonstrating viral antigens in cardiac tissues by immunofluoresence.[9]

Although viraemia following an influenza virus infection is rare or at least difficult to detect, both influenza A and B virus infections have been associated with myopericarditis.[10,11] Furthermore, electrocardiographic abnormalities in uncomplicated infuenza A and B virus infection have also been observed.[12]

Cytomegalovirus has also been implicated as a cause of heart disease[13] and atherosclerosis (see Chapters 6 and 8); more recently, attention has been drawn to the finding that patients with AIDS frequently have cardiac problems[14] (see Chapter 7).

Prospects for treatment of enterovirus infections

Over the past 6 years or so, a new generation of antipicornavirus compounds have been described by scientists at the Sterling-Winthrop Research Institute in the USA. Chemically, these anti-viral agents belong to the (oxazolinyl-phenyl) isoxazole class of compounds. They inhibit viral replication by binding to the viral capsid and either block virus uncoating as observed for poliovirus type 2 and human rhinovirus 2 (HRV-2), or inhibit virus attachment as demonstrated with human rhinovirus 14 (HRV-14).[15–17]

Figure 10.1 shows how one of these WIN compounds resides inside the pocket just underneath the 'canyons' present on the surface of the viral capsid. The drug interacts with amino acids lining the walls of the drug-binding pocket,[19] and either stabilizes the capsid and hence prevents virus uncoating or distorts the receptor binding site in the canyon and thus inhibits virus attachment to cells.

One of these compounds, WIN 54954, has a broad spectrum of anti-picornavirus activity, particularly against rhinoviruses, polioviruses, coxsackie B1–5 viruses, some echoviruses and coxsackie A9 virus, at very low concentrations (range 0.004–0.17 µg/ml, Table 10.1). In experiments in mice, both WIN 54954 and another WIN compound, WIN 51711, have been shown to prevent paralysis effectively when given either just before or after infecting

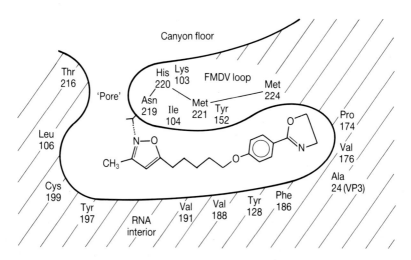

Fig. 10.1 Schematic representation of a WIN compound in the binding pocket just underneath the 'canyons' on the surface of a rhinovirus. Reproduced with permission. From Badger *et al.*[18]

Table 10.1 Activity of WIN 54954 against some picornaviruses.[20]

Virus	Serotype	MIC (µg/ml)*
Rhinovirus	1	0.009
	6	0.130
	9	0.075
	15	0.130
	20	0.056
	24	0.056
	30	0.040
	41	0.410
	54	0.650
	72	0.620
	86	0.140
Echovirus	3	0.010
	4	0.060
	5	0.430
	6	0.020
	7	0.004
	9	0.060
	11	0.360
	24	0.020
	30	0.250
Coxsackievirus	B–1	0.030
	B–2	0.007
	B–3	0.009
	B–4	0.020
	B–5	0.030
	A–9	0.004

*MIC = minimal inhibitory concentrations.

the animals with either poliovirus type 2, coxsackie A9 virus or echovirus type 9.[20,21] These results are encouraging and suggest potential *in vivo* efficacy. It would therefore be interesting to test the efficacy of WIN 54954 in preventing or treating, say, coxsackie B3 virus infections using the murine model of myocarditis.[22] If results suggest good *in vivo* efficacy, consideration should be given to evaluating this drug in humans in placebo controlled trials. However, before such trials are conducted information regarding the pharmacokinetics and tolerance of this drug in humans are required (it is most probable that such information regarding WIN 54954 has already been obtained by the Sterling-Winthrop group). However, it is anticipated that some considerable difficulties would be encountered when these drugs reach the stage of evaluation in humans. For example, it would be particularly difficult to establish criteria for patient selection in such trials or clinical and laboratory parameters needed to monitor progress and efficacy of therapy effectively. Indeed, the serological monitoring of an enterovirus infection has never been reliable or useful, especially since both subclinical infections and heterotypic immune responses are common. Virus may or may not be shed or detected in an enterovirus infection of the heart. Furthermore, unlike *Herpes simplex* or varicella-zoster virus infections, there are no vesicles or virus in vesicular fluids that have been so useful in measuring the efficacy of acyclovir and other anti herpes drugs. Whether efficacy could be assessed purely on clinical outcome remains to be seen, though this is unlikely to be satisfactory.

Yasin *et al.*[23] and Heinz *et al.*[24] have reported that picornaviruses develop resistance to anti-viral agents very rapidly. Further, it has recently been shown that rhinoviruses rapidly develop resistance to another capsid-binding drug following topical treatment in the nose.[25] More recently, in a specially designed controlled study, volunteers were challenged with both the drug-resistant and the parental wild-type virus. It was found that the drug-resistant virus, like the parental wild type, was able to infect and produce illness in a proportion of the challenged volunteers.[26] Furthermore, virus isolates from volunteers challenged with the drug-resistant virus remained resistant to the drug despite replication in the human body, suggesting that resistance to the drug was a relatively stable genetic trait.[26] It is therefore only reasonable to speculate that, like rhinoviruses, enteroviruses will most probably also develop drug resistance during the course of treatment of patients with entero-virus cardiomyopathies. The clinical significance of enterovirus drug resistance once established will, therefore, need to be determined at the time. Once an active anti-enterovirus compound is found, it would be important to determine how it could be most usefully applied. For example, whether it would be more useful to give it prophylactically, that is, to prevent an infection or therapeutically, to treat a recent ongoing or a chronic infection? Although anti-viral agents could be useful if they were to prevent an entero-virus infection, it would be difficult to identify individuals who may be at risk of being infected with an enterovirus infection and likely to develop heart disease. In addition, several serotypes of different enteroviruses may circulate at any point in different enteroviruses may circulate at any point in time in a particular community. Furthermore, although some of these anti-viral agents have some broad spectrum activity, they are unlikely to be equally active against all enteroviruses. Indeed, as has been observed with rhinoviruses, different enterovirus seroytypes are likely to show variable levels of sensitivity to any capsid-binding anti-viral agent.[27] More probably, these anti-viral agents would be used to treat an acute episode of a laboratory diagnosed enterovirus infection, perhaps with or without evidence of cardiac involvement. The object would be to prevent or at least reduce or limit the damage that such infection may cause to the heart tissues. Such treatment would be especially useful if it were actually to prevent an enterovirus from establishing a persistent or chronic infection of the heart tissues leading to the development of DCM. Furthermore, it would be particularly useful if these compounds were to penetrate cardiac tissues in sufficient anti-viral concentrations and 'cure' an established chronic enteroviral infection. However, penetration of the cardiac cells or tissues by these compounds, particularly at high enough concentrations to halt a viral infection, may also result in toxicity. The side effects, should they occur, would therefore need to be weighed very carefully against the beneficial effect of treatment. Perhaps the efficacy of these anti-viral agents in treating a persistent or chronic infection should first be assessed in an animal model system and/or in tissue cultures that are chronically infected with an enterovirus.

In summary, at the present time, a number of anti-picornaviral compounds, which are active against several enteroviruses, have been identified. Their potency has been demonstrated in both cell culture and in animal model systems. Their toxicity and efficacy in humans still need to be determined. It is anticipated that difficulties will be encountered when they are evaluated in humans.

Prospects for prevention of enterovirus infections

Preventing an enterovirus infection of the heart by inducing protective herd immunity through mass vaccination programmes is likely to prove very difficult. Infection with one enterovirus serotype does not generally confer immunity or protection against infection by an heterologous serotype. Because of the extensive serological cross-reactivity between serotypes, it would be difficult to establish susceptibility to a particular enterovirus infection. Indeed, even the presence of an antibody in the serum of an individual does not in itself always accurately predict immunity or protection from infection or reinfection. Because of this, any effective future vaccine will, most probably, have to be multivalent and contain representative members of the most common serotypes of each group of the enteroviruses (with some coxsackie B virus serotypes such as B4 and B3 being the most prominent components of such a vaccine). Generally, it would be difficult to prepare such a multivalent vaccine particularly for entereovirus. Many of these viruses, especially the coxsackie A viruses, do not grow well in cell culture. Furthermore, it would be difficult to ensure that all the viruses in a live vaccine are well attenuated and that they would not revert to virulence following replication in humans. Experience with the live-attenuated poliovirus vaccine showed that this was difficult to guarantee for all three serotypes in the vaccine and neurological complications including aseptic meningitis and poliomyelitis related to vaccination are well documented. Alternatively, one would confine the components of the vaccine to the two or three enterovirus serotypes that are most commonly involved in infection of the human heart. However, to test and assess the level of attenuation of these two or three viruses in this vaccine, one would still need to identify and establish a sensitive and reliable animal model system. For example, in the poliomyelitis vaccine, neurovirulence of the attenuated viruses in the vaccine is tested in monkeys. Whether a reliable 'universal' animal model system to test virulence of other enteroviruses, not only in relation to carditis but also to other conditions caused by these viruses, can be found, remains to be seen. Alternatively, 'high potency' inactivated vaccine against a selected group of enteroviruses may be developed. Such a vaccine would have the important advantage of safety. Furthermore, the question of monitoring and measuring the degree of virus attenuation would not arise. However, some enteroviruses, particularly the coxsackie A viruses, do not grow readily in cell culture let alone be produced in large enough concentrations for such a vaccine. Inactivated vaccines can be expensive to produce and unlike live vaccines, they do not produce local immunity in the gut which may be essential in preventing an enterovirus infection.

With the advent of recombinant DNA techniques, antigenic mapping and X-ray crystallography, it is now possible to identify and map the major immunogenic sites on the surface of at least some of the coxsackie B viruses. This has already been demonstrated with rhinovirus 14,[28] poliovirus[29] and recently mengovirus.[30] This will improve our understanding of the importance and position of the various protective epitopes on the surface of the coxsackieviruses, especially if possible 'common' and perhaps 'protective' epitope(s) were to be identified. The identification of such epitope(s) would allow the construction of a 'live' recombinant virus vaccine expressing all the relevant antigens. If nucleotides which are responsive to Coxasackie virus 'virulence' could be identified, it may then be possible to construct a virus which is capable of infection but not of producing diesease. Indeed, this is not entirely impossible to achieve. Thus recent work has shown that nucleotide changes in positions 480, 481 and 472 in the genome of poliovirus 1, 2 and 3 vaccine strains, respectively, affect the neurovirulence of these viruses directly.[31–35] Regions in the genome of coxsackieviruses that affect cardiotropism might also be identified and deleted by genetically manipulating the genome. Such a recombinant virus would have the desired property of expressing the relevant epitopes without producing disease. Indeed, recently van Houten *et al.*[36] isolated an escape mutant coxsackie B3 variant that showed reduced replication in myocardial cells in mice. The virus was clearly less pathogenic than the wild type since infection with this mutant virus resulted in only 10% mortality in mice compared with 90% by the wild type virus.[36] Sequencing the genome of this and the wild-type virus will allow the identification of specific regions in the genome that may induce cardiotropism of coxsackie B3 virus infection. Alternatively, relevant coxsackie B virus epithopes may be expressed as part of a future chimeric vaccine that would perhaps include the polioviruses. Such a chimera has already has already been shown to induce good and specific antibody responses in animals to a number of viruses including rhinoviruses, HIV-1, polioviruses and recently papillomaviruses.[37] Relevant epitopes, say, on coxsackie B viruses, may also be presented as a synthetic peptide vaccine containing a general amino acid sequence, representing major sites in the VPI of three different strains of foot-and-mouth disease (FMD) virus (another picornavirus), was capable of inducing high levels of serotype-specific neutralizing antibody in cattle and guinea pigs.[38] Furthermore, two of these peptides provided complete protection of guinea pigs against their respective virus challenges. More importantly, perhaps, is that two of the three peptides offered cross-protection against challenges with the heterologous virus.[38] The heterotypic protection observed appeared to be related more to the presence of cross-reactive anti-peptide antibody than to neutralizing antibody.[38] Although, it would be difficult to extrapolate this finding to enterovirus infection of humans, it nevertheless demonstrates the feasibility of such an approach, perhaps at some point in the future. Moreover, it also demonstrates the feasibility of such an approach, perhaps at some point in the future. Moreover, it also demonstrates that immunization with a synthetic peptide vaccine does not necessarily generate only high specific antibodies that will not protect against variant viruses possessing minor mutations in their protein sequences. Currently, little is known about the role of cell-mediated immune responses either in the recovery from an enterovirus infection or in the immunopathology of the disease particularly in relation to the development of dilated cardiomyopathies. Recent studies showed that mice infected with one enterovirus are more likely to develop myocardial inflammation following exposure to a second enteroviral infection (see also Chapter 6).[22] It was proposed that cell-mediated immune responses to a conserved antigenic epitope(s) among the enteroviruses may be involved in the exacerbation of myocardial inflammatory disease during a second enterovirus infection.[22]

Because of the complexity of enterovirus infections, prospects for successfully preventing such infections of the heart by vaccination are likely to be fraught with difficulties.

Prospects for treatment and prevention of other viruses that also cause infections of the heart

There are no specific treatments for rubella and mumps virus infections at the present time. Only influenza A virus infections are amenable to treatment with both amantadine and rimantadine. Indeed, extensive studies have clearly established that both these drugs are extremely effective when given either prophylactically or therapeutically.[39] Furthermore, medication with either of these drugs results in only minor central nervous system or gastrointestinal side effects which are transient and reversible upon withdrawal of medication. Unfortunately, neither of these drugs are widely used and their efficacy in preventing or treating an influenza A virus infection of the heart has never been determined. It is also noteworthy that influenza A viruses have recently been reported to develop resistance to rimantadine very rapidly during the course of treatment and that these drug-resistant viruses were able to infect and produce disease in individuals who were in close contact with the treated index cases.[40]

Both rubella and mumps virus infections can be effectively prevented by vaccination. A live-attenuated vaccine for each of the viruses or a combined measles, mumps and rubella (MMR) vaccine is available and widely used. On the other hand, the efficacy of the inactivated or subunit influenza A and B vaccines remains questionable.

References

1. Editorial. Dilated cardiomyopathy and enteroviruses. *Lancet* 1990; **ii:** 971–3.
2. El-Hagrassy M. M. O, Banatvala J. E., Coltart D. J. Coxsackie B virus specific IgM responses in patients with cardiac and other diseases. *Lancet* 1980; **ii:** 1160–2.
3. Banatvala J. E. Coxsackie B virus infections in cardiac disease. In: Waterson A. P. ed. *Recent Advances in Clinical Virology 3*. Edinburgh: Churchill Livingstone, 1983: 99–115.
4. Muir P., Nicholson F. N., Tilzey A. J. *et al.* Chronic relapsing pericarditis and dilated cardiomyopathy. *Lancet* 1989; **i:** 804–7.
5. Burch G. E., Sun S. C., Chu K. C. *et al.* Interstitial and coxsackie B myocarditis in infants and children. A comparative histologic and immunofluorescent study of 50 autopsied hearts. *J Am Med Assoc* 1968; **203:** 1–8.
6. Bowles N. E., Richardson P. J., Olsen E. J. G., Archard L. C. Detection of coxsackie-B-virus-specific RNA sequences in myocardial biopsy samples from patients with myocarditis and dilated cardiomyopathy. *Lancet* 1986; **i:** 1120–3.
7. Archard L., Freeke C., Richardson P. *et al.* Persistence of enterovirus RNA in dilated cardiomyopathy: a progression from myocarditis. In: Schultheiss H.-P. ed. *New Concepts in Viral Heart Disease*. Berlin: Springer-Verlag, 1988: 349–62.
8. Best J. M., Banatvala J. E. Rubella. In: Zuckerman A. J., Banatvala J. E., Pattison J. R. eds. *Principles and Practice of Clinical Virology*. Chichester: John Wiley, 1990: 337–74.

9. Leinikki P. In: Zuckerman A. J., Banatvala J. E., Pattison J. R. eds. *Principles and Practices of Clinical Virology*. Chichester: John Wiley, 1990: 375–88.
10. Karjahainen J., Nieminen M. S., Heikkila J. Influenza A myocarditis in conscripts. *Acta Med Scand* 1980; **207:** 27–30.
11. Verel D., Warrak A. J. N., Potter C. W. *et al*. Observations on the A2 England influenza epidemic. A clinicopathological study. *Am Heart J* 1976; **92:** 290–6.
12. Adams C. W. Post viral myopericarditis associated with the influenza virus. *Am J Cardiol* 1959; **4:** 56–67.
13. Schonian U., Maisch B. Cytomegalovirus DNA in endomyocardial biopsies of patients with (peri)myocarditis. *2nd International Symposium on Inflammatory Heart Disease*. Marburg, FRG, June, 1990.
14. Calabrese L. H., Proffitt M. R., Yen-Lieberman B. *et al*. Congestive cardiomyopathy and illness related to the acquired immune deficiency syndrome (AIDS). Association with isolation of retrovirus from myocardium. *Ann Int Med* 1987; **107:** 691–2.
15. Fox M. P., Otto M. J., McKinlay M. A. Prevention of rhinovirus and poliovirus uncoating by WIN 51711, a new antiviral drug. *Antimicrob Ag Chemother* 1986; **30:** 110–16.
16. Pevear D. C., Francher M. J., Felock P. J. *et al*. Conformational change in the floor of the human rhinovirus canyon blocks adsorption to Hela cell receptors. *J Virol* 1989; **63:** 2002–7.
17. Diana G. D., Treasurywala A. M., Bailey T. R. *et al*. A model for compounds active against human rhinovirus-14 based on X-ray crystallography data. *J Med Chem* 1990; **33:** 1306–11.
18. Badger J., Krishnaswamy S., Kremer M. J., Oliveira M. A., Rossmann M. G. *et al*. Three-dimensional structures of drug-resistant mutants of human Rhinovirus 14. *J Mol Biol* 1989; **207:** 163–74.
19. Smith T. J., Kremer M. J., Luo M. *et al*. The site of attachment in human rhinovirus 14 for antiviral agents that inhibit uncoating. *Science* 1986; **233:** 1286–93.
20. Woods M. G., Diana G. D., Rogge M. C. *et al*. *In vitro* and *in vivo* activities of WIN 54954, a new broad-spectrum antipicornavirus drug. *Antimicrob Ag Chemother* 1989; **33:** 2069–74.
21. McKinlay M. A., Steinberg B. A. Viral efficacy of WIN 51711 in mice infected with human poliovirus. *Antimicrob Ag Chemother* 1986; **29:** 30–2.
22. Beck M. A., Chapman N. M., McManus B. M. *et al*. Secondary enterovirus infection in the murine model of myocarditis. *Am J Pathol* 1990; **136:** 669–81.
23. Yasin S. R., Al-Nakib W., Tyrrell D. A. J. Isolation and preliminary characterization of chalcone Ro 09–0410-resistant human rhinovirus type 2. *Antivir Chem Chemother* 1990; **1:** 149–54.
24. Heinz B. A., Rueckert R. R., Shepard D. A. *et al*. Genetic and molecular analyses of spontaneous mutants of human rhinovirus 14 that are resistant to an antiviral compound. *J Virol* 1989; **63:** 2476–85.
25. Dearden C., Al-Nakib W., Andries K. *et al*. Drug resistant rhinoviruses from the nose of experimentally treated volunteers. *Arch Virol* 1989; **109:** 71–81.
26. Yasin S. R., Al-Nakib W., Tyrrell D. A. J. Pathogenicity for man of human rhinovirus type 2 mutants resistant to or dependent on chalone Ro 09–0410. *Antimicrob Ag Chemother* 1990; **34:** 963–6.
27. Andries K., Dewindt B., Snoeks J. *et al*. Two groups of rhinoviruses revealed by a panel of antiviral compounds present sequence divergence and differential pathogenicity: *J Virol* 1990; **64:** 1117–23.
28. Rossmann M. G., Arnold E., Erickson J. W. *et al*. Structure of a human common cold virus and functional relationship to other picornaviruses. *Nature* 1985; **317:** 145–53.

29. Hogle J. M., Chow M., Filman D. J. Three-dimensional structure of poliovirus at 2.9 A resolution. *Science* 1985; **299**: 1358–65.
30. Boege U., Kobasa D., Onodera S. *et al*. Characterization of mengo virus neutralization epitopes. *Virology* 1991; **181**: 1–13.
31. Evans D. M. A., Dunn G., Minor P. D. *et al*. A single nucleotide change in the 5′ non-coding region of the genome of the sabin type 3 poliovaccine is associated with increased neurovirulence. *Nature* 1985; **315**: 548–50.
32. Omata T., Kihara M., Kuge S. *et al*. Genetic analysis of the attenuation phenotype of poliovirus type 1. *J Virol* 1986; **58**: 348–58.
33. Van der Werf S., Bradley J., Wimmer E. *et al*. Synthesis of infectious poliovirus RNA by purified T7 RNA polymerase. *Proc Natl Acad Sci (USA)* 1986; **83**: 2330–4.
34. Pollard S. R., Dunn G., Cammack N. *et al*. Nucleotide sequence of a neurovirulent variant of the type 2 oral poliovirus vaccine. *J Virol* 1989; **63**: 4949–51.
35. Ren R., Moss E. G., Racaniello V. R. Identification of two determinants that attenuate vaccine type 2 poliovirus. *J Virol* 1991; **65**: 1377–82.
36. van Houten N., Bouchard P. E., Moraska A., Huber S. Selection of an attenuated coxsackievirus B3 variant, using a monoclonal antibody reactive to myocyte antigen. *J Virol* 1991; **65**: 1286–90.
37. Jenkins O., Cason J., Burke K. L. *et al*. An antigen chimera of poliovirus induces antibodies against human papillomavirus Type 16. *J Virol* 1990; **64**: 1201–6.
38. Doel T. R., Gale C., Do Amaral C. M. C. F. *et al*. Heterotypic protection induced by synthetic peptides corresponding to three serotypes of foot-and-mouth disease virus. *J Virol* 1990; **64**: 2260–4.
39. Dolin R. Rimantadine and amantadine in the prophylaxis and therapy of influenza A. In: De Clercq E. ed. *Clinical Use of Antiviral Drugs*. Boston: Martinus Nijhoff (Publishers), 1988: 277–87.
40. Hayden F. G., Belshe R. B., Clover R. D. *et al*. Emergence and apparent transmission of rimantadine-resistant influenza A virus in families. *N Engl J Med* 1989; **321**: 1696–702.

11

Virus infections in heart transplant recipients and evidence for involvement of the heart

T. Wreghitt and N. Cary

Introduction

Viral infections are a major cause of morbidity and mortality in solid organ transplant patients.[1,2] In this chapter viral infections will be briefly reviewed that occur in this group of patients with particular reference to heart and combined heart–lung transplant recipients and evidence for involvement of the heart will be considered. The protozoan organism *Toxoplasma gondii* will also be included as this infection is usually diagnosed serologically in virology laboratories and it shares many features in common with virus infection.[3]

The rate and severity of virus infections in transplant recipients are affected by a number of factors:

1. The severity of the basic immunosuppressive regimen and the agents used (particularly azathioprine, anti-thymocyte globulin, and the anti T-cell monoclonal antibody OKT3.
2. The rejection rates experienced and the associated enhanced immunosuppressive therapy.
3. The presence of concomitant infections.
4. The prevalence of the virus infection in the recipient and donor populations. The extent of donor/recipient virus or *T. gondii* mismatch (the most significant factor).

The herpesviruses, particularly cytomegalovirus (CMV), herpes simplex virus (HSV) and Epstein–Barr virus (EBV) are most frequently associated with clinically significant infection in transplant recipients. Less frequently, other viruses such as adenoviruses and papilloma viruses may cause morbidity. Rarely, cardiotropic viruses such as Coxsackie B virus may cause infection.[4]

Cytomegalovirus

Cytomegalovirus is the most important virus infecting solid organ transplant recipients.[1,5] It is a particular problem amongst heart and combined heart–

lung transplant recipients reflecting the necessarily high levels of basic and enhanced immunosuppression that these patients receive.[2] In addition, in combined heart–lung transplant patients this may be a reflection of the potentially lethal effects of CMV pneumonitis in the grafted lungs.

Amongst the heart transplant recipients transplanted at Papworth Hospital, Cambridge between 1979 and 1990, 51% had evidence of active CMV infection after transplantation. Cytomegalovirus antibody-negative patients receiving hearts from CMV antibody-positive donors (CMV mismatched) experience the most severe infections. Details of the rates of infection analysed by donor and recipient CMV status for heart transplant recipients are shown in Table 11.1. In addition, it has been shown that these CMV mismatched patients suffer a more severe form of primary CMV infection than those patients who acquire primary CMV from blood or blood products.[2] In our series, fatal CMV disease has been seen only in those heart transplant patients who acquired the infection from the donor organ.[2] Ten per cent of this group have died from CMV infection and those who survive have a much higher rate of complications requiring hospital readmission than other patient groups. Combined heart–lung transplant recipients may experience non-donor organ-acquired fatal CMV disease.[6]

The amount of CMV infection and disease experienced in CMV antibody-positive heart transplant recipients is significantly greater in those who receive organs from CMV antibody-positive donors (Table 11.1). This difference is not seen in combined heart–lung recipients.

Cytomegalovirus infection usually occurs within 4 to 8 weeks of transplant with primary infection occurring slightly earlier than reactivation or reinfection. Cytomegalovirus infections are associated with multiorgan involvement. In severe CMV infections, patients present with fever and leucopenia. They may also experience confusion, arthralgia and malaise, and a few will have the most florid complication, pneumonitis, which is frequently fatal. Outside the transplant setting myocarditis is a recognized, although rare, feature of CMV infection and it appears that this virus has a low cardiac virulence. The few case reports that exist in previously healthy individuals[7,8] have often based the diagnosis on clinical grounds without definite histological proof. Autopsy histology in the case reported by Tiula and Leinikki[9] showed a lymphocytic

Table 11.1 Summary of cytomegalovirus (CMV) infections in 351 heart transplant recipients.

| CMV status of | | | Number of patients with | | Number |
Donor	Recipient	Total	Primary CMV	CMV reactivation or reinfection	who died of CMV
+	−	60	48 (80%)		4
−	−	79	12 (15%)		0
+	+	109		72 (66%)	0
−	+	130		60 (46%)	0
Totals		378		192 (51%)	4

myocarditis without CMV inclusions, the latter feature being necessary to make an absolute histological diagnosis.

In the transplant setting, Baandrup and Mortensen[10] reported on 422 renal transplant recipients. Although in seven of 16 fatal cases of primary CMV infection cardiovascular problems were considered a major factor in the cause of death, in only one case was there histological evidence of myocarditis associated with CMV inclusions. Our experience in heart transplant recipients where there is abundant cardiac biopsy material available has been similar. In a 3-year period during which 2249 post-transplant endomyocardial biopsies have been histologically assessed, only one example of definite CMV myocarditis has been seen (Fig. 11.1), in spite of the fact that many patients have been known to be suffering from active CMV infection around the time of endomyocardial biopsy. Nevertheless, there is a suspicion that CMV myocarditis could occur in the absence of classical viral inclusions and the case report of Tiula and Leinikki[9] raises this question in the non-transplant setting where the confusing factor of myocardial lymphocytic infiltration associated with allograft rejection was not a consideration in the differential diagnosis. In the transplant population this possibility of undiagnosable CMV myocarditis is not simply of academic importance because significant allograft rejection will tend to be treated with enhanced immunosuppression, a therapy likely to worsen any CMV infection present. Stovin et al.[11] addressed this problem comparing the histological findings in serial endomyocardial biopsies from 22 heart transplant recipients up to the time of development of primary CMV infections with 21 recipients who did not develop CMV. They concluded that in spite of the fact that the donor organ was the most likely source of infection there was no evidence of increased cellular infiltration of the biopsies at the time of active CMV infection and on this basis suggested that it was unlikely

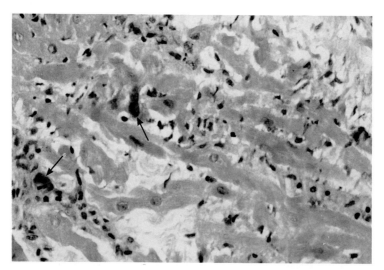

Fig. 11.1 Cytomegalovirus myocarditis, endomyocardial biopsy. This heart transplant recipient was suffering from CMV disease at the time of the biopsy with CMV pneumonitis and colitis. He died a few days later. Note the presence of large CMV infected cells (arrowed) and accompanying tissue damage and inflammation. Haematoxylin and eosin, high power.

CMV infection could produce a myocardial infiltrate that could be confused with significant allograft rejection.

More recently Bruneval *et al.*[12] have used *in situ* hybridization and immunohistochemistry specifically to look for evidence of CMV infection in endomyocardial biopsies from a group of heart transplant recipients selected because of severe infection. Even in this group only three out of 22 biopsies showed evidence of infection by one or other of these techniques and the cells involved were recognizable on the basis of morphology alone. Two of these three also showed inflammatory infiltration, but as this was clearly spatially separate it was interpreted as being due to rejection, the presence of a few CMV infected cells simply being an indicator of the generalized CMV infection present and not of active myocardial disease.

Dilated cardiomyopathy as a direct consequence of CMV myocarditis has been described for renal transplant recipients.[13,14] These reports may be criticized however on the basis that the evidence for myocarditis was clinical and there was not absolute proof of CMV-related cardiac disease in terms of the presence of inclusions in the heart associated with myocardial damage and inflammation. This is important because Baandrup and Mortensen[10] showed in their series of renal transplant recipients that whilst major cardiovascular problems were frequently contributory to death in primary CMV disease, in only one of 16 cases was there histological proof of CMV myocarditis.

The potential involvement of CMV in the pathogenesis of atherosclerosis and also in graft vascular disease has been considered in Chapter 8. Although the studies reviewed demonstrate an association between CMV infection and cardiac graft vascular disease, evidence for a direct role in the pathogenesis does not exist. Whilst it is attractive to suggest that the disease could be initiated by CMV infection of the vessel wall, the association could simply be a reflection of the relatively higher level of basic and enhanced immunosuppression in the CMV-infected group. These in turn are inextricably linked to higher rates of cellular rejection. Therefore it remains to be proven that the high rates of CMV infection in those who develop graft vascular disease are not merely an indirect measure of cellular rejection, this being the process responsible either directly or indirectly for vascular occlusion.

Treatment and prophylaxis

Ganciclovir (Cymevene, Syntex) is the drug of choice for treating CMV infections in transplant recipients.[15] It is well tolerated and few patients experience severe side effects necessitating cessation of therapy. In those who cannot tolerate ganciclovir, foscarnet (Fosavir, Astra) is a suitable alternative.

Since CMV can produce severe and sometimes fatal infections in heart transplant recipients, several transplant centres have investigated the use of prophylactic treatment with ganciclovir[16], acyclovir[17] or CMV hyperimmune globulin[18] or a combination of these. As yet, there have been no reports of prophylactic regimens which can reliably prevent CMV disease in heart transplant recipients, but it is likely that ganciclovir is the most effective therapy with the beneficial effect being dependent on an adequate duration of treatment. Acyclovir can reduce but not eliminate the impact of CMV disease in transplant recipients. Cytomegalovirus hyperimmune globulin has been shown to reduce the impact of CMV disease by approximately 50% in transplant recipients.[18]

Herpes simplex virus

Herpes simplex virus (HIV) infections are most frequently seen in the first few weeks after transplantation when patients are experiencing their most severe immunosuppression. Primary HSV infections in transplant recipients are rare and the vast majority of infections are the result of reactivation of the patient's own latent HSV.[19] Although most patients experience fairly mild symptoms, some have severe infections. Orofacial and genital lesions are most commonly seen, but more extensive infection of the upper respiratory tract and gastrointestinal system may also occur. Occasional life-threatening pneumonitis may be seen especially in combined heart–lung transplant recipients.[19] Cardiac infection does not appear to be a feature clinically and this is perhaps not surprising as HSV is a virus that primarily infects epithelia and neural tissue. If it occurs at all then it would be expected to be limited to those with severe disseminated infection where the diagnosis would be apparent from manifestations in other organs. Herpes simplex virus myocarditis however has never been diagnosed on post-transplant endomyocardial biopsy material at Papworth Hospital.

Acyclovir (Zovirax, Wellcome) is the drug of choice for treating HSV infections. Patients are treated with oral acyclovir if the infection is of mild or moderate severity, while more severe infections should be treated with the intravenous preparation. In those patients who are at high risk of developing severe and potentially life-threatening infection, for example, HSV antibody-positive combined heart–lung recipients, acyclovir prophylaxis is appropriate.

Epstein–Barr virus

Evidence of Epstein–Barr Virus (EBV) infections has been found after transplant in 23% of Papworth heart and heart–lung transplant recipients. Six per cent of patients experienced primary infection, which was most probably acquired from the donor organ (or blood) whilst 17.4% had evidence of reactivation of endogenous EBV or reinfection. Fifty-three per cent of patients with serological evidence of EBV infection were symptomatic. Symptoms were generally mild, most commonly fever, headache, sore throat and coryza. Clinical evidence of cardiac involvement has not been reported.

It has been suggested[20] that EBV may be responsible for the endocardial lymphoid infiltrates frequently seen in post-cardiac transplant endomyocardial biopsies. However, the study which suggested this used the extremely sensitive polymerase chain reaction to detect EBV and it is possible that the EBV detected was a 'passenger' in B-cell clones present in the lymphoid infiltrate which had been expanded by cyclosporine A therapy. Nakhleh et al.[21] carried out a study of endocardial lymphoid infiltrates using *in situ* hybridization methods to detect EBV genomic sequences. All 22 endomyocardial biopsies with endocardial infiltrates studied were negative and they therefore concluded that EBV was unrelated to their development. In a review of 2350 consecutive endomyocardial biopsies Forbes *et al.*[22] suggested that endocardial lymphoid infiltration in the absence of cellular rejection in the deep myocardium was most likely a manifestation of low-grade allograft rejection, possibly in relation to fluctuating cyclosporine A levels.

Epstein–Barr virus is implicated in post-transplant B-cell lymphoproliferative disorders.[23,24] Ten (67%) of the 15 Papworth heart and combined heart–lung transplant recipients, who have developed lymphoproliferative disease after transplantation, have had serological evidence of active EBV infection in the preceding few months/years. This increased incidence of EBV infection in this group of patients, compared with that in the whole series (23%), may be the result of several factors, including the association of EBV infection with the subsequent development of lymphoproliferative disease. However, it may simply reflect the fact that patients who are more profoundly immunosuppressed are both more likely to experience EBV reactivation and develop lymphoproliferative disease.

Involvement of the heart may occur in lymphoproliferative disease. In two heart transplant recipients, where the disease behaved in a malignant fashion and caused death, the neoplastic lymphoid infiltrate was seen in endomyocardial biopsy material. Atypical large lymphoid cells were present focally in endocardium with extension into the underlying myocardium (Fig. 11.2). This tendency to involve the grafted organ was a conspicuous feature in the five cases of lymphoproliferative disease in combined heart–lung transplant recipients who all showed intrapulmonary disease.

As a mild disease EBV reactivation does not usually require specific therapy. Many cases of post-transplant lymphoproliferative disease respond to a reduction in immunosuppression and this may be combined with acyclovir therapy although there is little evidence to suggest that this agent will be

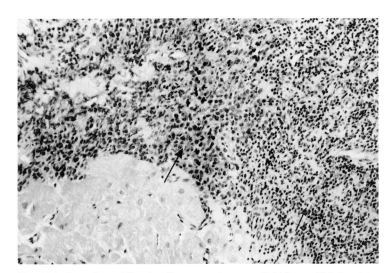

Fig. 11.2 Lymphoproliferative disease, endomyocardial biopsy. This heart transplant recipient developed lymphoproliferative disease 6 years after transplant. The disease behaved in a malignant fashion and he died with widely disseminated disease a month later. The endomyocardial biopsy taken around the time of diagnosis on lymph-node biopsy shows the atypical lymphoid infiltrate in the endocardium (large arrow) with extension into the underlying myocardium. This infiltrate lies adjacent to a non-neoplastic endocardial infiltrate (small arrow) of the kind commonly seen after cardiac transplant. Haematoxylin and eosin, medium power.

effective in a disease due to EBV transformation rather than simple infection. The more malignant examples of lymphoproliferative disease essentially behave like lymphomas and consequently need to be treated with appropriate cytotoxic chemotherapy.

Enteroviruses

There have been few reports of enterovirus infection in transplant recipients. These viruses are not known to be transmitted with donor organs, but this may occur. Amongst the Papworth heart recipients, only one patient, the first combined heart–lung transplant recipient, experienced a coxsackie B infection in the first few weeks after transplant. A positive histological diagnosis of viral myocarditis has never been made on post-transplant endomyocardial biopsy material other than for CMV infection already discussed. Even if enterovirus infection were in fact more common than recognized post-heart transplant, a definite histological diagnosis of myocarditis would not be possible due to the fact that any associated inflammatory infiltrate and myocyte damage would be indistinguishable from acute cellular rejection.

Toxoplasma gondii

Toxoplasma gondii is a coccidian parasite which is associated with clinical syndromes in congenitally infected infants and immunocompromised patients similar to those produced by CMV. Non-immunocompromised persons usually experience asymptomatic infection; rarely, they may have a glandular fever-like syndrome. Human immunodeficiency virus (HIV) antibody-positive patients and transplant recipients experience more serious infections.

In transplant recipients, *T. gondii* infection may be acquired from the donor organ. Prior to the introduction of pyrimethamine prophylaxis, the comparative risk of *T. gondii* antibody-negative patients acquiring the infection from *T. gondii* antibody-positive donors (mismatches) was 57% in heart, 20% in liver and <1% in kidney recipients.[25] A similarly high incidence of donor-acquired infection was seen in the Stanford heart transplant series, occurring in three out of four mismatches.[26] Infected patients develop symptoms within the first month after transplantation, usually beginning in the third or fourth week. All symptomatic patients present with fever. Infection in these circumstances produces serious and potentially life-threatening multisystem disease with myocarditis, pneumonitis or encephalitis, or a combination of these. Two of the four heart transplant patients who developed primary donor-acquired toxoplasmosis at Papworth died of the disease and in all four, toxoplasma cysts were seen in the heart in endomyocardial biopsy or autopsy material,[3] which were important in establishing the diagnosis and indicative of the propensity of this organism to infect the heart. As with viral infection of the transplanted heart, any associated inflammation may be indistinguishable from cellular rejection and indeed this may be the only diagnosis entertained if toxoplasma cysts are not adequately searched for in biopsy material. In order to maximize diagnostic yield from endomyocardial biopsies multiple haematoxylin and eosin-stained serial sections should be examined. Even when this is done only a very few myocyctes containing cysts may be seen. Fortunately the need for a painstaking search for toxoplasma cysts in all endomyocardial biopsy material from toxoplasma mismatches has to some extent been obviated with the introduction of pyrimethamine prophylaxis. Nevertheless, establishment of a tissue diagnosis of toxoplasma myocarditis may be necessary on occasion and it has been shown that as an alternative to conventional histopathological methods, the toxoplasma genome may be detected in endomyocardial biopsy material around the time of active infection in primary toxoplasmosis, using a polymerase chain reaction method.[27] Initial results suggest that this method may be more sensitive than histopathological detection.

Recrudescence of *T. gondii* infections in patients who were *T. gondii* antibody-positive before transplant has been described following heart transplantation.[3,26] In our series[3] this was comparatively rare, occurring in only three of 75 patients (4%). In contrast Luft *et al.*[26] reported an incidence of 53% in the Stanford heart transplant series. This marked difference may be a reflection of differences in serological methods used to detect recrudescence and it may be of relevance that none of the patients in the Stanford series developed symptoms attributable to *T. gondii* recrudescence compared to two of the three patients in our series. Recrudescence is generally associated with less serious clinical features than primary donor-acquired infection, although pneumonia has been seen in one case.[3] Toxoplasma cysts were not seen in any of the post-transplant endomyocardial biopsy material from our three patients who developed serological evidence of recrudescence suggesting that the myocardium was not involved.[3]

Prophylactic pyrimethamine (25 mg daily for 6 weeks) with folinic acid is now routinely given to all *T. gondii* antibody-negative recipients who receive hearts from *T. gondii* antibody-positive donors and this has dramatically reduced the incidence of primary donor-acquired *T. gondii* infection from 57 to 14%.[28] Those who develop evidence of infection in spite of pyrimethamine prophylaxis do so much later than those who never received prophylaxis (mean 53 weeks after transplantation compared to 4 weeks). Furthermore, only 20% develop symptoms and these are generally mild compared to 100% of those who did not receive prophylaxis in whom symptoms were severe or life-threatening. Patients with symptomatic *T. gondii* infection may be treated with a combination of pyrimethamine, sulphonamides and spiramycin.

References

1. Dummer J. S., Hardy A., Poorsattar A., Ho M. Early infections in kidney, heart and liver transplant recipients on cyclosporin. *Transplantation* 1983; **36:** 259–67.
2. Wreghitt T. G. Cytomegalovirus infections in heart and heart–lung transplant recipients. *J Antimicrobial Chemother* 1989; **23** (Suppl E): 49–60.
3. Wreghitt T. G., Hakim M., Gray J. J. *et al.* Toxoplasmosis in heart and heart–lung transplant recipients. *J Clin Pathol* 1989; **42:** 194–9.
4. Wreghitt T. G., Taylor C. E. D., Banatvala J. E. *et al.* Concurrent cytomegalovirus and coxsackie B virus infections in a heart–lung transplant recipient. *J Infect* 1986; **13:** 51–4.
5. Wreghitt T. G., Hughes M., Calne R. Y. A retrospective study of viral and *Toxoplasma gondii* infection in 54 liver transplant recipients in Cambridge. *Serodiag Immunother* 1987; **1:** 219–39.
6. Smyth R. L., Scott J. P., Borysiewicz L. K. *et al.* Cytomegalovirus infection in

heart–lung transplant recipients: risk factors, clinical associations and response to treatment. *J Infect Dis* 1991; **164:** 1045–50.

7. Wilson R. S. E., Morris T. H., Russell Rees J. Cytomegalovirus myocarditis. *Br Heart J* 1972; **34:** 865–8.

8. Wink K., Schmitz H. Cytomegalovirus myocarditis. *Am Heart J* 1980; **100:** 667–72.

9. Tiula E., Leinikki P. Fatal cytomegalovirus infection in a previously healthy boy with myocarditis and consumption coagulopathy as presenting signs. *Scand J Infect Dis* 1972; **3:** 57–60.

10. Baandrup U., Mortensen S. A. Histopathological aspects of myocarditis with special reference to mumps, cytomegalovirus infection and the role of endomyocardial biopsy. In: Bolte H. D. ed. *Viral Heart Disease*. Berlin, Heidelberg New York: Springer-Verlag, 1984: 13–25.

11. Stovin P. G. I., Wreghitt T. G., English T. A. H., Wallwork J. Lack of association between cytomegalovirus infection of the heart and rejection-like inflammation. *J Clin Pathol* 1989; **42:** 81–3.

12. Bruneval P., Amrein C., Guillemain R. *et al.* Poor diagnostic value of *in situ* hybridisation and immunohistochemistry in endomyocardial biopsies to detect cytomegalovirus after heart transplantation. *J Heart Lung Transplant* 1992; **11:** 773–7.

13. Shabtai M., Luft B., Walzer W. C. *et al.* Massive cytomegalovirus pneumonia and myocarditis in a renal transplant recipient: successful treatment with DHPG. *Transplant Proc* 1988; **20:** 562–3.

14. Ando H., Shiramizu T. Dilated cardiomyopathy caused by cytomegalovirus infection in a renal transplant recipient. *Jpn Heart J* 1992; **33:** 409–12.

15. Dunn D. L., Mayoral J. L., Gillingham K. J. *et al.* Treatment of invasive cytomegalovirus disease in solid organ transplant patients with ganciclovir. *Transplantation* 1991; **51:** 98–106.

16. Merigan T. C., Renlund D. G., Keay S. *et al.* A controlled trial of ganciclovir to prevent cytomegalovirus disease after heart transplantation. *N Engl J Med* 1992; **326:** 1182–6.

17. Balfour H. H., Chace B. A., Stapleton J. T. *et al.* A randomised, placebo-controlled trial of oral acyclovir for the prevention of cytomegalovirus in recipients of renal allografts. *N Engl J Med* 1989; **320:** 1381–7.

18. Snydman D. R. Cytomegalovirus immunoglobulins in the prevention and treatment of cytomegalovirus disease. *Rev. Infect Dis* 1990; **12** (Suppl 7): S839–48.

19. Smyth R. L., Higenbottam T. W., Scott J. P. *et al.* Herpes simplex virus infection in heart–lung transplantation patients. *Transplantation* 1990; **49:** 735–9.

20. Kemnitz J., Cohnert T. R. Lymphoma like lesion in human orthotopic cardiac allografts. *Am J Clin Pathol* 1988; **89:** 430 (abs).

21. Nakhleh R. E., Copenhaver C. M., Werdin K. *et al.* Lack of evidence for involvement of Epstein–Barr virus in the development of the 'Quilty' lesion of transplanted hearts: an *in situ* hybridisation study. *J Heart Lung Transplant* 1991; **10:** 504–7.

22. Forbes R. D., Rowan R. A., Billingham M. E. Endocardial infiltrates in human heart transplants: a serial biopsy analysis comparing four immunosuppression protocols. *Human Pathol* 1990; **21:** 850–5.

23. Ho M., Miller G., Atchison R. W. *et al.* Epstein–Barr virus infections and DNA hybridisation studies in posttransplant lymphoma and lymphoproliferative lesions: the role of primary infection. *J Infect Dis* 1985; **152:** 876–86.

24. Purtilo D. T., Tatsumi E., Manolov G. *et al.* Epstein–Barr virus as an etiological agent in the pathogenesis of lymphoproliferative and aproliferative diseases in immune deficient patients. *Int Rev Exp Pathol* 1985; **27:** 113–81.

25. Speirs G. E., Hakim M., Calne R. Y., Wreghitt T. G. Relative risk of donor-transmitted *Toxoplasma gondii* infection in heart, liver and kidney transplant patients. *Clin Transplant* 1988; **2:** 257–60.

26. Luft B. J., Naot Y., Araujo F. J. *et al.* Primary and reactivated Toxoplasma infection in patients with cardiac transplants. Clinical spectrum and problems in diagnosis in a defined population. *Ann Internal Med* 1983; **99:** 27–31.
27. Holliman R., Johnson J., Savva D. *et al.* Diagnosis of toxoplasma infection in cardiac transplant recipients using the polymerase chain reaction. *J Clin Pathol* 1992; **45:** 931–2.
28. Wreghitt T. G., Gray J. J., Pavel P. *et al.* Efficacy of pyrimethamine for the prevention of donor-acquired *Toxoplasma gondii* infection in heart and heart–lung transplant patients. *Transplant Int* 1992; **5:** 197–200.

Index